PSYCHODYNAMIC THERAPY

Psychodynamic Therapy

A GUIDE TO EVIDENCE-BASED PRACTICE

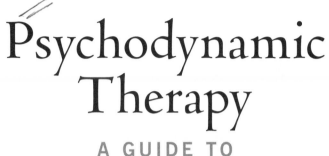

Richard F. Summers
Jacques P. Barber

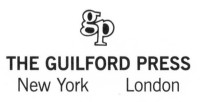

THE GUILFORD PRESS
New York   London

© 2010 The Guilford Press
A Division of Guilford Publications, Inc.
72 Spring Street, New York, NY 10012
www.guilford.com

Printed in the United States of America

This book is printed on acid-free paper.

Last digit is print number: 9 8 7 6 5 4 3 2 1

Library of Congress Cataloging-in-Publication Data

Summers, Richard F.
  Psychodynamic therapy : a guide to evidence-based practice / Richard F.
Summers, Jacques P. Barber.
    p. cm.
  Includes bibliographical references and index.
  ISBN 978-1-60623-443-3 (hbk.: alk. paper)
  1. Psychodynamic psychotherapy.   2. Evidence-based
psychotherapy.   I. Barber, Jacques P., 1954–   II. Title.
  RC489.P72S86 2010
  616.89′14—dc22

                                                          2009029455

To Ronnie, Sam, and Claire,
Smadar, Natalie, and Adam

About the Authors

Richard F. Summers, MD, is Clinical Associate Professor and Co-Director of Residency Training in the Department of Psychiatry at the University of Pennsylvania School of Medicine, and a faculty member of the Philadelphia Center for Psychoanalysis. Dr. Summers's clinical interests focus on combined psychotherapeutic and psychopharmacological treatment of mood and anxiety disorders, and adult life cycle development. His research interests include the contemporary revision of the theory and technique of psychodynamic psychotherapy, new approaches to psychotherapy training and education, the role of the therapeutic alliance in learning psychotherapy, comprehensive psychodynamic formulation, and positive psychology. Dr. Summers is the recipient of numerous teaching awards, including the Earl Bond Outstanding Teacher Award and the Outpatient Teacher of the Year Award from the University of Pennsylvania Department of Psychiatry, the Maestro Award from Pennsylvania Hospital, the Irma Bland Award for Excellence in Teaching Residents from the American Psychiatric Association, the Robert Dunning Dripps Award for Excellence in Graduate Medical Education from the University of Pennsylvania School of Medicine, the Psychiatric Educator of the Year from the Philadelphia Psychiatric Society, and Teacher of the Year from the Psychoanalytic Center of Philadelphia. He has been named a "Top Doc" by *Philadelphia* magazine numerous times since 1996; is President-Elect of the American Association of Directors of Psychiatric Residency Training (AADPRT) and chairs committees of

AADPRT and the American Psychoanalytic Association; is a member of the American College of Psychiatrists and a fellow of the American Psychiatric Association and the Philadelphia Psychiatric Society; was a Templeton Foundation Senior Fellow at the Positive Psychology Center at the University of Pennsylvania; and has served as an examiner for the American Board of Psychiatry and Neurology. Dr. Summers also maintains a private practice.

Jacques P. Barber, PhD, ABPP, is Professor of Psychology in the Department of Psychiatry at the University of Pennsylvania School of Medicine, Associate Director of the Center for Psychotherapy Research at the University of Pennsylvania, and Foreign Adjunct Professor in the Department of Clinical Neurosciences at the Karolinska Institute in Stockholm, Sweden. He was recently president of the Society for Psychotherapy Research. Dr. Barber conducts research on the outcome and process of dynamic and cognitive therapies for depression, panic disorder, substance dependence, and personality disorders. He recently finished a National Institute of Mental Health (NIMH)–funded randomized clinical trial of dynamic therapy versus selective serotonin reuptake inhibitors/serotonin–norepinephrine reuptake inhibitors for major depression, and is currently conducting another NIMH-funded randomized clinical trial of dynamic therapy versus cognitive-behavioral therapy for panic disorder. In the past, he was involved in a large National Institute on Drug Abuse–funded multisite randomized clinical trial comparing psychotherapies and drug counseling for cocaine dependence, and provided a detailed independent assessment of adherence and competence of therapists and counselors in that study. Dr. Barber has written extensively on the impact of the therapeutic alliance and of therapists' use of theoretically relevant interventions on the outcome of therapy. With Hadas Wiseman, he recently coauthored the book *Echoes of the Trauma: Relational Themes and Emotions in Children of Holocaust Survivors.*

Acknowledgments

Our residents and graduate students are the inspiration for this book. Their curiosity and intelligent skepticism gave us conviction that advances in science and changes in culture mean there are new and better ways to conceptualize psychodynamic therapy and better ways to teach it. Our students are the future of psychotherapy practice and we thank them for sparking our interest in this project and for pushing us to clarify, simplify, distill, and integrate traditional ideas with the burgeoning new empirical knowledge we have about psychotherapy.

We thank our patients who graciously agreed to have their stories told in this book with the hope that others will learn from their experiences. We have tried to convey the spirit of equality, collaboration, honesty, and closeness that we have felt with so many people with whom we have worked in psychotherapy.

There are so many people to thank. Hanita Sawney, Geoff Niemark, Matt Hurford, Dhwani Shah, Michelle Goldsmith, and Kevin McCarthy, as residents and psychology graduate students, went out of their way to encourage us, give us valuable feedback, and help us track our target audience for the book, and we are indebted to them.

George Vaillant was an early and consistent supporter; his encouragement and advice were taken to heart. We are thankful to him for reading chapters and reminding us to tell a story and not pontificate. Marty Seligman, Chris Peterson, and James Pawelski at the Positive Psychology Center at Penn encouraged this project and provided support for the notion that psychotherapy should include an emphasis on positive emotion. The Templeton Foundation gave R. F. S. a Senior Fellowship that allowed for uninterrupted writing time as well as the rare pleasure for a busy clinician—time to think and talk and not just listen. Alan Gruenberg gave encouragement and critiqued the chapter on psychotherapy and psychopharmacology, and he, Margaret Ann Price, and James Hetznecker made extra allowances when writing impinged on practice time. Emily Greenfield read and commented on early chapters. Ellen Berman coauthored Chapter 14 on combining psychotherapy and couple and family therapy, and Rob Garfield gave valuable feedback as well. Debbie Kim has asked every month or so for the last 6 years when the book will be done, and that has always been a spur to keep moving. Ron Rieder and Melissa Arbuckle provided a forum to discuss some of the ideas about dynamic psychotherapy and positive psychology with the psychiatry residents at Columbia University.

Six years of classes of Penn psychiatry residents read chapters as part of an ongoing seminar and made many constructive and encouraging comments. Shabad-Ratan Khalsa and Caleb Morfit read later versions of the chapters and made helpful edits, corrections, and suggestions. David Cleary and Rachel Chizke helped with the index. Brian Sharpless challenged us to articulate more clearly our ideas about change in psychotherapy. Robert Schweitzer at the University of Queensland graciously agreed to assign draft chapters to his psychology graduate students, who provided helpful reactions to the material. Tony Rostain has been wonderfully supportive of the book from its inception, with both words and support for protected writing time.

We thank our editor, Jim Nageotte, whose advice is subtle and correct.

Finally, we thank our families, who have given us their affection and enthusiasm despite the hours this work has taken us away from them. R. F. S. knows his parents' example helped inspire this effort. When our energies flagged, our wives, Ronnie and Smadar, expressed absolute confidence that we would complete the book and that it would be worthwhile; their faith and love is a great gift.

Contents

Introduction

We have had the extraordinary experience of seeing patients in psychodynamic therapy get better. They gain self-awareness, see others more clearly, and make changes in their lives. Dynamic treatment is hard to describe, but easy to understand when you watch it unfold.

Outmoded ideas about dynamic psychotherapy dominate in psychology, psychiatry, and social work teaching. Students often learn more through trial and error and personal experience than from formal teaching. We think this is more than a problem of pedagogy; rather, we think the theory and technique of the therapy needs to be updated.

Our goal, therefore, is to describe a clear, pragmatic model of therapy, and jettison much of unnecessary baggage of the past. We borrow from new findings in psychotherapy research and narrow and clarify the focus, aims, and goals of the treatment. Our model of dynamic psychotherapy is based on a developmental and conflict view of mental life, and relies on clearly defined core psychodynamic problems, case formulation, and goals that are coordinated with the formulation. In addition, our view of therapy calls for an engaged therapeutic stance with an emphasis on transparency, well-defined techniques for integration with other treatments, and an active approach to change. Ultimately, the treatment must be therapeutic, and we suggest these changes will increase the efficacy of the therapy. A better model will also be easier to learn.

We are a psychiatrist and a psychologist, both psychoanalytically trained, and both teaching in an academic psychiatry department. We realized on a brief walk to a Grand Rounds presentation in 2002 that we each dreamed of writing a book proposing a current and contemporary

1

model for dynamic therapy. In a rush of words we explained our ideas, and agreed in a few minutes that we wanted to write a book. We each felt we had learned an old model for treatment in training and that over the years we had gradually updated it in our minds and in our work. We realized that what we were teaching was very different from what we ourselves had learned. We thought that by trying to codify our approach we could improve our practice, and that our trainees would benefit as well.

One of us (RFS) is Co-Director of Residency Training in the Department of Psychiatry at the University of Pennsylvania. Having trained as both a general psychiatrist with an interest in diagnostic evaluation and as a psychoanalyst in a traditional analytic institute, RFS found a challenging and satisfying role teaching psychodynamic therapy to residents. He felt he was able to take the knowledge and experience gleaned from his psychoanalytic training and years of practice and make it relevant to a new generation of residents that had come of age after the bruising debates about biological psychiatry versus psychotherapy. He conceptualized his role as someone who was able to bridge the great tradition of psychoanalysis and the intellectual ferment of a modern psychiatry department.

One day in a resident and psychology interns' seminar, RFS described how he explained to patients the mechanism of change in dynamic psychotherapy. A resident politely but pointedly commented that the explanation sounded a lot like the explanation given by the cognitive therapy expert who lectured regularly in the following seminar hour. This insightful comment made RFS realize that he had gone from translating to reinventing. He was teaching an adaptation of the traditional psychodynamic approach, enriched by new developments in psychotherapy research and current concepts of mind and brain. RFS realized he was not translating something old into a language understandable in the contemporary world, but like others who had traveled the same path from psychoanalytic training to academic psychiatry, he had a more concise and focused model of psychodynamic treatment in mind.

JPB, a psychologist and psychotherapy researcher, is a principal investigator in studies of dynamic therapy for major depressive disorder and panic disorder funded by the National Institute of Mental Health (NIMH). His research on dynamic therapy focused on the Core Conflictual Relationship Theme (Luborsky & Crits-Christoph, 1990) and the supportive–expressive model developed by Lester Luborsky and his colleagues (Luborsky, 1984; Barber & Crits-Christoph, 1995). He studied manualized versus nonmanualized supportive–expressive dynamic psychotherapy (Vinnars et al., 2005), dynamic treatment for patients with avoidant and obsessive–compulsive personality disorder (Barber, Morse, Krakauer, Chittams, & Crits-Christoph, 1997) and cocaine dependence (Barber et al., 2008), and supportive–expressive psychotherapy for depression and personality disorders (Barber & Crits-Christoph, 1995). Through JPB's diverse clinical and research experiences and his interest in defining the core mechanisms of therapeutic change, he began to envision a new psychodynamic model that built on the conceptual advances in the psychotherapy literature.

As a teacher of residents and psychology trainees, JPB has several concerns. Many trainees, especially in psychology programs, lack significant exposure to the psychodynamic model. Those who are exposed often learn using the same method and the same clinical material that were used to teach not only JPB's generation, but even that of his own teachers. He was also concerned that although many of the early developers of cognitive-behavioral therapy (CBT) approaches had learned much from dynamic therapy, their writings emphasized CBT techniques without explaining their psychodynamic context. Essential techniques for connecting with patients, listening to them, and developing a therapeutic alliance originally developed in psychodynamic therapy. To the first generation of CBT therapists, these techniques were a given. That generation tended to distance themselves from their former psychodynamic teachers and training, and the second and subsequent generations of CBT practitioners were not trained exhaustively in many relational (nonspecific or common) aspects of psychotherapy.

The empirical database on the efficacy of cognitive therapy and interpersonal therapy became a juggernaut that determined subsequent popularity and funding opportunities, and made it more difficult to study dynamic therapy. JPB became convinced that trainees simply were not being adequately exposed to psychotherapy based on the dynamic model and what this model had to offer for all forms of psychotherapy. The question for him became: What are the core principles we really believe in, and what data do we have to build the foundation of a modern approach to dynamic psychotherapy? His goal is to make dynamic psychotherapy be as efficacious as possible while recognizing its potential limitations (e.g., Barber et al., 2008).

Our convergent paths led to this effort. In this book we describe a contemporary psychodynamic therapy model that we believe is practical, effective, and easily integrated with other treatment modalities, such as family and systems interventions and psychopharmacology. We are not outlining a fundamentally new theory, but eliminating redundant and unhelpful ideas, and assimilating timely concepts and findings from other models. Our emphasis is on a new pragmatic technique, rather than a new theory.

Some have wondered whether the days of psychodynamic therapy are numbered. The American Psychiatric Association and American Psychological Association have both convened panels to determine whether psychodynamic therapy is an evidence-based treatment. Without more data, we believe this prematurely opens the door to delegitimatization and defunding of the practice by third-party payers. The accrediting body for residency training programs has questioned whether dynamic therapy is a necessary competency for psychiatric residents. A *New York Times* article quotes the authors of a long-term dynamic psychotherapy study as "strongly [urging] scientists to undertake more testing of psychodynamic therapy, as it is known, before it is lost altogether as a historical curiosity" (Carey, 2008, p. A18).

We argue for the currency and value of dynamic therapy. In an age of scientific scrutiny, where many question its value, this is both a how-to book about psychodynamic therapy and a guide for its survival. The empirical evidence base for psychodynamic treatment is stronger than its critics maintain (e.g., Leichsenring, Rabung, & Leibing, 2004), and there is very little evidence for its lack of efficacy. Evidence-based practice in psychotherapy (e.g., APA Presidential Task Force for Evidence-Based Practice, 2006) requires that relevant research inform clinical practice. The clinician must employ a wide range of research findings, including randomized clinical trials but also including other types of data such as naturalistic studies, to help an individual patient in a specific clinical encounter. Our focus in this book is on just such a broad conception of research-informed clinical practice.

The case vignettes included in this book come from our clinical practices as well as from trainees we have supervised. All have been altered and disguised to protect the privacy of these individuals. Several examples are amalgams of more than one person. Those patients on whom we base the more extensive cases have reviewed the text and given feedback and suggestions to make the descriptions as accurate as possible. Psychotherapy is a personal experience for both the patient and the therapist. Therefore, we have often narrated the examples in the first person in order to include the therapist's thoughts and feelings. In these descriptions, the narrator could be either of us or one of our trainees.

Our task in describing our model is to balance the immediacy and face validity of our clinical experience with the data that are available about it. However, to keep this book readable, we have not attempted to provide comprehensive references for all our claims.

PART I

CONTEXT

CHAPTER 1

Why Dynamic Psychotherapy?

PSYCHIATRIST: We are here to understand your unconscious.
MASON: My unconscious is none of my business.
—JACKIE MASON, "The World According to Me"

Some trainees have the intuitive sense that the dynamic model allows an entrée into human issues that are universal and deep. They are struck by the immediacy of their own emotional experiences, and their patients', while doing the therapy. They sense the pervasiveness of patterns and repetitions from the past. These trainees personally resonate with the deeper meanings suggested by the dynamic model. Other students think psychodynamic therapy is wildly subjective and lacking any scientific basis whatsoever. Students need the opportunity to process these gut reactions. It takes a while for trainees to immerse themselves in the ideas and feel and discuss their emotional reactions in order to reflect on the treatment more dispassionately.

Students react negatively to pronouncements made by dynamic practitioners about what is true. They want evidence and explanation. Traditional psychodynamic teaching methods can be more like catechism than intellectual exploration, and there can be a clash of paradigms between evidence-based practice (which includes empirically supported psychotherapies) and clinical anecdotes about psychodynamic work. Adding to the difficulties in learning about dynamic therapy, trainees are exposed to disagreements among faculty about the value of the treatment. For every pearl of psychodynamic wisdom that is taught, there is a critical comment made by another esteemed faculty member. Tanya Luhrmann's

(2000) study of psychiatry training in the early 1990s, *Of Two Minds,* documented the conceptual strains psychiatry residents feel between the objective, medical, and scientific approaches to patient care associated with psychopharmacology, and the intuitive, empathic experience of dynamic psychotherapy.

What is the best way to learn about psychodynamic therapy? We think that a pragmatic focus on patients and an experience of the therapeutic process helps to break down these barriers and tensions. The story of Beth, narrated by her therapist, illustrates many of the features of an effective dynamic therapy.

> Beth was a 31-year-old single woman who came for treatment because of depression, loneliness, and problems with men. She was a clinical nurse specialist who was recognized for being compassionate and competent. She had an edge of insecurity that was partly obscured by her assertive manner and tall, imposing presence.
>
> Beth came for the appointment because she had been jilted by her boyfriend of 2 years and had quickly developed depressive symptoms, including typical neurovegetative symptoms, as well as self-hatred and social isolation. Beth's story, which tumbled out over the first few sessions, was upsetting to hear. Her father was an alcoholic who had been abusive to her mother, and her parents had divorced when she was 6 years old. Shortly after the separation, she was abducted by her father and taken to stay with him for several weeks in another city. She was physically safe during this time, but only after repeated pleading did he relent and allow her to return to her mother's home.
>
> Beth's mother struggled to take care of her and her younger sister. When Beth was 10 years old, her mother was remarried to a rigid man who kept the household under strict control. She felt her mother was elsewhere and that no one really cared about her. In her adolescence, she drank too much and took hallucinogens a number of times. She went to college, but felt lonely and sad. After her sophomore year, she enlisted in the armed forces and was stationed abroad for 3 years. Although these were more stable years, Beth still felt aimless and alone. She had several boyfriends, and each relationship ended with either rejection or the discovery that they were unfaithful. She had a few female friends, but the relationships were not very close, and she seemed to keep herself at a distance.
>
> I quickly forgot Beth's mildly intimidating manner and appearance as I felt more and more compassion for her, and respect for how she had coped with what she had been through. My initial impression was that she had had a very traumatic childhood and that the early strife in her family made it difficult for her to trust

closeness. The abduction and the rigid stepfather probably contributed to her fears about men. In her world, women were preoccupied and men were potentially dangerous. Substances and travel helped her get away, but then there was just emptiness.

After 2 months of therapy, Beth revealed that she had been date-raped at the age of 17, and that her most recent boyfriend had hit her. Although I had already felt disturbed by Beth's life of danger and neglect, at this moment, our connection deepened. Up to now, she had been reporting about what had happened, and we were making some connections between her early feeling of fear and loneliness and her later isolation and problems with men. But these new revelations were different. As she described them, her fear and anger were in the room. Now I felt like I was immersed in the story, not just hearing about it.

Soon Beth returned to talking about the recent breakup and ensuing depression. The abuse from the boyfriend seemed to have triggered her early memories of the divorce and abduction—she felt out of control with the boyfriend and had an old feeling of guilt and responsibility. Making the connection between the boyfriend and the father was frightening to her, but after discussing this several times, she began to feel some relief and an unaccustomed sense of calm. She grasped that her upset about the breakup and being hit was even more intense because of her childhood experiences, and this gave her more strength to deal with the present.

In one session Beth tearfully recounted a phone call from the former boyfriend. He tried to seduce her into rekindling their relationship, and at the same time, berated her for not being loyal and affectionate. She was confused about this. She felt badly about his claims, wondering whether she had been at fault for the breakup, and questioning her ability to love and be loyal. She was excited by the prospect of seeing him again, but knew this was a bad idea. She was angry at his manipulation and frightened that she could fall back into the relationship.

I pointed out (perhaps a little too quickly) how destructive the relationship had been and how important it was that she keep her distance from him. Suddenly there was a palpable shift in the room, and she seemed to treat me with suspicion and resentment. Up until then, Beth seemed to regard me like a good uncle, helpful and wise. Now, she accused me of being controlling and giving advice when I did not know what it felt like to be her. She told me it was easy to tell her to be strong and independent, as I was not there to help her pick up the pieces when she was lonely or afraid. I saw a return of the imposing demeanor I had seen initially; she seemed tall and cold and angry.

This shift happened quickly, and I was taken by surprise. I just listened, nodding. I was not sure what to say, so I played for time until I could understand what was happening. Soon I realized that I had become the next person (after the father and boyfriend) in a repetitive scenario in which she felt dependent on an authoritative and controlling man. She felt I could help her and take care of her, but I could also be untrustworthy, selfish, and possibly dangerous. My encouragement to reject the boyfriend had triggered a strong reaction.

We continue to discuss this case throughout this chapter. This vignette captures the essence of dynamic psychotherapy—exploration of current conflicts and relationships in order to understand how they relate to the past, the search for recurring patterns, and a focus on the therapeutic relationship to see how conflicts are repeated. The treatment challenges the therapist to be warm and empathic in understanding the patient's feelings, but keep cool as the relationship deepens and old patterns are replayed.

There is no doubt that Beth's distant mother and scary father had something to do with why she had trouble with men and why she came for therapy. When she began to talk about her traumatic experiences and feel intense emotion in the sessions, the therapist became even more deeply engaged. When she suddenly became angry with the therapist, he recognized that her pattern of feeling and relating to others based on a traumatic scenario from her past was now being enacted with him. What was he supposed to do now? This moment is an interpersonal crisis, but also a psychodynamic opportunity. The task of the therapy is to elucidate what is going on in this moment. The patient did not come to therapy to solve her problem with the therapist, but rather to decrease her depression. However, the enactment in the therapeutic relationship makes it possible to understand the underlying issue better and therefore helps her solve it.

DEFINING DYNAMIC PSYCHOTHERAPY

Although widely practiced, the definition of psychodynamic psychotherapy is vague. Typically it has been regarded as a more efficient but watered-down psychoanalysis; that is, it is usually seen as lying along a continuum, with psychoanalysis at one end and supportive psychotherapy on the other. Many writers have used this fundamental conception (Rockland, 2003; Luborsky, 1984). Clustered at the psychoanalytic or expressive/interpretative end are the classical parameters and techniques, including frequent sessions, therapist neutrality and abstinence, interest in the past, the use of interpretation, and attention to resistance (the patient's difficulty in talking about problems), transference (the patient's feeling toward the therapist), and countertransference (the therapist's feeling toward the patient). We discuss each of these concepts later as we describe our pragmatic model. At the supportive end are ego support, advice, guidance, and a greater focus on the present. Psychoanalytic or psychodynamic psychotherapy (we regard these terms as synonymous) mixes and melds these approaches, typically during once- or twice-weekly meetings. Ironically, the treatment has been more defined by what it is not—psychoanalysis or supportive psychotherapy—than what it is.

Contemporary writers suggest other definitions. Kernberg (1999) regards dynamic psychotherapy as the judicious use of traditional psychoanalytic techniques. He observed that psychodynamic psychotherapy and psychoanalysis are convergent with respect to their interest in transference, countertransference, unconscious meanings in the here and now, the importance of analyzing character, and the impact of early relationships. He collaborated with colleagues (Kernberg, Selzer, Koenigsberg, Carr, & Appelbaum, 1989) on a manualized form of psychodynamic therapy with specific techniques for treating borderline personality disorder.

Gabbard emphasizes the central goal of increasing the patient's understanding and the focus on the therapist–patient relationship, but describes it differently. He defines psychodynamic psychotherapy as "a therapy that involves careful attention to the therapist–patient interaction, with thoughtfully timed interpretation of transference and resistance embedded in a sophisticated appreciation of the therapist's contribution to the two-person field" (Gunderson & Gabbard, 1999, p. 685).

Luborsky's pioneering work on systematizing the theory and technique of psychodynamic psychotherapy, conceptualized by him as supportive–expressive psychotherapy (Luborsky, 1984), has had a widespread influence on modern dynamic therapy. This dynamic treatment model has been further defined by Book (1998) as appropriate for a wide range of patients and conditions. Supportive–expressive psychotherapy, like most manualized psychodynamic treatments, does not prescribe therapist interventions on a session-by-session basis; rather, it provides general principles of treatment and guidelines for therapists. For example, symptoms such as depression are understood in the context of interpersonal/intrapsychic conflicts, which in supportive–expressive psychotherapy are called Core Conflictual Relationship Themes (CCRT; Luborsky & Crits-Christoph, 1990).

McWilliams (2004) characterizes the essence of psychodynamic psychotherapy differently—she describes the sensibility of the therapist. For her, the attitudes of curiosity and awe, respect for complexity, a disposition to identification and empathy, valuing of subjectivity and affect, appreciation of attachment, and a capacity for faith are the fundamental ground on which the dynamic therapist's approach rests. Although the essential enterprise is exploratory and reflective, she is less interested in the details of the technique than in the process the therapist attempts to stimulate.

In summary, we see the current practice of psychodynamic psychotherapy as an amalgam of techniques (see Table 1.1), some of which are exploratory, and some supportive, employed in the context of an important therapeutic relationship. Sessions are held often enough that the therapeutic relationship develops sufficient intensity to be a factor in its own right. The attention to the transference and countertransference is common to all of the definitions we surveyed and is a unique and identifying aspect of psychodynamic psychotherapy.

These features were represented in Beth's treatment. The therapist has the challenge of figuring out how to respond to Beth's anger and mistrust. He could soothe and support, reminding Beth that the therapy was a safe place and that he certainly did not mean to criticize, control, or judge her. This would be a supportive approach, and common to a variety of psychotherapies. He could note that there is a perceptual distortion and ask the patient to evaluate the evidence for this perception.

TABLE 1.1. Essential Features of Psychodynamic Psychotherapy in Current Practice

- Use of exploratory, interpretative, and supportive interventions as appropriate
- Frequent sessions
- Emphasis on uncovering painful affects, understanding past painful experiences
- Goal is to facilitate emotional experience and increase understanding
- Focus on the therapeutic relationship, including attention to transference and countertransference
- Use of a wide range of techniques, with variability in application by different practitioners

This is a cognitive therapy intervention. Or the therapist could keep the patient's angry feelings in the room, helping to contain them and not argue them away. He could help her observe the feelings and connect them with the themes they have already discussed. This latter approach is unique to psychodynamic psychotherapy.

THE VALUE OF DYNAMIC PSYCHOTHERAPY

Although we do not seem to have to argue the value of psychodynamic psychotherapy in psychiatry training settings, it has nevertheless almost disappeared from many psychology training programs. The standing of psychodynamic psychotherapy reflects both scientific controversy and sociocultural forces. Dynamic therapy is the subject of cultural and style pieces in the *New York Times,* and it is the focus of contentious dialogue between outpatient mental health providers and their utilization reviewers. It is all too infrequently the focus of interest in our professional journals. There are four responses to those who question the value of psychodynamic psychotherapy.

Empirical Database

First, the question of psychodynamic therapy's effectiveness often devolves into a simplistic comparison with other treatments, most often cognitive-behavioral therapy. We consider this to be one aspect of the question of dynamic therapy's value, certainly a crucial one, and an empirical issue that is far from settled. We will address this question, but we will also broaden it and revise it.

There are relatively few empirical studies (summarized in Chapters 5 and 6 on core psychodynamic problems), relatively few funding sources, and few studies in the pipeline, although there may be a recent uptick (see Leichsenring et al., 2004; Høglend et al., 2008; and Milrod, Leon, Barber, Markowitz, & Graf, 2007). The most recent meta-analysis of long-term psychodynamic psychotherapy provided preliminary evidence for its efficacy in treating complex problems (Leichsenring & Rabung, 2008). Our conclusion about the current state of the literature is that there is some support for psychodynamic psychotherapy as an effective treatment for certain conditions, and certainly very few instances showing that dynamic therapy is less effective than other treatments.

In recent years a major controversy has raged among psychotherapy researchers regarding how one evaluates the efficacy of treatments. The randomized clinical trial, with appropriate control groups, is regarded as the gold standard. Cognitive and behavioral therapists tried to establish the efficacy of their treatments from the beginning, understanding that this was missing in psychodynamic research. They valued the experimental method highly, and this led them to emphasize randomized clinical trials. The American Psychological Association's Presidential Task Force on Evidence-Based Practice (2006) concludes more broadly that "research, clinical expertise, and patient characteristics are all supported as relevant to good outcomes" (p. 271). Anecdotal and clinical case studies are compelling because of the inferential nature of psychodynamic concepts and the unique relational component of the treatment. Psychodynamic practitioners value case studies for these reasons and have tended to eschew involvement in empirical research. Alternative approaches, such as qualitative case studies, naturalistic follow-up, and process studies, are regarded with less favor by researchers; however, randomized clinical trials are not sufficient to provide the base needed for comprehensive evidence-based practice (Barber, 2009).

Like many therapies in long-standing use, what constitutes "the treatment" is hard to characterize and therefore hard to test. Several investigators developed manuals for dynamic therapy, including Luborsky for supportive–expressive therapy (Luborsky, 1984; Book, 1998), Kernberg and his colleagues for transference-focused psychodynamic psychotherapy for borderline personality disorder (Kernberg et al., 1989), and Milrod for panic disorder (Milrod, Busch, Cooper, & Shapiro, 1997). These protocols are an important step forward, but they raise many questions. Do these manualized treatments reflect all aspects of psychodynamic psychotherapy technique, or do they select out certain ones? Indeed, what are the most important aspects of the technique, what promotes change most effectively, and what kind of change?

The evidence-based approach to psychotherapy research has, under the influence of the NIMH and pharmaceutical companies, focused on patients with a clear-cut primary phenomenological diagnosis such as phobias, panic disorder, posttraumatic stress disorder (PTSD), or depression. This contributes to the dearth of psychodynamic therapy studies. Many psychodynamic therapists do not pay close attention to the phenomenology of Axis I disorders. Instead, they base their treatment interventions on psychodynamic formulations that include the phenomenological data along with other variables such as self-esteem, relationships, and life cycle issues. Because psychodynamic treatments focus relatively less on symptoms and more on other aspects of well-being and mental functioning, then assessing only symptoms may underestimate the efficacy of the treatment.

Grants submitted to study the efficacy of psychodynamic therapy often meet an additional hurdle. They must justify why we should study the efficacy of the treatment when we already know that CBT is effective. By missing the boat to be first treatment to show efficacy, it is more difficult to gain the resources to meet this standard for subsequent treatments.

Depth

Second, psychodynamic therapy is valuable because it has been an incubator of psychotherapeutic innovation for almost a century. Most of the contemporary psychotherapies, and many developed and discarded along the way, have emerged from it. Later treatments were derived conceptually from the Freudian legacy, or developed by individuals who were trained in or exposed to it. We suggest that the depth of the treatment, intensity of the interpersonal engagement, and the intrinsic sense of meaning that arises when discussing issues of great personal importance stimulates creative thought. Perhaps this is why dynamic therapy has been so effective in spinning off new ideas. It attracts those with empathy and provides a meaningful model for a deep emotional exchange with a patient. Working with Beth was challenging and emotionally engaging for the therapist. Following a tightly prescribed protocol may not have provoked the same personal involvement and curiosity in the therapist.

A deep treatment is one that embraces fundamental problems and essential solutions. It aims to reshape the individual in some profound way and gets close to the idea of cure. A deeper therapy speaks for itself and provides its own feeling of justification. Psychodynamic therapy may carry the torch for depth in the psychotherapy arena today.

The observation has been made that that only psychodynamic psychotherapy among the psychotherapies retains the ambition to cure or help patients transform themselves in a profound way (Seligman, 2002). Indeed, we recognize that a deep treatment may not be required for all patients. Much of the success of behavioral therapy is thought to reside in its focus on symptoms and in its parsimonious and directed use of therapeutic resources to decrease symptoms. It does not aim to be a therapy of depth, and this is one of its strengths. In contrast dynamic psychotherapy, which facilitates a patient's rewriting of his life narrative, his picture of himself, his past, present, and future, seems uniquely positioned to address the depth of a individual's experience.

Psychodynamic Narrative Is Part of Our Culture

Third, dynamic therapy is valuable because Freudian ideas permeate contemporary Western culture. The unconscious, the effect of early childhood on later experiences, internal conflict as a normal state of affairs, phases of development, and the ubiquity of anxiety are ideas we practically find in our drinking water. They are integral to our culture's picture of the individual, the life cycle, and interpersonal relationships. Because they inform and shape our worldview, our treatments must somehow involve, refer to, and embrace these beliefs. Indeed, Jerome Frank (Frank & Frank, 1991) said that therapy must reflect the prevailing values of the culture and address the individual through this language. At the same time that its importance is waning in therapeutics, the upsurge of interest in psychoanalysis and Freud in the humanities reflects how deeply embedded these ideas are in our cultural and intellectual tradition.

We suggest that psychodynamically based treatments have a special focus on the rewriting of a personal narrative. The need to develop a narrative understanding is essentially human, reflected in storytelling traditions, literature and art, and the autobiographical urge that strikes virtually everyone at some point in time. Dynamic psychotherapy takes this fundamentally human task as its challenge. We believe that psychodynamic psychotherapy retains its currency because it encourages patients to tell and rework their stories in an intensive way.

Therapy for Therapists

Fourth, therapists tend to choose psychodynamic psychotherapy for their own treatment, as documented in a recent study of psychiatry trainees (Habl, Mintz, & Bailey, 2009). Our impression is that other trainees tend to choose dynamically oriented treatments, as well. Why this occurs during a time when other psychotherapies are proliferating is an interesting question. Therapists often enter treatment early in their careers and are influenced by their teachers and mentors, and their treatment choice may simply reflect a cohort effect. As newer psychotherapies achieve greater dominance and their proponents fill the ranks of mentors and teachers, this is likely to diminish.

But perhaps therapists enter psychodynamic psychotherapy because it is particularly useful to them. Perhaps therapists themselves prefer the depth and explicit attention to narrative intrinsic to dynamic psychotherapy. The emphasis on affect and ways of understanding intense affective experiences, provides therapists with the clarity and resilience needed to work with distressed and suffering individuals. The intense focus on the therapeutic relationship also helps us understand our enactments, transferences, and countertransferences.

THE CHANGING FACE
OF PSYCHODYNAMIC PSYCHOTHERAPY

We have summarized current definitions of psychodynamic therapy and argued for its currency and value. But to stay current, the treatment must evolve. There are new ideas and new knowledge that suggest changes in theory and technique, and powerful social forces that are shaping its use (see Table 1.2). Some of the most current influences are detailed below.

Research on the *demand characteristics of social situations* and psychotherapy outcome and process research have demonstrated the importance of educating and socializing the patient into the process of psychotherapy, and have shown improved efficacy when this occurs (e.g., Greenberg, Constantino, & Bruce, 2006). Confusion, lost time, and uncertainty can result when patients start psychotherapy without adequate explanation and education. Orientation to psychotherapy and greater *transparency* about its processes and goals offer the potential of greater efficacy.

The impact of the *therapeutic alliance* on outcome is one of the most consistent findings in the field of psychotherapy research (Messer & Wampold, 2002), despite the fact that it accounts for only a small amount of variance in outcome (Barber, 2009). Different types of psychotherapy show precious little difference in outcomes. Rather, the development of a strong therapeutic alliance provides a path to success common to all psychotherapies. Increased awareness of the importance of the alliance and techniques for addressing rupture of the alliance have generated new ideas about how this factor can be optimized in psychodynamic psychotherapy, especially with reference to clinician abstinence and neutrality.

There is a convergence between the psychoanalytic concept of *unconscious fantasy* and the CBT concept of *schema*. Arising primarily in the CBT literature, schemas are the deep cognitive structures that develop out of early life experiences and are maintained by the subsequent distorted perceptions; their persistence is the essence of psychodynamic pathology. This concept shares similarities with Luborsky's CCRT (Luborsky & Crits-Christoph, 1990), which is an example of an interpersonally anchored schema. Slap's (Slap & Slap-Shelton, 1991)

TABLE 1.2. New Ideas, Knowledge, and Social Forces Shape Change in Psychodynamic Psychotherapy

New knowledge, social forces	Changes in psychotherapy theory and technique
Demand characteristics of therapy	Education, orientation, explanation
Increased recognition of the importance of the therapeutic alliance	New techniques for developing alliance and repairing ruptures
Convergence of concepts of fantasy, schema, pathogenic thoughts	Emphasis on schema resulting from traumatic experiences
Importance of narrative	Rewriting of narrative a focus of therapy
Reality of trauma; therapeutic relationship a result of patient and therapist factors	Less hierarchical treatment relationship, closer attention to minute-to-minute aspect of process
Positive psychology	Attention to character, positive emotion, and enhancement
Need to understand psychotherapy in combination with other treatments	Clarification of role of psychotherapy in overall treatment plan
Neurobiological understanding of psychotherapy	May provide additional scientific evidence for psychoanalytic concepts
Patient advocacy and empowerment	Education, transparency, informed consent
Concern about efficiency	Time-limited treatment; changes in technique, goals

reformulation of psychoanalytic theory around a schema model conceptualizes a central traumatic scenario in childhood that gives rise to symptoms. Control–mastery theory (Weiss, Sampson, & the Mount Zion Psychotherapy Research Group, 1986) is a related psychoanalytic model developed by the Mt. Zion Research Group that holds that symptoms arise from "unconscious pathogenic beliefs," which are inferences about traumatic events. All of these contributors point to deep mental organizing principles that are cognitive and ideational. These schemas, or traumatic scenarios, influence subsequent perceptions, feelings, and thoughts.

Just as the critical study of texts forms the basis for analysis in academic humanities departments, methods for using *narrative in healing* have gained currency in medical circles and have been studied by psychoanalysts for some time (Spence, 1982). There is increased interest in narrative medicine (Charon, 2006), which emphasizes the importance of the patient's personal story as a way of understanding, managing, and healing. These developments have led to an increased focus on the role of narrative in psychotherapy. We see the central task of psychotherapy as the rewriting of a more complex and useful narrative of the patient's life and experience.

Awareness of the *importance and prevalence of trauma* has resulted in an increased interest and focus on the real experience of the patient. There is greater interest in the importance of external factors and less emphasis on internal fantasy in determining the impact of the traumatic experience. This shift makes for less hierarchy in the relationship between patient and therapist. When the patient's experience is understood to have actually occurred, and is not just a result of his or her construction of reality, then the reality of who the therapist is and how he behaves is real and important as well. This has led to more interest in the intersubjective elements in the therapist–patient dyad, a focus on the concept of enactment as opposed to transference, and a loosening of some of the constraints on therapist behavior. These developments parallel the increased interest in relational or interpersonal psychoanalysis, which conceives of the therapeutic relationship as a newly constructed entity created by patient and therapist. Relational psychoanalysis puts greater emphasis on the here and now of minute-to-minute interactions. Techniques suggested by these recent developments include greater therapist self-disclosure and close attention to the aspects of the therapeutic process generated by the therapist's attitudes, thoughts, and feelings (Mitchell, 1988).

The field of *positive psychology,* which explores positive emotion, happiness, and techniques for enhancing positive experience, provides a new perspective to psychotherapy (Seligman, 2002; Peterson, 2006). The contribution includes an emphasis on the concepts of character and virtue, the relative independence of positive emotions from negative emotions, and interventions for enhancing subjective satisfaction. The importance of positive experiences in promoting increased self-reflection and change suggest new therapeutic techniques.

Traditionally, psychotherapy was studied within its own "silo," separated from its frequent integration with other treatments, for example, psychopharmacology, couple and systems therapy, and educational and behavioral treatments. The likely synergy (and also tension) with these treatments is just beginning to be studied. An example of this is the data showing that *psychotherapy and psychopharmacology may be syner-*

gistic in moderate to severe depression, but not be more effective than either treatment alone in mild depression (Thase, 1999). Findings like this clarify the role of psychotherapy in general and also, perhaps, of specific psychotherapies in the real naturalistic settings in which they are employed.

New neurobiological findings bear witness to the changes in the brain resulting from psychotherapy (Etkin, Pittenger, Polan, & Kandel, 2005) and open the door to understanding psychotherapeutic change and the specific changes resulting from specific psychotherapies (Goldapple et al., 2004). Although we cannot test and improve interventions using neuroimaging data yet, this is a possibility in the future. Several contemporary neuroscientists suggest that there are neurobiological data to support traditional psychoanalytic concepts (Westen & Gabbard, 2002; Kandel, 1999), including the theory of dreams (Solms, 1995).

There are a number of social forces generating change in the practice of psychodynamic psychotherapy. *Patient advocacy organizations* have reminded us of the importance of knowledge about illnesses for patient empowerment. This encourages educational interventions about the nature of symptoms and illness, and about treatment alternatives and treatments themselves. The need for informed consent for treatment has spread beyond medical and surgical treatments to include psychotherapy and has contributed to a more open, transparent process of diagnosis and treatment selection, and also of initiation of psychotherapy. Some anticipate that an explicit informed consent process, which includes spelling out the risks of psychotherapy, will become the standard for psychotherapy as it is for other procedures in the medical care system.

Greater *concern about efficiency* has led to time-limited treatments (e.g., Barber & Ellman, 1996; Crits-Christoph, Barber, & Kurcias, 1991). Both patients and payors are more focused on the speed of treatment. The resulting push to target symptoms and focus on goals has resulted in changes in both technique and objectives. This has been an impetus for technical innovation and reevaluation of goals. The interest in pruning the length and expense of treatment has sharpened interest in whether psychotherapy should decrease symptoms or promote healthy development, with the recognition that different therapies may have different goals. This has resulted in the development of psychodynamic treatment focused on specific disorders (e.g., Milrod et al., 1997, for panic disorder; Crits-Christoph, Connolly Gibbons, Narducci, Schamberger, & Gallop, 2005, for generalized anxiety disorder). It has also clarified the continuing need for treatment of other problems such as developmental and lifecycle issues that are not symptom based, such as identity formation, intimacy and relationship problems, and loss and grieving. Common clinical scenarios include teenagers in conflict with their parents as they try to "find themselves," young adults with difficulty committing to intimate relationships, and middle-aged adults struggling with adapting to new limitations in career or health.

A PRAGMATIC PSYCHODYNAMIC PSYCHOTHERAPY

We have argued for the value of psychodynamic psychotherapy and at the same time described some of the new ideas and social forces that suggest how it has to change.

> Beth continued weekly psychotherapy for 2½ years. She became convinced that her inner experience of loneliness and mistrust of others, especially men, was triggered by repeated memories of her very painful childhood experiences. She developed a new, clearer picture of her childhood. At the same time, she started to realize that her current life was not so bad. She began dating, and enjoyed it more than before. After a while she met a man who was much more kind, stable, and psychologically healthy than the men she had been with before. She also began to develop more friendships with women.
>
> Beth's relationship with me was rocky at times, and in addition to trying to understand it, much time was spent helping Beth feel safe and comfortable in the therapy. This included education, explanation about the therapy, and attention to particular moments of mistrust. Beth seemed to alternate between trusting, positive feelings and sudden anger, suspiciousness, and withdrawal. She became more and more aware that these reactions reflected her old feelings, which alternated between childlike trust and then betrayal and fear. I became better at anticipating when the shifts would occur and could interpret and clarify them more clearly. We developed a kind of rhythm—discussion of her new relationship, her periodic interactions with her parents, and feelings and thoughts about me. As she moved from one to the other and was able to apply her understanding of the old relationship templates that played out in each situation, she became stronger and more confident. She also seemed looser, more playful, and wittier than before. This flexibility was evident in her description of her daily life. She said she felt more attractive, too.
>
> Beth was pleased with her new relationship and expected that it might develop into marriage. Ultimately she decided it was time to

try to live life on her own and end therapy. She had one last spasm of fear and doubt just before the end of treatment when she was unsure if she could manage on her own. This upset resolved quickly when she realized that it was, again, a replay of the same old pattern of loneliness and fear. With her new self-awareness, clearer perceptions of others, and more adaptive behavior, she was ready to move on.

Beth's treatment was successful, and it incorporated traditional ideas about dynamic psychotherapy (emphasis on experiencing affects, exploring the past, looking for patterns, increasing awareness, working on the therapeutic relationship) as well as many of the new ideas we have discussed here (attention to the therapeutic relationship, education and explanation, transparency, rewriting the narrative). The next chapter sets out the basic theory and technique of the updated model, referred to as pragmatic psychodynamic psychotherapy, and the subsequent chapters will elucidate these ideas, explaining, giving examples, and providing specific practical tips.

CHAPTER 2

Pragmatic Psychodynamic Psychotherapy

Conceptual Model and Techniques

It is the theory that decides what we can observe.
—ALBERT EINSTEIN

Pragmatic psychodynamic psychotherapy (PPP) is based on a developmental and conflict model of mental life and involves clearly defined psychodynamic diagnosis and formulation, a focus on education and transparency, integration with other synergistic treatment modalities, and an active, engaged therapeutic stance. It differs from classical psychodynamic psychotherapy, which has tended to be open ended, hierarchical, not diagnosis specific, inadequately integrated conceptually and technically with psychopharmacology and other concurrent treatments, less active, and less focused.

The reader's therapeutic urge (and anxieties about what to do with patients) will probably be somewhat frustrated by reading about theory and technical principles. This chapter does not tell you specifically what to do—that comes next. But it will provide the larger framework for the rest of the book, which will focus on the concrete, specific, and practical application of these ideas.

23

CONCEPTUAL MODEL AND ASSUMPTIONS

This section addresses the theoretical underpinnings of PPP (summarized in Table 2.1), including the assumptions and central conceptualizations, while the next section discusses the primary psychotherapy techniques.

Conflict, Conflict, Conflict . . .

The essential and perhaps most enduring legacy of Freud and psychoanalysis is its emphasis on the centrality of unconscious conflict in men-

TABLE 2.1. PPP Model and Assumptions Compared with Traditional Psychodynamic Psychotherapy

PPP assumptions and conceptualization	Traditional psychodynamic psychotherapy assumptions and conceptualization
• Mental life involves ongoing conflict and compromise formation. Behavior is multiply determined.	• Mental life involves ongoing conflict and compromise formation. Behavior is seen as secondary phenomenon.
• Mental processes—affect, cognition, drives—operate in parallel.	• Affect and drive have primacy; cognition is secondary.
• Behavior is determined by thoughts and feelings and in turn shapes thoughts and feelings.	• Behavior and symptoms are secondary to conflict.
• Traumatic experiences in the past prefigure later perceptions and experience. Traumatic scenarios are repeated.	• Unresolved conflict leads to developmental fixation and repetition of conflict.
• There is an interweaving of dynamic factors with biological, psychological, and social factors in wellness and in the development, maintenance, and resolution of psychopathology.	• Psychodynamic factors are essential factors in development of pathology, and other factors are epiphenomenal or associated.
• Change occurs in therapeutic relationship with increase self-awareness and insight, emotional reexperiencing, specific empathic attunement between patient and therapist, and development of alternative perceptions and new behaviors.	• Change occurs in therapeutic relationship as a result of insight and new experiences.

tal life (Freud, 1916, 1917a; Brenner, 1974). All elements of mental life can be viewed as part of the ongoing turmoil arising from competing wishes, fears, and prohibitions, and attempts to resolve these contradictions.

Drives and impulses, whether conceptualized as sexual and aggressive in the original psychoanalytic formulations, or intense urges for attachment, bonding, mastery, and affiliation in subsequent thinking, are the motivating sparks that initiate intrapsychic conflict. Drives and impulses appear in consciousness (make themselves known) in derivative form as fantasies, thoughts, feelings, and perceptions. *Fantasies* involve wishful scenarios, either conscious or unconscious, that are stirred up by these drives and impulses, and are an attempt to find an expression and a fulfillment of these needs. *Cognition* is a domain seemingly less directly affected by impulses; it refers to our attempt to find reliable, valid, and persisting ideas about ourselves and our world. Many aspects of cognition are affected by conflict, such as pessimistic assessments and negative attributions arising from early loss. Our *feelings,* which refer to the conscious subjective experience of our emotional or affective states, are a more immediate dimension of our sense of ourselves and our environment.

Each of these aspects of mental experience is involved in intrapsychic conflict, and the conflict model elucidates and identifies the warring elements. The conflict could be between different drives (love and aggression, for example) or between a drive and cultural values (a common conflict in our Western culture is between the wish to be close vs. the need for independence). The conflict could also be between a drive and reality, as in the tension between the need for intimacy and the lack of a partner.

The concept of conflict, as originally formulated in the psychoanalytic literature, assumed the classic form of impulse (drive), prohibition (fears or conscience), and defense (means of coping), all of which lead to a compromise formation (symptom, character trait, behavior, attitude) (Brenner, 1974). Object relations theorists focus instead on conflict between internally constructed representations of self and others (Greenberg & Mitchell, 1983; Kernberg, 1988). The feelings engendered by a good and loving mental representation of the mother might conflict with the feelings stimulated by a coexisting representation of the mother as harsh and vindictive. The essence of the psychodynamic model, whatever subtype, is looking at urges, their imagined consequences, and the associated fantasies, thoughts, and feelings—the diverse constituents of mental life—through the lens of conflict and compromise.

Conflict is mistakenly equated with pathology. It is normal for there to be chronic conflict. Compromise formations, the result of vectors of conflicting mental urges, are ubiquitous. Better compromise formations are, or should be, our life goal, and they are certainly our therapeutic goal (Waelder, 1936). Any aspect of a person's life can be examined through the lens of compromise formation. Examples of compromise formations include important life decisions, a person's characteristic interpersonal style, beliefs, attitudes, creative productions, and psychological symptoms. For example, a juvenile-onset diabetic who struggled with fear, anger, and frustration about the deprivations and effects of her dietary requirements and injections might choose to become a doctor or nurse. This compromise formation is an adaptive defensive process that helps master the frustration and anger about the illness by becoming a provider of care—in control and not suffering, helping others with problems. An effective teacher who was adopted in childhood after several foster placements and subsequently has trouble committing to an intimate relationship is managing his fears of abandonment by protecting himself from getting hurt again through avoidance of a close relationship, but expresses his need for closeness through mentoring relationships with his students. Artistic productions are an attempt to express (and sublimate) conflict by portraying them for an audience. Picasso's *Guernica* expresses the horror of an attack on a defenseless Spanish town by transforming it into something deeply engaging, beautiful, and memorable. Thus the painting is a compromise formation, expressing the outrage and fear about what happened and creating something universal and heroic, adding beauty to the pain. Rap music gives voice to the harsh realities of street life expressing both the artist's power and deep vulnerability.

From the conflict perspective, how is a symptom different from these successful examples of conflict and compromise? Like the difference between a weed and a prize botanical specimen, a symptom is a dysfunctional, maladaptive, or unwanted compromise formation, while a successful compromise is a source of strength. Unfortunately, poor compromises are often maintained, as they are the patient's best attempt at resolving conflict at a particular point in time, and they persist long afterward.

The psychodynamic perspective allows us to analyze and deconstruct patients' compromise formations. We look at behavior, symptoms, and feelings and break them down into their constituent parts. But therapy must also help patients rebuild, and the analyzing focus on the conflicted roots of any bit of mental life is balanced by a healthy appreciation for the carefully constructed compromise formations patients bring us.

Joan was an affectionate and insightful woman in her early 50s whose mother suffered depressive episodes during her early school years. She complained of anxiety and a strong need to please and care for her parents and children during their frequent vacations, family occasions, and holidays. Joan was uncomfortable discussing this problem because she felt she was a good daughter and mother, and it was confusing for her to regard the need to please as a problem. But at the same time she knew there was something excessively pressured in her need to care for her family in these circumstances.

Through her psychotherapy, Joan recognized her conflicted wishes for love and closeness with her mother, and her sadness and loneliness when she felt abandoned by mother during her periods of depression. She could not specifically remember feeling angry with her mother because of her frustrated needs, but she knew she often felt guilty. She was amazed when she recognized how often time spent with her family in the present stirred up these old feelings.

She saw, too, the compromise formations she had evolved to adapt to her abandonment—helpfulness, compartmentalization of feelings, and a demeanor of optimism and effectiveness. She hoped that being helpful might help her mother feel better so that she would be more available.

To some extent, Joan's behavior was a maladaptive compromise. Although it allowed her to feel more closeness, stave off her fears of loss, and convince herself she was good and loving, it took an enormous toll on her. She was tired, often irritated, and stretched thin. She realized she felt chronically angry with her mother, and this probably prevented her from feeling closer to her.

Situation after situation was discussed in which Joan employed this compromise—helping in order to deal with feelings of abandonment. The therapist helped her deconstruct the feelings, thoughts, and behavior associated with each. As she came to see the conflicts behind each of these situations—fear of loss, anger and resentment, guilt, resolution to help and protect, distorted ideas about the mother's illness and what caused it, and behaviors designed to prove her own goodness—she felt less compelled and driven, more relaxed, and more aware that her fears were based on an old and outdated scenario. She became much less anxious. She began to feel more deeply loving toward her mother. She was less saddled by anger and hurt and had the sense that she could use her helpfulness to good purposes when she wanted to, and not be helpful when she did not want to.

Conflict and the resolution of conflict through development and experience, or through therapy, is the mantra here. Of the theoretical assumptions of PPP, this probably is the most similar to traditional psychodynamic practice and may be the feature that distinguishes it most from CBT and other types of psychotherapy.

Parallel Processing: Drive, Affect, Cognition, Behavior

In our pragmatic model of psychotherapy, affects, thinking, and behavior are conceptualized as operating in parallel, without one having primacy over the others. These features of mental life influence one another, rather than operate in a linear sequence. Affects, thoughts, and behavior are derivative of drives, and reflect them.

This perspective contrasts with the traditional psychodynamic view and also with the paradigm of cognitive therapy. In traditional dynamic psychotherapy, the focus is on understanding drives, affects, fantasies, and how they relate to one another. Relatively speaking, there is less interest in cognition and less focus on behavior. The traditional psychodynamic approach has been to amplify and elucidate feelings over all else.

However, the systematic distortions in thinking that develop over time can have a profound effect on a patient's experience, perceptions, and behavior and have an autonomous life of their own. For example, the repeated negative attribution that a patient may make to each new social contact involves not just a feeling, but also a belief. There is a specific conviction about what will occur next, and what the patient has to do to avoid shame, disappointment, or whatever the feared outcome is. PPP includes a focus on these pathogenic cognitions as well as the affects and fantasies.

CBT gives primacy to disturbances in thinking (Beck, 1976; Lazarus & Folkman, 1984). This approach views affect as a result of cognition ("I think, therefore I feel"), and therefore spends much time at rectifying "wrong" cognitions. A primary focus on cognition risks losing the immediacy and conviction that comes with a focus on feelings and the access to this important data about the patient's mental life. In our view, affect and cognition are two different aspects of the same process. There may be contexts in which feelings drive thoughts, and other situations in which thoughts shape feelings. The implication for our treatment approach is that we emphasize both affect and cognition in treatment. In fact, we may even recommend to a therapist that if a patient tends to emphasize affect, maybe he or she should emphasize cognition, whereas if the patient tends to emphasize cognition he or she should emphasize affect a bit more. Barber and Muenz (1996) have used the term the "theory of opposites" to characterize their finding that depressed patients with obsessive–compulsive personality disorder do preferentially better with an interpersonally based therapy than a cognitively based therapy. They speculated that it is helpful for patients to receive treatment that somehow works against their defensive and personality style.

Behavior and Change, Behavioral Change

In the traditional psychodynamic model, behavior was seen as the downstream effect of where the real action is—in the patient's head. Behavior was caused by conflict and would change when the conflict was untangled. Some believed that resolving the conflict was the only way to permanently modify behavior. At times, traditional psychoanalytic and psychodynamic education showed a surprising lack of interest and concern about patient's symptoms (and behavior), seeing them as almost epiphenomenal.

PPP regards behavior as equally important as subjective experience and intrapsychic conflict. Behavior is multiply determined by mental events as well as by somatic and neurobiological factors. Behavior results from mental conflict, but it also has the power to change experience and thus affect intrapsychic conflicts and mental life. This two-way causality is a crucial theoretical aspect of PPP and distinguishes it from the traditional psychodynamic model. New behaviors and the new experiences that result from them may need to be encouraged long before the patient will spontaneously generate new experiences and new perceptions of him- or herself. In this sense, we build on Wachtel's (1997) insight about cycles of behavior and experience, for example, the dynamics of shyness. If one is anxious about being rejected, one tends to avoid meeting new people. This impedes the development of social skills and reinforces the sense of isolation. Therefore if one is shy, one is likely to become more shy. To break the cycle, one must find a way to do something different, such as learning new social skills that will enable more social opportunities. Traditionally, dynamic therapists have waited for insight that might open up possibilities of behavioral change, whereas we suggest that the patient's behavior may not change on its own.

> Chris was a tall, thin man in his 30s, whose wife struggled with a chronic recurrent depression. He complained that she was not interested in him, and he felt rejected and depressed. They spent little

time together. He was very involved with their three young children and felt himself to be an exemplary father, in contrast to his feeling that his wife was not very involved. Chris had many opinions about her emotional problems and criticized her for not doing things that he thought would make her feel better. His attitude and demeanor frequently had a patronizing quality as he spoke about her in sessions and, it seemed, when he spoke to her at home. Chris's somewhat dismissive attitude helped him deal with his pain and disappointment about her condition and manage his own chronic neediness and sense of emptiness.

Although he could begin to see all of these conflicting feelings in himself and how his attitude was defensive, he was absolutely at a loss to see how he could behave differently with his wife. He was aware of the historical roots of this problem—his mother had panic disorder and agoraphobia. He had four siblings, and his mother was often very stressed and unavailable during his childhood. But, he kept feeling, what else could he do but try to be helpful and reasonable? After all, he felt, he really was doing a good job helping a depressed wife, and he was great with the kids. There was a gap between his intellectual insight about the patterns, and his ability to step away from his need to protect himself from pain by being exemplary.

In order to increase his awareness and find ways of experiencing the family situation differently, together we came up with specific "scripts" that allowed him to express his concern and empathy, but did not offer as much specific help. For example, when his wife complained about feeling exhausted, Chris simply made an empathic comment such as, "You've had a long day," and did not offer to take over unless she specifically asked for it. This made it easier for Chris's wife to get more involved. She felt he was more respectful and she was able to exercise more autonomy. He felt relieved at not having to help as much.

Chris noted that not only did his wife seem to be more responsive, but there was something different in how he felt after one of their arguments. He was a little more distant from her, saddened perhaps, but felt less of a sense of responsibility, less "controlled" by her unhappiness, and less like her difficulties were the cause of his unhappiness. Noting all of these feelings, which were a consequence of new behavior, afforded him a new perspective on himself. Chris could see more clearly his old adaptation to his childhood situation and felt less need to respond reflexively to his current family the same way. He was more introspective about the various conflicted feelings he had about his wife, and surprisingly, less dependent on her.

Attention to how patients think and feel in psychotherapy helps promote self-awareness. However, behavior is more than a downstream effect of intrapsychic change; rather, it may also be causal in patients' problems. Changes in behavior can result in changes in feelings and perceptions.

"What's Past Is Prologue"

Shakespeare's (2005) pithy phrase is a sound-bite explanation for the formation and perpetuation of psychodynamic problems. Earlier life experiences that are overwhelming and cannot be absorbed, integrated, or metabolized result in conflicted compromise formations. They are the basis for the patient's subsequent repetitive difficulties. Originally, Freud hypothesized that psychosexual conflict and the development of the "infantile neurosis," a flare of symptomatology associated with sexual and aggressive conflict in the young child, was the basis for later neurotic developments (Freud, 1918). He saw the adult neurosis as a reactivation of the childhood problem.

This aspect of traditional psychodynamic theory was the rationale for the extensive historical explorations and reconstructions that are the hallmark of psychoanalytic treatment, where the past is prologue to the present, and all understanding is historical understanding. An interest in the past and its effect on the present led Freud and others to the question of childhood trauma. Trauma has been central to the psychodynamic perspective, both informing it and also generating some heated controversy and confusion. The contemporary recognition of the frequency of severe traumatic events, including childhood violence, abuse, and serious neglect, required revision of some of the early excessive focus on the intrapsychic factors in response to trauma (Herman, 1997). The field has become much more aware of the importance of social, cultural, and indeed, realistic and practical factors in the response to trauma, and posttraumatic illness has become an important focus of current study.

PPP embraces the kernel of the original Freudian model—earlier trauma generates pathology that is reactivated later in life—but in a more generic mode. Traumas may be acute, externally evident, obviously overwhelming and destructive, or they may be subtle. These more subtle but nevertheless serious problems may include a mismatch between needs and opportunities, between temperaments of child and caregiver, or struggles with neurobiologically driven extremes of experience (anxiety, mood lability, perceptual distortions). At the same time that trauma is important, we recognize that memory is actively constructed and can be misleading and distorted; much care must be taken to avoid forcing definitive conclusions about what happened in childhood.

The schema concept, which refers to a deep organizing structure in the mind, is particularly relevant here (Bartlett, 1932; Slap & Slap-Shelton, 1991). Developing out of overwhelming and traumatic experience, the child forms a relatively fixed perceptual pattern with an associated solution or adaptation to this. This pattern is focused into a schema, or traumatic scenario, that is finite and relatively specific, including perceptions of others, feelings, associated thoughts and ideas, fantasies, and the attempted solutions to the traumatic situation. The schemas formed in the wake of traumatic experiences, great and small, become repetitive scripts, activated over and over again later in life. The perceptions, drives, fantasies, thoughts, and feelings are repeated, as are the compromise formations developed to adapt to them.

Bowlby's (1958) attachment model provides an excellent example of one kind of traumatic experience that becomes the basis for future difficulty. Problems in early caregiver attachment result in insecure attachment that manifests itself in either clinging or avoidance. Subsequent relationships are experienced and managed according to this old scenario. New intimate partners, who may in fact be highly stable and affectionate, are experienced with the same insecurity as the earlier relationship, and the same clinging or avoidant adaptations show themselves.

Traumatic scenarios or schemas are reactivated by subsequent associated situations, and the same old pattern is enacted over and over again. For example, Chris's powerful reaction to his wife was based in part on his traumatic experience with his preoccupied agoraphobic mother.

The Biopsychosocial Model and Psychodynamics

The repetition of the traumatic past, which distorts and reshapes the present in a Groundhog Day–style reliving, is only one explanatory factor in a complex system. A danger of the psychodynamic perspective is that it can become an all-inclusive explanation (Popper, 1962). One can almost always find a conflict-based explanation for a problem, and this can cause the therapist to diminish the importance of other contributing factors. For example a patient may be depressed because her daughter is ill, and this reminds her of her own childhood illness and the losses that accompanied it, or because of another cycle of her bipolar spectrum illness, or because of her fatigue and sleeplessness associated with a medical problem.

The biopsychosocial model (American Psychiatric Association, 2000) provides the conceptual basis for including the major biological, psychological, and social factors that must be entertained in understanding individual pathology. However, this umbrella concept is somewhat loose in characterizing what data and what kinds of formulations are relevant within each of these three main areas (bio, psycho, and social), and how these factors are specifically related.

The psychodynamic factors are those that affect the meaning of current events because of prior traumatic events. This is as opposed to many nondynamic factors, such as purely cognitive factors that affect the information-processing capacities of the mind, neurobiological factors like temperament, genetic factors in personality, subsyndromal and syndromal psychiatric illnesses, and social factors such as family system, culture, and political power.

Although it is difficult to sort out the relative effects of the various potential causes for symptoms, the PPP model regards the dynamic factors as only one in a series of parallel causal factors. These various considerations form a continuing chain over the life cycle, with dynamics affecting neurobiology, which affects the social milieu, which affects the dynamics, and neurobiology, and so on. The case formulation (discussed in Chapter 7) is the vehicle for focusing these different perspectives in an individual case. The rich literature on formulation (Perry, Cooper, & Michels, 1987), and more recent contributions (McWilliams, 1999; Summers, 2002), discuss the best format for accomplishing this. The formulation is central in PPP because it allows the clinician to focus on what the psychodynamic factors are, and how they are related to the nondynamic factors, paving the way for effective goal-setting, treatment planning, and integration with other treatments when necessary.

Therapeutic Change

PPP promotes change in how people experience themselves, their relationships, and their world, through three mechanisms. Patients (1) develop increased self-awareness and insight into themselves, which includes reexperiencing painful affects, thoughts, feelings, and memories; (2) develop an empathic close relationship with the therapist that is different from other relationships past and present (Alexander & French, 1946); and (3) find new ways of perceiving old situations that allow them to try new behaviors in response to them. We summarize the model for change here, and the techniques for facilitating it in the next section. A more detailed discussion of these issues is provided in Chapter 10.

Change begins first by facilitating increased self-awareness and insight. This is both a cognitive and an emotional process and involves helping patients reexperience the painful feelings they have worked hard to ward off. By reexperiencing old feelings and understanding their context, patients begin to work through the meanings (sometimes unconscious) attached to these events. Slowly, the old feelings and perceptions reenter consciousness, and once they are conscious, patients' natural problem-solving capacities can be engaged. This process unites insight or self-understanding and emotional reexperiencing. Some have characterized this aspect of therapy as habituation or desensitization to the painful feelings (McCullough et al., 2002).

Feelings of loss, separation, fear, worry over the impact of angry urges, loneliness, insecurity, and shame are intensified by the expectation that experiencing these feelings will make things worse. Usually, the opposite is true. Roosevelt's famous encouragement to Americans in the midst of the Great Depression, "The only thing we have to fear is fear itself," reminds us that the feeling is not the fact. Believing in the truth of a feeling leads to trouble if it is an old feeling replayed. Indeed, confronting old feelings and reexperiencing them is viewed as therapeutic in therapies ranging from behavior therapy (Foa & Rothbaum, 1998) to experiential therapy or gestalt (Greenberg, 2002).

The accepting atmosphere created in therapy and the open-ended interviewing style of the psychodynamic approach help to guide the patient gently to these painful recollections. Childhood traumatic scenarios are expressed either through recalling and discussing memories, or through derivatives of these earlier situations, that is, current situations that contain the same patterns and same feelings. Becoming distant from (or habituated to) these feeling or thoughts is therapeutic, increasing the patient's sense of mastery, control, and autonomy. The patient is no longer afraid of them and can be more emotionally open and flexible.

Second, almost all psychotherapies rely on the development of a safe, trusting, and open relationship between therapist and patient, and many posit that the relationship itself is part of what brings about the therapeutic effects of the treatment. This is true despite the significant differences in theory and technique. We suggest that psychodynamic psychotherapy, and PPP, depends not just on the development of a general trusting relationship, but on an attuned and empathic bond between the patient and the therapist. The therapeutic effectiveness of PPP depends on the patient's feeling that the therapist understands and accepts her specific feelings, needs, thoughts, and history. The therapist, in turn, feels that the patient knows that she knows these things. This loop of mutual awareness and understanding is what we mean by the specific attunement and empathic bond. We see this type of therapeutic closeness as an essential component of what facilitates change in the patient.

Third, understanding one's problems opens the door to learning how to experience them differently. Through correction of the inaccurate perceptions implied in old scenarios and recognition of alternative ways to perceive the same situations, patients can see new aspects to repetitive experiences that they were previously unable to change. From that recognition emerges what may be the most solidifying aspect of therapeutic change—a new behavioral response. Patients often need to reexperience painful old scenarios to begin the process of detoxifying them and move on to see alternative perceptions, more reality-based and from multiple points of view. With this, they are often able to consider new and different behavioral responses. These new behaviors, perhaps never previously considered, often reflect the patients' therapeutic goals and allow for new experiences. These new experiences create a positive feedback loop, bringing new emotional growth and still more opportunities. They bring new experiences of self and other and allow for stronger contemporary, reality-based perceptions and development of ever-better and more effective compromise formations. PPP's emphasis on new behavior and its mutative effects reflects the effectiveness demonstrated by recently developed behavioral treatments.

TECHNICAL PRINCIPLES

Streamlining the conceptual basis for PPP allows for a clearer and easier-to-learn set of therapeutic techniques. All too often, in our own training, we were confronted with a bewildering array of interesting, seemingly very important, but often conflicting therapeutic techniques. Our teachers encouraged us with the hopeful words, "it takes experience," to tell us which technique to use when. It does require experience to coax a therapeutic relationship into existence and support an open-ended free-association process. But we think there are guidelines that define, facilitate, and constrain the process to help trainees to set it in motion. Summarized in Table 2.2, these techniques are articulated below and discussed extensively in the rest of the book.

TABLE 2.2. PPP Technique Compared with Traditional Psychodynamic Psychotherapy

PPP technique	Traditional psychodynamic psychotherapy technique
• Free association allows for emotional exploration, reexperiencing of important feelings, fantasies, and thoughts.	• Same focus, but more open-ended, unstructured interaction.
• The therapist focuses on the development and maintenance of the therapeutic relationship, with consequent focus on current reality, and an active, engaged, empathic therapeutic stance.	• Development of therapeutic alliance is important, but more abstinent and less reactive stance allows for less confusion in observation of transference reactions.
• Equal attention is paid to various derivatives of conflicts, including but not focused on transference and the past.	• Important to focus on transference, countertransference, and past.
• Identifying the core psychodynamic problem and developing a comprehensive case formulation is essential; this is done early, shared with the patient, and is the basis for collaborative goal setting and treatment planning. Psychotherapy technique is problem specific. Formulation is consistent with the ongoing process of patient developing a life narrative.	• Case formulations focus primarily on psychodynamic factors, are developed later in treatment, and not shared with patient. Patient develops insight and awareness of conflicts through therapist's clarifications and interpretations. Psychotherapy technique does not vary across problems.
• Goals drive the treatment and are the basis for integrating dynamic psychotherapy with other modalities of treatment.	• Elucidation of psychodynamic conflicts and their resolution is the primary focus in treatment; symptom relief is less emphasized. Integration with other treatments is not systematically planned and implemented.
• Alternative perceptions and new behaviors are proposed in response to derivatives of traumatic scenarios.	• Through self-awareness, patients change perceptions and try new behaviors.
• The therapist's role, the rationale, and the goals of treatment are discussed in a transparent manner.	• Concern about effects on transference and ability to effectively analyze transference results in less direct orientation, education, and explanation about the psychotherapeutic process and maintenance of a more "mysterious" therapist persona.

Association: Free, but Not Too Free

Like play, which occupies a space between reality and fantasy, psychotherapy provides the patient with an opportunity to dream while awake, let her mind go, permitting thoughts, feelings, memories, and images to bubble up. This is meant in the metaphorical sense, since of course the patient is awake and sitting in a chair looking at the therapist. But the patient is encouraged to put her associations (spontaneous thoughts) into words. Of course, this is difficult to do; it is a skill that develops over time and it is subject to the same conflicts the patient is trying to explore.

To this end, PPP uses traditional open-ended interviewing techniques, facilitating the patient's uninhibited expression of emotions, private thoughts, urges, and fantasies (Gabbard, 2000). Sessions begin without a specific agenda, and patients are encouraged to put their thoughts and feelings into words. The technique is to focus on the here and now (in the sense of what the patient is genuinely feeling and spontaneously thinking about) because that is the road to deeper self-awareness. Although the therapist will carefully remember previously discussed material, including an emerging picture of the patient's problems, the patient is given relatively free rein to talk about what is on her mind in the moment.

The therapist attempts to connect the patient's current feelings and thoughts with others that constitute a pattern. If the therapist believes an important issue from the previous session or earlier in the same session has not been addressed, the patient is encouraged to address that topic. Increasingly over a session connections will be made, and there is an ebb and flow between spontaneous associations and directed exploration of important thoughts and feelings.

The PPP therapist allows for enough open-endedness to help the patient bring new material into the sessions, and experience feelings and thoughts in an unforced and natural way. But he or she maintains a hand on the tiller, gently steering the session in the direction of fleshing out and working on the central psychodynamic problems, allowing for them to be reexperienced and reconsidered.

The Therapeutic Relationship

Perhaps the most robust finding in the psychotherapy outcome literature, which cuts across types of psychotherapy, is the observation that the strength of the relationship between a patient and her therapist is associated with good outcome (Martin, Garske, & Davis, 2000). This is true from early in the process, by the second or third session, according to some work (Martin et al., 2000; Barber, Connolly, Crits-Christoph, Gladis, & Siqueland, 2000). There is an extensive literature on the development of the therapeutic relationship and its maintenance and repair in the case of the inevitable ruptures (Safran & Muran, 2000). PPP defines the development of an effective therapeutic relationship and the skills for maintaining it as central.

Techniques for facilitating the development of the therapeutic alliance include (1) consistent empathic and affective attunement—paying attention to and inquiring about what the patient is feeling in the here and now; (2) clearly defining and negotiating therapist and patient roles (Bordin, 1979); (3) an active and engaged therapeutic stance, including ongoing reaction and interaction, questions, probing, preliminary observations, feedback; and (4) careful attention to the moments of disappointment, frustration, or disengagement that occur in any continuing therapeutic relationship (Safran & Muran, 2000).

Traditional psychodynamic psychotherapy certainly attends to the therapeutic alliance as well, but it has a tendency to leave the patient and therapist roles less defined out of concern about making transference manifestations harder to see. The traditional psychodynamic therapist maintains a more mirror-like and abstinent attitude. When therapeutic ruptures do occur, they tend to be understood as related to transference reactions, and important "grist for the mill" of understanding. PPP, too, sees ruptures as partly reflective of transference issues, but also of current problems in the alliance; repair and resolution of ruptures, with resumption of a dominant positive tone to the therapy, are regarded as critical.

> Nicholas was a successful businessman who came for psychotherapy in the wake of his wife's announcement that she wanted a separation. Apparently, she could not tolerate his emotional distance and his controlling, infantilizing behavior toward her. He was in his early 40s, tall, balding, suntanned, and genial. His description of the situation was articulate and logical, and he had a strategic attitude and approach toward the separation, almost like it was a business negotiation. But he was desolate apart from his wife and children, and felt he had no purpose in life.
>
> Nicholas wanted to engage the therapist in a nuanced discussion of how to lure his wife back and persisted with a chess-like analysis of what he should say to her and when. He wanted the therapist to be a relationship consultant and help him achieve his defined goal—resuming the relationship as it had been. The chal-

lenge in developing the therapeutic relationship was not simply to help Nick reconstitute the relationship as it had been, but to help him see the problems had led to the split. He would never get back with his wife unless he gained some understanding of the emotional issues involved in the separation, his contribution to it, and his reactions to it. In fact, he was angry and ashamed about what had happened.

By consistently empathizing with his feelings of loss, there was some space in the therapy for Nicholas to talk about his deeper feelings, not just his strategy to get his wife back. After clarifying the therapist and patient roles, specifically the therapist's role in listening, understanding, reflecting, and formulating, and the patient's role in exploring, articulating, taking responsibility, and changing, Nicholas was able to discuss the conflict with his wife without slipping back to seeking advice and help. He took some responsibility for seeing the impact his needs had on others. Of course, he did not change this attitude and behavior simply because of an educational discussion about the roles of patient and therapist, but it did give him some awareness of his constant tendency to relate to others as staff who were disappointing him. Patient and therapist developed a shorthand, each of them commenting at times that he was back into "chess-playing mode," as opposed to thinking about what was really going on.

With this intelligent but concrete and practical man, an active give and take between patient and therapist was essential. He rapidly became anxious and frustrated without ongoing interaction in the therapy, and frequent comments questions and encouragement from the therapist were very helpful. There had been some discussion about his difficult relationship with his father, and the therapist connected his frustration when the therapist was quiet to his anger at his father, who left his mother when he was 12 years old.

Nicholas continued to get frustrated when I could not give him advice and answers—should he compromise and offer to do more of the household chores, should he push back when his wife said she wanted to go out with her friends? I did not tell him what to do, and then shortly afterward I went on vacation and had to cancel two appointments. When I returned, he seemed preoccupied and much less engaged. He could not explain why, and seemed to get angry when I asked about this. Instead of exploring the transference reactions at that point (his feeling of anger and rejection by me) I reassured him and was a little more active than usual.

In this case, the principle was to meet the patient where he was, and the therapist's judgment was that adopting a more traditional aloof therapeutic stance might have generated some additional insight, but it would compromise the working relationship. When the therapeutic alliance is threatened, the rupture must be repaired; sometimes this means reassurance and reality, sometimes this means interpretation.

All Derivatives Are Created Equal

Sometimes referred to as a "three-legged stool," psychodynamic therapy focuses on incidents in the present reality, the past, and in the relationship with the therapist. In the traditional model, attention to one of these domains should be matched by attention to the others; neglect of any area is seen as a resistance. Although this is consistent conceptually with the PPP model, the pragmatic focus of our treatment model dictates that priority be given to the present derivatives of conflict. All three legs of the stool are not always necessary, and historical reconstructions and feelings about the therapeutic relationship are not regarded as ultimately more important than derivatives of conflict present in everyday reality.

Transference is the carryover of old feelings, perceptions, and ideas about early relationships onto later ones. Countertransference refers to the feelings, perceptions, and ideas the therapist has about the patient that derive from the patient's presentation and the actual therapist–patient relationship, as well as from the therapist's earlier life experiences. These two fundamental psychodynamic concepts are discussed in much greater detail in several later chapters. The therapist typically recognizes transference reactions by listening and observing, but also by noting countertransference reactions and relating these to ongoing enactments with the patient. Like the transference, countertransference may be more of a focus in traditional psychodynamic treatment than in PPP. We wish there were more data on which patients benefit from a focus on the present, the past, or the transference.

The bread and butter of PPP is the detailed exploration of and discussion about the many current reality situations, especially those involving narratives about meaningful interpersonal relationships. When the free-associative process leads to memories of the past, or when the discussion of the transference becomes immediate, then these elements become the focus. The exploration of these areas adds depth and a sense of conviction to the process, but this is not absolutely necessary to the therapeutic process. Some patients naturally shift their focus to the past and recall essential memories that help to buttress their understanding of their repetitive scenarios. Some have a particular affinity for seeing how they play out in the relationship with the therapist.

Core Psychodynamic Problems, Comprehensive Case Formulation, and Narrative

Traditional psychodynamic psychotherapy did not focus on diagnosis, either from a psychodynamic or descriptive perspective. It did not matter so much what the diagnosis was, because you went ahead and did the same treatment either way. Psychodynamic formulation, when it was done, was an activity of the therapist and not shared or discussed with the patient; it was almost parallel to the therapy rather than central to it.

PPP starts by identifying the core psychodynamic problem the patient is suffering with. We propose that there are six core problems that are effectively treated with psychodynamic therapy: depression, obsessionality, fear of abandonment, low self-esteem, panic anxiety, and trauma. These problems are discussed in detail in Chapters 5 and 6. Along with setting up the therapeutic alliance, the therapist's job is to assess the patient and determine which one of these problems (if any) best characterizes the patient. This seems quite simple, but it was not how prior generations of psychodynamic practitioners were taught.

Identifying the core problem allows the therapist to anticipate the typical descriptive characteristics of the problem and quickly consider the common psychodynamics that go with each. Treatment goals, dilemmas in developing the therapeutic alliance, specific therapy techniques, and common transference and countertransference reactions all revolve around the core problem. If you know the core problem, you will know what to expect in each of these areas, and the road map for the treatment will be quite clear.

Individuals are not reducible to core problems, and this is where comprehensive case formulation comes in. The formulation is the bridge between the core problem and the specifics of the patient's life and history. A comprehensive and pragmatic psychodynamic formulation includes the core psychodynamic problem and the essential psychodynamics (the primary repetitive pathologic scenario), but also nonpsychodynamic neurobiological factors such as temperament, syndromal and subsyndromal disorders, and the social and cultural context (McWilliams, 1999; Summers, 2002). Chapter 7 shows how to develop a formulation from a patient's history.

A comprehensive formulation includes an articulation of the two-way causality that links dynamic factors and the symptoms associated with psychiatric syndromes. It hypothesizes how the dynamic factors influenced the development of symptoms and syndromes and how the syndromal illnesses affected the dynamics. It is based on a longitudinal history that begins in childhood and includes symptoms, important environmental experiences, life cycle developmental factors, traumatic experiences, medical factors, and the effect of treatments.

Although different aspects of psychodynamic formulation have been written about and studied empirically in the last two decades, they have probably only had an impact on clinical practice in the area of development of brief psychodynamic treatment. Unfortunately, formulations are not widely used in everyday practice.

The PPP approach to formulating patients' problems differs from the traditional one not only in the breadth of the factors included, but also in its centrality and transparency. By the second or third session, the core problem should be clear and the beginnings of a formulation should emerge. A few sessions later the core problem and initial formulation can be discussed with the patient. The formulation becomes the shared focus of therapist and patient and can be developed, extended, and amended for the remainder of the therapy. The traditional psychodynamic model rarely diagnoses core problems and takes the position that not enough data are available to make for an accurate formulation early in treatment.

Defining the problem and making a comprehensive formulation often allows for the development of a good collaborative therapeutic alliance. It leads to the effective targeting of symptoms that will potentially respond to psychotherapy and identification of possible obstacles to treatment. The formulation also helps to plan the coordination of the psychodynamic psychotherapeutic interventions with other interventions, such as psychopharmacology, couple or family counseling, or behavioral treatment.

While the ideas that go into the core problem and formulation are based on a collaborative give and take with the patient, the task of formulation is the therapist's. By contrast, the development of a life narrative (Spence, 1982; McHugh & Slavney, 1998) is both the therapist's and the patient's responsibility. A narrative understanding of lifetime events, how they relate, and how they come together in the person the patient is now allows a patient to appreciate her strengths, opportunities, advantages, disadvantages, skills, and vulnerabilities. Like a handmade quilt that is pored over, discussed, and worked on together, this careful and collaborative construction is the main work of therapy and also a goal. The narrative is the tangible product of therapy that the patient will appreciate and use. A life narrative will help a patient anticipate how she will react to situations in the future and will help her effectively solve problems and make decisions. It is a basis for realistic and healthy self-esteem (Strupp & Binder, 1984).

A Sharper Tool

Traditional psychodynamic psychotherapy was often described by critics as a "blunt instrument." This means that the technique and the power of the approach are applied to a wide range of problems and done the same way every time. Thus the therapeutic impact is broad based and not targeted. PPP tries to focus the treatment where it will have the greatest impact and titrates the intensity to the nature of the problem and the goals of the patient.

What does this actually mean? Two key steps in treatment planning are helping patients define their goals and then designing a treatment that will get them there. Directly asking patients about what they hope to achieve is the place to start. Guidance and advice about what can be done realistically helps to set the stage for a successful enterprise. Of course, most patients will not be able to make the extent of change they hope for, but they may be surprised by what they are able to accomplish. A crucial aspect of treatment planning is determining how much to focus on symptoms or areas of difficulty, and how much to work on personal growth and facilitation of life cycle developmental tasks. The distinction between these two areas is not always clear, but our experience indicates that most patients have a strong sense of which of these they are working on, and it is important to maintain the focus where the patient desires.

With a clearer picture of what the patient hopes to achieve, and with the therapist's awareness of the conflicted basis for these treatment goals (remember that even treatment goals are a compromise formation), it is possible to design the treatment using the comprehensive case formulation. This guides patient and therapist to the particular psychodynamic scenarios that should be the focus of treatment.

Because our model identifies nonpsychodynamic dimensions of the patient's problem, targeting the treatment means delivering the psychodynamic aspect of the treatment when the patient is maximally ready. The classic example of this is the severely depressed patient with multiple life stressors and a dysfunctional pattern of dealing with loss, who initially benefits from a symptom-focused treatment, such as psychopharmacology or a highly targeted dynamic or cognitive psychotherapy. Then the patient will benefit from longer-term psychodynamic treatment when the severe depressive symptoms have remitted somewhat. The anxiety-generating aspects of psychodynamic treatment make its use in the initial period contraindicated, but later dynamic work may be effective when the patient is stronger and less symptomatic.

PPP is easily combined with other treatment modalities (e.g., psychopharmacology) using the comprehensive formulation as the blueprint. Although the course of treatment is difficult to predict, the core problem and formulation provide a basis for anticipating the course of treatment, including potential symptom relief, maturation, and growth, as well as potential resistances and obstacles. Thus PPP allows for a more rational basis for combining dynamic and other approaches and recognizes that there are phases of treatment that require more or less psychodynamic attention.

Promoting Change

The techniques used to promote change take advantage of the three mechanisms of change described in the theory section earlier. Each technical approach reflects one or more of these mechanisms. The first approach is exploration of painful affects, memories, thoughts, and feelings. This requires a host of traditional psychodynamic interviewing techniques (Brenner, 1974; Greenson, 1967). Emotional exploration helps the patient develop insight and self-awareness and decrease the intensity of old frightening feelings. PPP is not very different from traditional psychodynamic psychotherapy in this area.

The second technique is helping the patient develop alternative perceptions to troublesome situations based on a here-and-now, more objective, multidimensional view of reality. PPP techniques include clarification of old scenarios and exploration and open-minded discussion of alternative perceptions. These discussions often have a kind of "detective work" feel to them, with collaborative back-and-forth about possibilities, weighing and accepting or rejecting perceptions, responses, and realities. The therapist asks about and encourages speculation about the motivation and experiences of others in the stories patients tell, helping to consider a variety of ways of understanding difficult situations, noting the differences between the patient's repetitive experiences and the realities they find themselves in. For example, Beth reconsidered how she viewed men she was dating. Did they seem exciting because they were unreliable and this reminded her of her father? Nicholas thought about whether his wife was indeed as unavailable as he experienced her to be. Was his perception accurate, or was he interpreting her behavior this way because of his old experiences?

The third technique is trying new behaviors. We encourage new behaviors and want the patient to assess their impact. With new and more contemporary perceptions of the repetitive trouble situations and discussion about alternative responses to these situations, you can consider new actions and responses the patient could make. The new responses will often call upon social skills and capacities that may be evident in areas of the patient's life less caught up in conflict.

Patients frequently will discover the new strategies or ideas themselves. In PPP we are not afraid to suggest new behaviors to consider. Thus we might suggest that a patient try to avoid the same old critical entanglement with an aging parent and keep some distance while recognizing the ongoing hurt or loss he may feel. The traditional concerns about stimulating power struggles, infantilizing the patient, or reproducing earlier traumatic situations by "telling a patient what to do," must be taken into account. New behaviors are considered, not pushed, and we do worry that we not deform the treatment relationship in a way that will undermine the alliance. But the potential therapeutic impact of working actively to develop a new behavioral repertoire often outweighs the risk of making it more difficult to see and work with transference manifestations.

> Jackie learned that her college-age daughter was gay, and she was distraught. She knew it was important to be supportive; this revelation was not a choice her daughter was making, but rather an aspect of who she was. But it was so disappointing to Jackie, and she was ashamed and confused about why she felt so badly about it. There were times her daughter dressed in an especially masculine way, and this particularly bothered Jackie. Her upset about this progressed to the point where she avoided being alone with her daughter, despite their history of many shared activities and interests.
>
> Through the therapy Jackie realized that not only was she dealing with the loss of some cherished fantasies about her daughter and how she and her husband would spend time with her and a future family, but there were also some specific conflicts of her own. She was the only child of a loving but somewhat demanding mother whom she found oppressive at times. She was covertly angry and never expressed it. It turned out that Jackie interpreted her daughter's lesbian identity as a rejection of herself as a mother. She often interpreted her daughter's behavior as being angry and rejecting of

her, just as she felt at times about her own mother. Her daughter, of course, behaved as she did for her own reasons—her sexual identity was clear to her, and it had little to do with her feelings for her mother. The daughter, it turns out, thought Jackie was avoiding her since her revelation. This made her feel rejected and angry, and she had behaved defiantly and rudely a few times.

After Jackie got clearer about why she was so upset and realized that her interpretation of her daughter's anger and rejection was wrong, she felt better. But, she was still locked in a negative cycle with her, and when together, she had to do a lot of mental work to remind herself that her daughter was not rejecting her.

In therapy, she was encouraged to confront her fears head on and try some new behavior, such as speaking with her daughter about her concerns. At her daughter's next visit home, she arranged to spend as much time together as possible and asked her about her dating life, friends, and even about her plans in the future about having children. Jackie was worried she would find out how bad their relationship really was, but the opposite turned out to be true.

When Jackie stepped aside from her old perceptions (angry daughter, insensitive mother) and tried a new behavioral response (interest and engagement), Jackie's daughter melted and explained that she was afraid of being criticized and rejected. She did not choose to be a lesbian, and she wanted to be close and have a family in the future. Jackie felt immeasurably better. She was able to put aside her more traditional dreams for her daughter once she knew that her relationship with her daughter was different from her relationship with her own mother.

Transparency

The relationship between patient and therapist is a necessary (but not sufficient) vehicle for therapeutic change in PPP. It is the medium in which the techniques take place, but it also is an irreducible element in healing. The empathic and affective bond between patient and therapist must have a real and immediate element, as well as a transferential and countertransferential dimension. The pragmatic psychodynamic therapist is professional and relatively anonymous in demeanor, but understands the need for engagement and the inevitability of enactment in the fantasies and needs of the patient. For example, the bias is in favor of responding to patients' inquiries and attempts to engage the therapist. Respond to questions first, and you can analyze and understand the interaction later; but do not forget to inquire about how your response was heard and integrated. It is surprising how patients are able to respond to direct

Red head

communication from the therapists and also maintain curiosity and interest in the transference.

We find transparency about the treatment to be quite helpful. An explanation of the core problem, formulation, treatment methods and alternatives, and even elements of treatment technique is an important element in therapeutic success. This approach is not only consistent with contemporary medical–legal requirements such as informed consent (Beahrs & Gutheil, 2001), but also increases the degree of reality in the psychotherapy relationship and supports the patient's healthy adult functioning. It includes educating the patient about her problem and the life cycle issues that may be salient. Traditional dynamic therapy involves a more "mysterious" role for the therapist and lacks the emphasis on explaining to patients what is happening with them and with the treatment.

In medical care in general, the empowerment of patients through increased knowledge, although resisted by some clinicians because it can be upsetting, time-consuming, and sometimes inaccurate, more often than not turns out to be helpful. Providing information is a nonspecific intervention that decreases the frequent sense of being out of control and helps patients select more appropriate treatments that they pursue with more full compliance. Transparency refers to open and full disclosure about issues that are central to the patient's condition, prognosis, and treatment. This does not necessarily refer to therapists' personal reactions that need to be monitored and used carefully. Needless to say, openness to consultation and outside input is also part of a transparent approach to psychotherapy.

SUMMARY

PPP has clearly delineated theoretical principles and techniques. It emphasizes a developmental and conflict model of mental life and organizes treatment around psychodynamic diagnosis and formulation. This treatment approach encourages patient education, greater transparency in the therapist, integration with other synergistic treatment modalities, an active engaged therapeutic stance, and specific attention to change. These characteristics differentiate PPP from traditional psychodynamic psychotherapy and other psychotherapies.

CHAPTER 3

The Other Psychotherapies

We are healed of a suffering only
by expressing it to the full.
—MARCEL PROUST

In this chapter, we summarize the sweep of psychotherapy history, as it helps to put our pragmatic model in context. First, we give an overview of the main schools of therapy in the 20th and 21st centuries and comment on the emphasis each psychotherapy places on cognition versus emotion, technique versus relationship experience, and the development of a narrative of the patients' life. Second, we describe in some detail the three main psychoanalytic theories as they provide the language used in formulating individual patients' dynamics. Third, we compare CBT with psychodynamic psychotherapy to illustrate the similarities and differences.

PSYCHOANALYSIS

Psychoanalysis was founded on the centrality of drive, unconscious conflict, and fantasy. Other ideas fundamental to this model are the developmental perspective, as played out in normal and pathological developmental struggles, and the insight that psychological symptoms are neurotic solutions to intrapsychic conflict. Although Freud longed for an overarching biological theory, his work on hysteria led him to conclude that there was no biological map that could explain the clinical phenom-

48

ena he observed. Instead he developed a psychic map that explained the pathology.

Because neither biology nor conscious awareness could explain patients' symptoms, Freud postulated the existence of the dynamic unconscious. To make the unconscious accessible, Freud had the patient lying on the coach, coming for daily sessions for several months, with encouragement of free association, saying whatever comes to mind. Unlike the Freudian caricature of cold therapist anonymity, lonely free association, and relentless interpretation of conflict, the actual early practice was warm, personal, often even overinvolved by today's standards. Advice and support were ubiquitous. Patients would go on walks with Freud, eat with him on occasion, and even go on vacation with him.

Framed in scientific language and mechanical metaphors, the classic psychoanalytic technique emphasized catharsis and emotional expression and attempted to pair this with insight. It emphasized techniques designed to increase insight and regarded the actual relationship between analyst and patient as less important. A new picture and different understanding of the patient's early and current life was the gold nugget patient and analyst searched for, and this new insight was regarded as the new truth.

Psychoanalysis is interested in ideas and understanding as well as emotion. It is both a well-described procedure and a new relationship experience for the patient. Narratives are important, although there is the implication that the story developed is true and based on historical reconstruction. Some analysts focus more on cognition and insight than emotion, while some certainly emphasize the new relationship experience.

Psychoanalytic thinking branched successively into three main directions over the next 75 years. These schools of psychoanalytic thought—ego psychology, object relations, and self psychology—form the backbone of ideas about psychopathology then and now. Each is a worldview replete with assumptions, observations, and terminology, all plausible but not proven. Together the three perspectives make a rich web of connections for understanding a person's life. Our clinical experience leads us to suggest that the core psychodynamic problems are best understood with a multidimensional perspective, but there is usually one psychoanalytic model that seems to "fit" each problem and each patient best.

Each of these three theories may speak to you professionally and personally, and may strike you as intuitively accurate or not. As is true with your patients, this affinity likely reflects something about your own background, personal and developmental, and your intellectual experiences. Often people become interested in psychodynamic psychotherapy because they have been exposed to one or another of the theories and they resonate with the depth of understanding which is conveyed. But as searching and evocative as these theories are, they can rapidly become overly complex, arcane, and difficult to penetrate. Students tend to pick just one and run with it. Our approach is more patient specific: each core problem is best understood using one (or sometimes two) of the theories. We explain the six core problems and associated theories in Chapters 5 and 6.

EGO PSYCHOLOGY

This is the classic theory that earned psychoanalysis respect; it became particularly established in North America. Ego psychology focuses on the theoretical concepts of intrapsychic conflict, the unconscious, and the constant pressure of drives seeking expression. These concepts were the original creative wellspring of psychoanalysis, and sometimes they are also the focus of criticism and jokes about psychoanalysis, as they present a particularly deterministic and reductionist view of the role of base instinct in human life. In this model, the mind contains warring drives (sexual and aggressive impulses) and reactions to these drives coming from the conscience, or superego. The ego attempts to arbitrate, prioritize, plan, and compromise among the impulses, conscience, and the demands of reality. All thoughts, feelings, fantasies, and behavior are conceptualized as resulting from the complex interweaving of these demands and the attempts to resolve them. The ubiquity of conflict and compromise is the major contribution of this model, while its view of the individual as a solely drive-satisfying organism is its downfall.

Superego is the aspect of mind that represents the conscience, that is, the rules and prohibitions about what is forbidden. Thoughts and feelings, as well as behavior, can be forbidden and can be the source of guilt and shame. Conflicts between the drives and the superego are many, and defenses such as repression, displacement, and sublimation are used to manage these seemingly clashing internal needs (Freud, 1926). The ego is the part of the mind that employs defenses, attempting to continuously develop solutions to conflicts. Ego function is the capacity to flexibly and effectively make compromises, and the ego must take account of external reality and the demands and constraints it requires (Freud, 1926).

Ego psychology also focuses on psychosexual development. The distinction between the oral, anal, and genital (or oedipal) phases determines both the form and content of conflicts. Here the sexual and aggressive impulses unfold over time in a predictable sequence and dominate the individual's experience. They represent developmental challenges that must be addressed and resolved. For example, the child in the anal stage must find a way to satisfy the powerful urges to retain control over his or her bodily functions while obeying the demands of the parents for toilet training, resolving competing feelings of love and hate, autonomy and submission. Later, oedipal libidinal urges toward a parent can result in complicated problems of guilt. Problems encountered during a developmental phase leave a fixation, or scar. Defenses patch or contain the unresolved conflict, and these scars are carried forward and express themselves in subsequent situations reminiscent of the earlier ones. Erikson's work extended these ideas from childhood through the entire adult life cycle (Erikson, 1964). The term *derivative* refers to thoughts, feelings, or behavior that derive from major conflicts. Derivatives are the bits of experience that are often the focus of therapy.

According to the ego psychology model, pathology occurs when compromises do not work very well (A. Freud, 1936). Instead of a smoothly flowing mental life with comfortable and consistent mental functioning, pathology is like lumpy batter, with globs of punitive conscience, slippery impulses, and unstable and dysfunctional behavior.

OBJECT RELATIONS

Whereas the ego psychology model conceptualizes a mental apparatus directed toward satisfying instinctual needs and compromising between internal and external demands, object relations theory emphasizes the primacy of the need for closeness and relationships. The essential urge is toward satisfying and close relationships, not toward sex and war. For the object relations theorist, sex is the sublimation of the love relationship, while for the ego psychologist love is the sublimation of the sex drive. The suckling infant certainly needs food but wants closeness more. Eagle (1984) argues for this theory, citing Harlow's work in the 1950s on young monkeys' preference for soft, yielding cloth "mothers" over wire "mothers," even when the wire "mother" provides food. This line of investigation was further developed by Bowlby in his work on attachment. According to the object relations model, relationships, and the fulfillment and frustration they bring, determine everything. Winnicott (1953), Mitchell (1986), and Kernberg (1975) are major clinical contributors to this model.

The term "object"—an unfortunately cold word—refers to another person who is the object of one's interest and impulses. But this theory with the cold-sounding name is really quite warm, organized around understanding the patient's early experiences with parents and other caregivers and how those relationships are internalized.

If you close your eyes now and begin thinking of your mother, the visual representation that you summon will be associated with feelings, recollections, and ideas from the past. This is an internalized image, or as the theory calls it, an object representation of your mother. Children internalize those who take care of them. These internal images are called introjections when the child is young. It is like the whole of another person gobbled up and lodged in the child's mind. When the child grows older, these introjections become identifications, and the internal images become more abstract and based on the parents' qualities and attributes—now, along with the image and feeling about the person, the ideas and beliefs the person stands for are in the individual's mind.

Introjects are very different from identifications. An introject might live on if there is a parent who was aggressive, frightening, and abusive. One hears and experiences the introjected parent almost as real, but stuck in one's head. In a healthy relationship, the introject becomes transformed into an identification. Identification is a gentler process; an example of this is the feeling that one is like one's father. According to object relations theory, humans inevitably form introjects and then identifications with important early caregivers, and they live on in us as sources of nurturance, satisfaction, criticism, or guilt.

Healthy object representations are like loving companions. However, when there has been serious conflict, the object representation may be split into a good object invested with loving feelings and perceptions, and a bad object representation invested with hate and negative perceptions. Object constancy is a developmental achievement. It means that important objects are not split, and loving feelings and aggressive feelings toward these individuals are integrated and synthesized. When the caregiver is gone, the child is able to remember the caregiver and feel confident that the goodness and care will return. Object constancy means the individual trusts others. Lack of object constancy means that when the caregiver is gone, the child feels alone and lost because the remembered hate and negativity drowns out the memories of love and affection.

Developing a stable representation of the self is a developmental achievement, too. This is a synthesized, multidimensional picture of one's self that allows for imperfections and incompleteness, but also includes one's best side. Under the stress of powerful feelings of fear and abandonment, or of anger and aggression, there is a tendency to develop a split self-representation, analogous to the split object representation. This would allow for preservation of a good sense of self, but it would result in alternating, dysfunctional, and uncoordinated responses to others in relationships. We discuss this idea further in the section on the core problem of fear of abandonment in Chapter 6.

Like a play in the theater of the mind, object relations theory emphasizes the internal interactions and conflicts between self and objects, and identifications and introjections. Every new relationship stimulates old scenes, old interactions, and old feelings. Although this sounds highly theoretical, the theory fits with intuitive observations we all make: "That person reminded me of my father, and so I was upset and just reacted."

The central question in ego psychology is: What is the conflict and what is the compromise? The central question in object relations theory is: What earlier relationship is being replayed, and what self- and object representations are stimulated? The goal of therapy from the object relations perspective is to help patients get in touch with feelings about these old relationships and notice their influence on the present; this helps the patient develop a more comprehensive, realistic, and flexible sense of self and others. Turning old, rigid, and person-like representations into new, flexible, abstract identifications is the goal. The story of Beth, the 31-year-old nurse, was told using the language of object relations. The therapist's conceptualization and the patient's narrative are about the repetition of old dysfunctional relationships and how current relationships stimulate old introjects and identifications and result in painful emotion and dysfunction (e.g., father, boyfriend, therapist). Beth's self-representation and object representations were formed long ago, and her current relationships triggered those old experiences. Her therapy allowed her to rework and reinterpret her past so that these old identifications had less impact on her current experience.

SELF PSYCHOLOGY

If ego psychology is about impulses, prohibitions, and defenses, and object relations is about the repetition of old relationships in the form of introjections and identifications, self psychology focuses on the development and maintenance of self-esteem. Kohut (1971, 1977, 1984) and subsequent contributors (see, e.g., Baker & Baker, 1987) recognized that the development and maintenance of self-esteem is a separate line of life cycle development. Kohut defined the new term, selfobject, as an ideal relationship between parent and child where there is optimal empathy and support. For Kohut, narcissism is the problem that develops when there is not enough selfobject function, that is, when the growing child does not receive the empathy needed to deal with the inevitable frustrations of life. The selfobject relationship protects the child from too much disappointment; it provides validation of emotional experiences and guides the child with an optimal mixture of dependence and independence. The selfobject relationship also allows the child to experience some frustration, as this promotes the ability to master life's disappointments. In Kohut's formulation, healthy self-esteem results from this optimal balance of empathy and frustration.

When there is not sufficient empathy and validation, or if there is excessive empathy that does not allow the child to learn to manage problems, the child struggles with terrible feelings of anger, fear, and inferiority. He or she is unable to contain and modulate these frightening experiences without lasting feelings of shame. Alternatively, there is so much protection that the child never experiences the optimal degree of frustration needed to develop strength, confidence, and independence. Grandiosity and elation are reactions to the child's feelings of inferiority and shame, and this is how impaired self-esteem can show itself in narcissism.

The need for selfobjects is greatest during childhood, but this need continues through adulthood and finds its expression in intimate love relationships, close friendships, and close family relationships. Early problems with selfobjects make it harder to perform the selfobject function for others later in life. In other words, it can be difficult to empathize if one has not been deeply empathized with.

The three major psychoanalytic theories (summarized in Table 3.1) used to be primary routes for learning about psychoanalysis and psychodynamic therapy. We propose a more delimited role for the theories. We recognize the depth, complexity, and rich picture each theory paints of the mind and its pathology, and we regard each as a language that can be used to articulate the nature of individuals' problems. Each theory is particularly valuable for describing particular core psychodynamic problems. For example, the object relations model fits the experience of those with fear of abandonment, ego psychology is especially helpful for panic and obsessionality, while the self psychology model usefully explicates low self-esteem.

TABLE 3.1. Psychoanalytic Theories

Ego psychology	Object relations	Self psychology
	Key terms	
Drive, superego, defense, ego function, compromise formation	Identification, introjection, self- and object representation	Selfobject, self-esteem, narcissism, grandiosity
	Model of conflict	
Drive–defense conflict, derivatives, compromise formation	Conflict between internalized object representations, use of characteristic defenses, such as splitting, projection, introjection	Struggle to achieve healthy self-esteem, loss, and frustration with caretakers
	Developmental aspect	
Psychosexual development	Object constancy	Healthy self
	Psychopathology	
Conflict between impulses, superego; development of compromise formations that limit function	Split self- and object representations, chronic conflict and anxiety in relationships, use of primitive defenses for managing internal conflict, dysfunctional attempts to solve relational conflict	Intense feelings of inferiority and defectiveness alternating with grandiosity, idealization, and devaluation in relationships, inability to tolerate frustration
	Concept of health	
Effective compromise formations which minimize anxiety and allow for flexible functioning and satisfaction of needs	Object constancy, more well-rounded self- and object representation, stable and satisfying object relationships, less conflicted identifications	Good self-esteem, vigorous assertiveness and tolerance for frustration
	Focus of psychotherapy	
Elucidation of conflicts, defenses, compromises, development of more effective defenses and compromises	Awareness of self- and object representations and their conflict, increased integration of split objects, more satisfying relationships and less conflicted identifications	Development of selfobject relationship with therapist, which allows for repair to self-esteem and increased capacity for closeness in context of optimally empathic relationship

SHORT-TERM DYNAMIC PSYCHOTHERAPY

From the earliest days of psychoanalysis, a movement to keep psycho-analytically inspired psychotherapy brief and concise arose in response to more complex theoretical notions and extended treatments. Ferenczi (1926), Rank (1929), and Alexander and French (1946) were the pioneers who recommended an active stance in therapy to hasten the exploration of unconscious material. In spite of their efforts, however, most psychoanalysts and psychodynamic clinicians responded to these ideas by regarding brief dynamic therapy as inferior to the lengthier psychoanalytic treatment.

Not until Malan (1976a, 1976b), and Mann (1973), Sifneos (1979), and Davanloo (1980) was brief psychodynamic psychotherapy deemed a valuable treatment option. Malan's emphasis on the importance of careful patient selection through the screening of inappropriate referrals and trial interpretations attracted therapists to the effectiveness of brief dynamic therapy for a subset of the patient population. Malan and Sifneos were also among the first to stress the significance of defining and maintaining a therapeutic focus.

Condensing the often theoretically complicated and vaguely described psychoanalytic model, Malan explicitly defined the essence of psychodynamic treatment through the description of two triangles. The "triangle of conflict" has apices corresponding to defense, anxiety, and underlying feeling or impulse. The second triangle, known as the "triangle of person," has relationships with current figures, relationship with the therapist (representing transference), and relationships with important figures from the past (e.g., parents) on its three corners.

According to Malan, the therapist's task is to expose the underlying feelings and impulses that the patient has been protecting via defense mechanisms and elucidate the role of the defenses in reducing the anxiety that the feelings create. He posited that the patient's hidden feelings were originally experienced in relation to the parental figures at some time in the past, and since then have frequently recurred with other significant figures in the patient's life, including the therapist. During therapy, the patient must understand the hidden impulses underlying each of the relationships described in the triangle of person. Typically, insight into a current relationship (either with a significant other or the therapist) is achieved first and is then related back to the parental figures. Crits-Christoph et al. (1991) considered the writings of Malan (1976a, 1976b), Mann (1973), Sifneos (1979), and Davanloo (1980) the four "traditional" approaches to brief dynamic therapy.

In the last 30 years, a new generation of brief dynamic therapists appeared on the clinical scene. Among the most important are Luborsky (1984), Horowitz et al. (1984), Strupp and Binder (1984), and Weiss et al. (1986). This new group, like the emerging cognitive therapists, (e.g., Beck, Rush, Shaw, & Emery, 1979), can be distinguished from previous generations by their greater interest in the empirical status of their treatment approaches. Perhaps resulting from their interest in research, this new generation has written intricately detailed descriptions of their clinical approaches that are very helpful for training and monitoring clinicians in the adequate use of their techniques. In fact, many of these books are considered treatment manuals and have been used in empirical research addressing the efficacy of these therapeutic methods.

CORE CONFLICTUAL RELATIONSHIP THEME

The CCRT method was developed by Lester Luborsky (1977) as a way to formulate and formalize core conflicts or central issues, and this can be included in a more comprehensive dynamic formulation of the patient's problems. The CCRT has received a great deal of research attention (see Luborsky & Crits-Christoph, 1998).

At the center of the CCRT are data extracted from patients' spontaneous narratives about their interactions with other people. The CCRT has three components: what the patient wanted or desired from the other person (wish); how the other people reacted (response of other, RO); and how the patient, or "self," reacted to their reactions (response of self, RS). The following example of a CCRT formulation is provided by McAdams (1990): "a man['s] first memory was that of being held in his mother's arms, only to be summarily deposited on the ground so that she could pick up his younger brother. His adult life involved persistent fears that others would be preferred to him, including extreme mistrust of his fiancée" (p. 441). In this man's narrative recollection of an early interaction with his mother, the wish expressed is "wanting to feel securely loved by mother"; the mother's response (RO) is "rejection," and the boy's response to this rejection (RS) is "mistrust" (Thorne & Klohnen, 1993).

The recurrence of CCRT components (wishes, ROs, and RSs) across relationships forms the person's overall CCRT. The assumption is that these recurring themes capture the central relationship patterns or schemas that underlie a person's typical ways of relating to other people. These central relational patterns are thought to be the product of highly

ingrained patterns of relationship with significant others, especially emotionally laden interactions with parental figures in the earliest years of
life (Bowlby, 1988). Thus CCRTs can be considered to be components of
dynamic character structure (Wiseman & Barber, 2008), and are highly
relevant to the formulation.

The CCRT and other short-term dynamic psychotherapies have
a strong influence on our pragmatic approach because they distill the
essential features of the psychoanalytic tradition—a balance between
the cognitive and emotional aspects of treatment, and an interest in both
technique and a new relational experience for the patient—and they
explicitly recognize the development of a new narrative (see, e.g., Strupp
& Binder, 1984). Short-term dynamic psychotherapies also attempt to
focus on the problems needing the most attention, with the understanding that effective work on those key problems will allow the individual
to regain a healthier developmental pathway.

COGNITIVE-BEHAVIORAL THERAPY

CBT integrates aspects of both behavior and cognitive therapies and
emphasizes changes in both cognition and behavior. The Skinnerian and
Pavlovian behavioral models and learning theories are the conceptual
basis of behavior therapy, which identifies dysfunctional behavioral strategies for managing anxiety and other unpleasant experiences. According
to this model, the symptom is the focus of treatment, rather than some
underlying condition or "disease." Treatment involves the systematic
dismantling of these dysfunctional behaviors and their replacement with
more effective and adaptive behaviors. A detailed examination of subjective experience and behaviors is the basis for designing treatments where
new behaviors can be tested, learned, and routinely applied.

Behavior therapy is the epitome of an emotional, experientially based
treatment, because it is the new experience itself that allows for change.
No new narrative is developed, because the treatment does not focus on
the meaning of thoughts and feelings. In this model, the new behavior
precedes new thinking and feeling. Thus behavior therapy emphasizes
both the technique and the experience of treatment and regards narrative understanding as less important.

Whereas behavior therapy emphasizes the primacy of behavior,
cognitive therapy regards cognition as central. From a psychodynamic
perspective, Aaron Beck et al.'s (1979) cognitive therapy seems to con-

tinue the tradition of ego psychology by further emphasizing the "rational" aspect of human nature, and deemphasizing its "irrational" counterpart. But for Beck, the irrational is not motivated by unconscious forces, it is the result of faulty thinking that can be corrected. Furthermore, Beck added aspects of activity and transparency to the therapy by being very goal-directed during the session and explicit with clients about what he intends to do. He initially focused on the treatment of a single disorder, depression, and included a variety of helpful behavioral interventions, such as the scheduling of pleasurable activities, in order to get the patients active. One of his significant contributions was to use evidence from systematic research to elaborate his theory and to evaluate the efficacy of his interventions. Most recently, Beck's cognitive therapy has been applied successfully to anxiety disorders, personality disorders, and even schizophrenia (Rathod, Kingdon, Weiden, & Turkington, 2008). Not unlike early psychoanalysis, the scope of cognitive therapy is widening, and now includes more complex and difficult cases (J. Beck, 2005). Therefore, the treatments are not always short.

Cognitive therapy departed from the psychodynamic tradition by emphasizing the role of cognitions and attitudes in the genesis of feelings and behavior. Furthermore, Beck suggested that the best way to change cognition is to provide the individual with new data. Cognitive therapy's standardized assessment, outcome, and training techniques have led the way to modern empiricism in the field of psychotherapy. Because of its focus on empirical validation, cognitive therapy has been able to clearly define its target and its methods and consequently demonstrate effectiveness in a wide variety of conditions. Compared to the psychodynamic psychotherapy, as its name suggests, cognitive therapy clearly relies on a more cognitive and less emotional understanding of psychotherapy process. It is more focused on technique than on the therapeutic relationship experience and has little interest in the development of a new narrative.

CBT is the umbrella term for therapies that involve aspects of either behavior therapy or cognitive therapy, or both. We refer to CBT throughout this book, rather than cognitive therapy or behavior therapy, as the work in this area increasingly involves the amalgamation of these approaches. For example, some contemporary behaviorists (see Foa & Rothbaum, 1998) have reformulated their exposure work into a more cognitive language. It is interesting to note that behavior and cognitive therapy together encompass attention to both cognition and emotion and emphasize both procedure and new experience, while the development of new narrative is still not of great importance in these therapies.

PSYCHODYNAMIC PSYCHOTHERAPY
COMPARED WITH COGNITIVE THERAPY

Because CBT is the predominant alternative to dynamic therapy, it is especially important to understand the differences and similarities between them. However, because CBT includes a wide range of theories and techniques, we decided to focus our comparison of dynamic therapy to only one model of CBT, namely to cognitive therapy. Both psychodynamic therapy and cognitive therapy aim to reduce painful affects, bringing out aspects of the patient's experience that were heretofore unclear, and both treatments aim to make perceptions more accurate. But their approaches are quite different. We contrast the two techniques in a variety of domains (summarized in Table 3.2).

Both psychodynamic and cognitive therapies regard patients' understanding of their situations as essential data. How patients perceive and process their experiences and the meanings they attribute to them are central. The cognitive therapist focuses on identifying core beliefs, cognitive rules and assumptions, and the repetitive automatic thoughts they generate. The traditional psychodynamic therapist deals in associations, feelings, wishes, fears, and fantasies, and includes thoughts, but regards them as likely secondary to feelings. Relationships and feelings about relationships are pay dirt for the psychodynamic therapist. However, as we noted above, some dynamic models are more cognitive than others (e.g., control mastery theory) and some therapists put a greater emphasis on cognitions than others.

In cognitive therapy, the *therapeutic relationship* is a vehicle for facilitating learning for the patient, not an important focus in and of itself. Following the dictum of "If it ain't broke, don't fix it," the cognitive therapist does not focus much on the therapeutic relationship unless it is threatened or the pathogenic beliefs cause a rupture. Beck recommends a good ongoing collaboration, which he calls "collaborative empiricism" (Beck et al., 1979, p. 7). The psychodynamic therapist has an active interest and a focus on the therapeutic relationship. It is an opportunity to observe repetitive patterns and also allows the patient a new kind of positive relationship experience. In Beth's treatment, the therapist was interested in her sudden upsurge of suspicion when he suggested a course of action with her boyfriend. This became a window for examining her tendency to be dependent and then angry and mistrustful. The therapist was careful to let this reaction blossom and then explore it. A cognitive therapist would most likely have maintained the collaboration by encouraging a thoughtful evaluation of the reality of

TABLE 3.2. Comparison between Psychodynamic and Cognitive Therapies

Cognitive therapy	Psychodynamic therapy
Therapeutic relationship	
• Relationship rarely the focus of discussion	• Relationship may be important focus of discussion
• Relationship required to enable learning	• Relationship required to enable learning
	• May observe patterns in transference
	• Relationship is corrective emotional experience
Focus	
• Automatic thoughts	• Associations
• Thoughts and cognitions	• Feelings, motivation
• Core beliefs about the self and world	• Wishes and fears
• Schemas	• Fantasies, traumatic scenarios, mechanisms of defense
• Symptoms	• Present and past, character or long-standing traits
• Beliefs about others	• Interpersonal relationship patterns
Main techniques	
• Identification of automatic thoughts and schema	• Looking for repetitive patterns
• Exposure	• Uncovering meaning
• Evaluating evidence for beliefs, homework	• Interpreting defenses, resistances, transference
• Problem solving, developing skills	• Understanding, working through
Process of treatment	
• Highly structured to maintain focus	• Less structured to access less conscious material
• Transparent	• Abstinent
• Education, therapist is explicit	• Minimal education about treatment
Mechanisms of change	
• Changing underlying beliefs	• Increasing self-awareness
• Teaching compensatory skills or strategies	• Working through, developing new perceptions
• Changing behaviors	• Improving relationships, trying new behaviors
Underlying assumptions	
• Problems = symptoms	• Problems are not necessarily the symptoms
• Remove symptoms = remove the problem	• Improving adaptation to conflict is solution
• Sometimes changing underlying beliefs is required	

the mistrust; from the cognitive perspective, healthy evaluation of relationships is an important social skill that needs to be developed, especially for people with troubled relationships or social phobias.

The cognitive and psychodynamic perspectives *focus* on different aspects of mental life. Where the cognitive therapist sees automatic thoughts, cognitions, and core beliefs, the dynamic therapist sees associations, feelings, motivation, wishes, and fears. In CBT, schemas are the legacy of the past and the driver of perceptions and current ideas, causing symptoms and beliefs about others. In a parallel fashion, fantasies, conflicts and defenses are the vehicles through which the past influences the present in psychodynamic therapy, and they determine character traits, attitudes, and relationships. Beth's therapist let her associate and tended to let her flow of thoughts and feelings structure the sessions. A cognitive therapist may have organized the time and led the patient through a sequence of activities that would help to demonstrate pathogenic schemas and their reflection in the patient's automatic thoughts and facilitate the ability to correct these.

The main cognitive *techniques* are identifying automatic thoughts and pathogenic thought patterns reflected in the content of the sessions, behavioral homework, and the use of special questionnaires like the triple-column thought record. Exposing the thought patterns allows for evaluating their accuracy and reality, and thus decreases their power. Once the automatic thought is exposed, cognitive therapists ask the three basic questions: (1) what is the evidence for the belief, (2) is there an alternative way of looking at the situation, and (3) what are the implications of the belief? Because cognitive therapy also involves behavioral techniques, assignment of behavioral activation tasks helps to decrease depression, while exposure to feared stimuli is used to decrease anxiety (through desensitization, habituation, or cognitive reframing). The psychodynamic therapist looks for painful emotions and elicits the thoughts, feelings, memories, and associations to these painful experiences, searching for repetitive patterns and uncovering their meanings and historical roots. The work aims to expose to conscious awareness a repetitive pathogenic scenario through interpreting resistances, defenses, and transference, allowing the patient to work through old experiences and change feeling, perception, and behavior. Beth's therapy revolved around her increasing understanding of a recurring scenario involving dangerous men and abusive experiences. She became aware of this repeating pattern and how it played out in her relationships. This understanding was elicited through observing Beth's associations and memories and by helping her sort through her various defensive strategies for minimizing her painful recollections. Cognitive therapists may also target the recurring pattern, but would access it via distortions in thinking and then use cognitive techniques for correcting inaccurate thoughts.

Cognitive therapy is relatively more structured than PPP, and the therapeutic *process* is transparent, with explicit education about the treatment. Psychodynamic therapists tend to avoid too much structure, preferring instead to facilitate patients' access to less conscious material by giving them support, empathy, time, and space. The therapist's traditional abstinence and neutrality help this. Minimal explanation about the procedures and mechanisms of psychodynamic treatment is given for the same reason. Beth's therapist provided enough support that she felt comfortable expressing her deeper and less rational feelings; the therapist was open-ended and unstructured, which allowed for some regression and a greater ability to observe the transference. There was less education and description of the treatment and why these techniques were used—the therapist wanted to let the relationship unfold. If Beth were in cognitive therapy, the tasks of therapy and the reasons for them would have been more clearly specified and transparent.

The hypothesized primary *mechanism of change* in cognitive therapy is modification of underlying beliefs and assumptions. Changes in core or surface beliefs are thought to lead to changes in emotions and in perceptions of self and others. Compensatory skills and strategies are also taught (Barber & DeRubeis, 1989, 2001) with the goal of bolstering new, more adaptive, and accurate beliefs. In CBT in general, the symptoms tend to be the problems, and when the symptoms are removed or decreased, the problem is solved. However, in some forms of CBT, and in most accounts of cognitive therapy (e.g., J. Beck, 2005), there is a belief that the underlying schemas need to be changed to prevent relapse. The mechanism of change in psychodynamic psychotherapy emphasizes increasing awareness of repetitive patterns regarding self and others, leading to less painful affects, new and more adaptive perceptions, and new behaviors with others (especially improved relationships). The problem is the power of the old, partly unconscious, repetitive patterns that are reflected in symptoms, and the problem is solved when the maladaptive power of the pattern is decreased, not only when the symptoms are decreased. Thus, to the extent that cognitive therapy emphasizes change in deep structures such as core beliefs or underlying assumptions, it shares commonalties with PPP. It is noteworthy that there is not much empirical evidence that changes in schemas are responsible for change in cognitive therapy (e.g., Barber & DeRubeis, 1989). In cognitive therapy, Beth most likely would have been seen to suffer from depression. In psychodynamic therapy, her problem is the destructive feelings stirred up in close relationships arising from her traumatic past; better relationships and getting better from depression depend on working though these feelings.

INTERPERSONAL PSYCHOTHERAPY

With its historical roots in the interpersonal psychoanalytic perspective of Harry Stack Sullivan (1947), interpersonal psychotherapy (Klerman, Weissman, Rounsaville, & Chevron, 1984) was empirically derived by looking for factors that predicted successful resolution of depression from psychotherapy. Interpersonal psychotherapy conceptualizes depression as a result of neurobiological vulnerability and role transitions that require flexibility and adaptation. This therapy includes education about depression and was designed specifically for depression. Some see interpersonal psychotherapy as a modified form of focused psychodynamic psychotherapy, while others regard it as a unique format. It has a strong narrative component and offers the same specific narrative to all patients: the patient has an illness (depression), and it has affected her life in many negative ways. The patient has had losses that need to be mourned in order to make a new adaptation to the new circumstances. Interpersonal psychotherapy involves both cognitive and emotional elements and emphasizes technique more than new experiential elements. In interpersonal psychotherapy Beth would have seen the cause of her depression as resulting from her biological vulnerability and the breakup with the boyfriend. Her difficulties in developing a new adaptation to being single would be the primary focus.

HUMANISTIC PSYCHOTHERAPIES

Other modalities of individual psychotherapeutic treatment, including client-centered therapy, developed by Carl Rogers (1959, 1961), Milton Erickson's unique psychotherapeutic technique (Erickson & Rossi, 1981), gestalt therapy (Perls, Hefferline, & Goodman, 1951; Greenberg & Watson, 2005), experiential therapy (Elliot, 2001), and existential psychotherapies (May 1969a, 1969b; Yalom, 1980), have generated significant interest and activity. These approaches have influenced many practitioners, but they do not seem to have become dominant forces on their own. Some of their ideas seem to have been integrated into eclectic practice. For example, the importance of therapist empathy and the need to communicate sincerity and acceptance to patients is an important and lasting legacy of client-centered therapy, while flexibility and an active and engaged, almost playful, attitude was encouraged by the Ericksonian tradition. Similarly, experiential therapies, such as gestalt therapy, emphasized the intensity of experience in the present, and have been assimilated by some therapists in their focus on patients' experience during therapy. In the last decade or two, a group of clinical researchers has generated much enthusiasm about process experiential therapy and gathered promising empirical evidence (Greenberg & Watson, 2005). Existential psychotherapies have identified certain universal aspects of experience but have failed to develop a significant following, except for Frankl's work on logotherapy (1946) and meaning and Yalom's on group existential therapy (1980).

SYSTEMS THEORY, COUPLE THERAPY, AND FAMILY THERAPY

Systems theory, and its impact on marital, couple, and family therapy, represents another major development in psychotherapy in the modern era. The recognition that dysfunction and pathology reside in relations between people and not simply inside people resulted in the development of systemic treatment models. Schools within systems treatment include (1) structural family therapy (e.g., Minuchin & Fishman, 2004), which aims to change systems and individuals by altering the roles of family members; (2) family support and educational models; and (3) psychodynamically oriented couple and family treatment. These approaches are powerful as the primary treatment and in conjunction with individual psychotherapies. Depending on the approach, cognition and emotion may each be a primary focus, and the patient's experience of treatment, though perhaps not the therapeutic relationship, is more important than specific technical procedures. A new narrative picture of the family system is an important goal of these treatments.

RECENT TRENDS

The development of diagnosis-specific psychotherapy has been of increasing interest. Instead of honing an effective therapeutic technique helpful for all comers, this trend reflects an attempt to elucidate the key aspects of a certain type of pathology and design a treatment to address those problems. Interpersonal psychotherapy for depression (Klerman et al., 1984), prolonged exposure treatment for PTSD (Foa & Rothbaum, 1998), and cognitive behavioral analysis system of psychotherapy (CBASP), an integrative cognitive therapy for chronic depression (McCullough, 1999), are examples of this trend. This trend has not bypassed dynamic therapy, as evidenced by the work of Kernberg et al. (1989) on borderline personality disorders, or the treatment developed by Crits-Christoph et al. (2005, 2006) for generalized anxiety disorders.

One cannot discuss modern-day psychotherapy without considering the role of psychopharmacology. Every new psychopharmacological development has advanced our thinking about the mind and about psychotherapy. The effectiveness and frequent use of psychopharmacology challenges psychotherapy theory and technique by raising questions about the essential nature of psychopathology, which modes of intervention are most effective, and how and when psychotherapy and psychopharmacology should be combined. Practical and theoretical questions are still unsettled about how these two approaches can be integrated to optimize the effectiveness of each. There is surprisingly little evidence supporting the use of combined treatment (Keller et al., 2000; Thase et al., 1997). Indeed, in anxiety disorders, there is evidence that CBT in combined treatment has less enduring effect than when delivered on its own (Barlow, Gorman, Shear, & Woods, 2000).

SUMMARY

An aerial view of the evolution of psychotherapy over the past 100 years helps to place PPP in a larger context (summarized in Table 3.3). Our review shows there has been a trend from more generalized techniques to more specific ones, that is, from one size fits all to treatments that are customized for diagnoses and symptoms. Emotionally based treatments and those that are more focused on cognition and thinking are both strongly represented, and it is hard to say that there is a trend toward dominance of one or the other. Each seems to speak to real problems. There is an emphasis on the specific techniques of treatment and also a lively interest in the patient's experience of the therapeutic relationship and treatment setting. There is a trend toward directly treating symptoms, and a trend away from depth or comprehensiveness of treatment. Narrative has become important in some psychotherapies, but among the more symptom-focused treatments there is less attention to the patient's life story.

TABLE 3.3. Essential Elements of the Psychotherapies

Psychotherapy	Cognitive versus emotional	Procedure/technique	Role of narrative
Pragmatic psychodynamic psychotherapy	Cognitive = emotional	Experience = technique	++
Freudian psychoanalysis	Cognitive = emotional	Experience < technique	++
Ego psychology	Cognitive = emotional	Experience < technique	++
Object relations	Cognitive < emotional	Experience = technique	++
Self psychology	Cognitive < emotional	Experience > technique	++
Short-term dynamic psychotherapy	Cognitive = emotional	Experience < technique	+
Cognitive therapy	Cognitive > emotional	Experience < technique	+
Behavioral therapy	Cognitive < emotional	Experience > technique	
Interpersonal psychotherapy	Cognitive = emotional	Experience < technique	++
Couple and family systems therapy	Cognitive = emotional	Experience > technique	+
Group therapy	Cognitive < emotional	Experience = technique	+
Interpersonal psychoanalysis	Cognitive < emotional	Experience > technique	++
Gestalt therapy	Cognitive < emotional	Experience > technique	+
Humanistic–Rogerian psychotherapy	Cognitive < emotional	Experience > technique	

PART II

OPENING PHASE

CHAPTER 4

The Therapeutic Alliance

Goal, Task, and Bond

I felt it shelter to speak to you.
—EMILY DICKINSON

The therapeutic alliance is the holy grail of psychotherapy effectiveness because of its special role in the empirical literature on outcome and its intuitive appeal to practitioners. The therapeutic alliance is a relationship created by the patient and therapist that cuts across many types of psychotherapy. It begins even before the first contact with the feelings and fantasies the patient and therapist have about each other. Like the citizens of Lake Wobegon in Garrison Keillor's storytelling, we clinicians all think we are above average in our ability to develop a therapeutic alliance; after all, most of us were told for years before becoming therapists that we are "good with people."

What is this generic interpersonal skill? Is it something that can be taught, or something given? We suggest that the ability to form a therapeutic alliance starts with social and emotional intelligence, one of the multiple intelligences defined by Gardner (1993) and later elaborated by Goleman (2006). It includes the ability to read others' emotions, identify their motivations and conflicts, and the capacity to feel and express appropriate emotions in response. These skills lead to positive interpersonal experiences.

Like the songbirds that need to hear songs at critical periods to develop the ability to sing, we need early relationship attunement and subsequent rich interpersonal lives to develop and hone this ability. There is probably also a neurobiological component to the ability to form an alliance. Recent research in the area of autism, Asperger's syndrome, and nonverbal learning disabilities has clarified that there are hard-wired aspects of brain function that involve facial recognition and the ability to evolve a "theory of mind," that is, the capacity to conceptualize others as thinking, problem-solving, emotional entities (Baron-Cohen, 1997). Mirror neurons fire in the same areas of our brains that neurons are firing in the brains of those with whom we empathize, and this wiring gives us access to important data (Rizzolatti, 2005). Social and emotional intelligence is built upon these capacities.

But what makes one good at flirtation, easygoing with new acquaintances, and judicious and reasonable with loved ones, is not what allows one to develop a therapeutic alliance. The ability to balance closeness and separation, nurturance and reflectiveness, and ambition and acceptance marks the sensibility of a therapist who has a strong therapeutic alliance with a patient. We believe that learning how to develop a therapeutic alliance is like learning to play a sport; the basic materials must be there, but the ability can improve over time with attention and practice. We maintained in an earlier paper on this subject that there are some data to support this view (Summers & Barber, 2003).

It is usually apparent to the therapist when a strong therapeutic alliance fails to develop. Something falls flat in the interaction, and there is a feeling that you and the patient are missing each other. You feel that you are not reaching the patient and not meeting his needs; or the patient seems satisfied, but you have no idea why, and you do not feel that you are really contributing anything.

This chapter reviews the concept of the therapeutic alliance, gives clinical examples, reviews the literature on learning how to develop a therapeutic alliance, and concludes with specific techniques and approaches you can use to facilitate it.

CONCEPT OF THE THERAPEUTIC ALLIANCE

Referred to variously as the therapeutic, working, or helping alliance, the idea that the therapeutic relationship is important for therapeutic success was foreshadowed by Freud's (1912b) comments on the positive feelings that develop between doctor and patient. Subsequent psycho-analytic writers such as Greenson (1967) and Zetzel (1956) articulated this concept more fully, distinguishing between the "real" and adaptive dimension of the treatment relationship and the transferential and fantasy-laden aspect. In his client-centered therapy, Rogers (1965) identified the empathic bond between the patient and therapist as the essential therapeutic agent in treatment.

Although the concept of the alliance has emerged historically in the psychodynamic literature, the strength of the collaborative relationship between patient and therapist has been recognized as crucial by therapists from different theoretical backgrounds. Most theorists, including Beck et al. (1979), emphasize the establishment of the patient–therapist relationship as an important first step of treatment. There is evidence suggesting that the therapeutic impact of the alliance is similar across diverse forms of treatment (Barber, Khalsa, & Sharpless, in press; Martin & Garske, 2000, Horvath & Symonds, 1991), although it might differ as a result of which alliance measure is used (Martin & Garske, 2000).

Goal, Task, and Bond

Seeking to operationalize this concept and apply it more generally across psychotherapies, Bordin (1979) identified three components of the therapeutic alliance: goal, task, and bond. He saw the therapeutic alliance as a mutual construction of the patient and therapist that includes shared goals, accepted recognition of the tasks each person is to perform in the relationship, and an attachment bond. He saw the therapeutic alliance as developing in the relationship between the two and as the vehicle through which psychotherapies are effective. He noted that different psychotherapies call upon different aspects of the therapeutic alliance at different points over the course of treatment.

Bordin's (1979) clarification of the components of the therapeutic relationship breaks down this ineffable idea and is helpful in thinking about how therapists can build their skills by developing the therapeutic alliance. Interestingly, very few studies have examined this question (see, e.g., Crits-Christoph et al., 2006). Developing the goal and task components of the therapeutic alliance are procedural skills, and it is easier to see how they could be learned and practiced. Improving one's ability to develop a bond may require more emotional and personal exploration and a history of positive relationship experiences.

George was a 42-year-old man who came for consultation in a crisis. His wife was 3 years older than he, and they had been married for 15 years. She had just told him she was having an affair with a colleague following a long-standing and close work relationship. The two had traveled to meetings together, often working late into the evening. George had been unhappy and worried about that relationship, discussing it often with her over the preceding several years. His wife had always reassured him that the relationship was platonic. Recently, she had revealed that the other relationship had become sexual, and she wanted to leave the marriage. George and his wife parented well together, and were both devoted to their three preteenage daughters.

George was open, honest, and likeable in the initial interview. It was easy to empathize with his plight. He was tearful, angry, and shocked. He expressed righteous indignation about the wrongs his wife had committed, and seemed to be realistic and brave about bearing up to the loss of his marriage. He was very angry, and the end of the marriage seemed inevitable. He was distraught about his children and the impact this would have on them. His father had died when he was 10 years old, and he had grown up with his mother as the sole parent.

George was very open, and the first two or three sessions were full of information and emotion. There was the sense of a patient starting an active and engaged therapy, but I kept having a feeling in the session that when he finished a topic there was a long pause until I asked a question. I was not sure what to ask him about and what to explore.

He told me he had a lifelong best friend, and he spoke with him often and told him about what he was going through. He was not sure that he needed to come to the therapy just to feel things and express himself; he was doing plenty of that already. He did not think that his marriage was repairable, and even if it was, it was pretty clear to him that his wife did not want to repair it. He felt he was going to try his best to work with her to minimize the impact on the kids, and develop a plan to coparent while living apart.

I kept asking myself, what are we doing together in the sessions? He was accepting the losses, had plenty of supports, seemed to be functioning well, and was practical and realistic about how to work with his wife to take care of his daughters. He was talking about all of this. Was he too well adjusted to really need therapy, or were we missing something?

From Bordin's perspective, what was happening in the therapeutic relationship in terms of goal, task and bond? *Task* refers to each person's role in the therapeutic dyad. The patient's job is to come to the appointment, describe his thoughts and feelings honestly and openly, reflect on them, and try to listen to and accept the therapist's observations. When the time comes, it is also his job to try to employ the understanding he has gained and consider how he could change and then work on implementing it. The therapist's job is to listen hard, use all of his resources to understand, put aside biases, develop an understanding of the patient, and effectively share this understanding (Luborsky, 1984). He should facilitate new perceptions, new approaches to solving problems, and new potential behaviors. The therapist must be open to the patient, but provide input and assistance.

With George, the task component of the working relationship was going well. He was certainly doing all that one would hope for. He was describing what was going on, both emotionally and practically, trying to understand the events, and maintaining an open interest in anything the therapist said.

Bond refers to the attachment between patient and therapist. It is the emotional link. Does the patient feel safe in the therapy and feel a sense of warmth and empathy from the therapist? From the therapist's perspective, is there a feeling of emotional engagement or the particular feeling of caring with objectivity and separation that allows us to do our best work? Here, too, George and the therapist seemed to be doing well. He expressed a sense of comfort and trust and seemed to feel that the therapist liked him, cared about his situation, and felt engaged with him in his troubles.

Goal refers to the shared goals of the therapist and patient. What is the patient working toward, what does he want to understand or change? What is his ambition in therapy? What area of his life does he want to do something about? The therapist must understand the patient's goals and work toward them as well. For example, if the therapist sees the problem as depression and difficulty with closeness, and the patient thinks the problem is a parenting issue with a difficult child and an unhelpful spouse, not only are the pictures of the difficulty different, but the goals will be also. The therapist will address the depression, expecting the other problems to improve as a result, but the patient will feel blamed and misunderstood by the therapist.

I realized that what was missing in the developing therapeutic alliance was clarity about George's goals of therapy. What were his goals, and what was in my mind? I had asked him in the first session what he wanted to get out of therapy, and he said that he needed help "talking it out" and surviving the ordeal. I had agreed that this was a reasonable and sensible goal, but now I wondered whether we meant different things by this.

Toward the end of the second session, and then several times again in the following two sessions, I commented that he seemed to have put up with a lot from his wife over a long period of time. He knew there was something wrong in the marriage, and he had known that her close relationship with her colleague was a symptom of that. She continued that relationship despite his repeated expressed concerns. I said it was striking that he had felt upset and frustrated but had gone along with the relationship as it was for years. Why was this, and what had he known or worried about all along, yet kept trying to ignore? What were his disappointments with her, his contributions to the marital unhappiness, his ideas about what could have been done, or should have been done, to alleviate their problems?

When I suggested this he became suddenly more alert and looked me directly in the eye. Up until now, he had been talking in sessions, but I realized that I felt it was not really to me. When I wondered aloud about his feelings and his role in the marital breakup, he responded that he did not know exactly what I meant, but he thought there was something true about it. He had always been agreeable, and maybe he tried harder than most people would have to meet his wife's needs. Maybe he tended to be this way in general, but what was the matter with that?

By the fourth session, the therapeutic alliance seemed more set. It seemed that the consolidation of the alliance had to do with the development of clearer shared goals. The therapy would be partly about expressing the hurt, loss, and fear George was experiencing, but it would also focus on his way of experiencing relationships, his characteristic way of handling his upsetting feelings, and perhaps what this had to do with his own childhood. Answering the question of why he kept going the same way in the marriage when he knew there were such serious problems was a new shared goal.

This example illustrates how the therapeutic alliance is more than just having a relationship with the patient. It shows the close interrelationship between the three components and how the therapeutic alliance was cemented when the goal was clarified. Effective performance of tasks and shared goals will facilitate the bond because the patient feels closer when the work is going well. The bond in turn facilitates the development of the tasks and goals because the patient feels safe enough to share deeper concerns. This allows for more ambitious goals because the bond helps a patient persist at the difficult task of being in therapy during emotional and upsetting periods.

Another brief example illustrates the task component of the therapeutic alliance and the importance of helping the patient say what is on her mind.

Jen was an attractive 29-year-old woman with long dark hair and a slightly disheveled appearance. In her first appointment, she looked like a college student rushing out to class in the morning, but she had finished law school 4 years before.

Jen had been an associate at a prestigious law practice and had been laid off as financial pressures hit the firm. Shortly thereafter she had a serious motor vehicle accident with multiple injuries requiring an extended rehabilitation. Her convalescence was complicated by depression, binge drinking, and demoralization. She seemed far from the successful young lawyer she had been just 3 years before, and I thought that she was like Humpty-Dumpty—she had fallen and could not put herself back together. After the layoff, accident, and rehab, she could not get back on track. She had distanced herself from her former friends, and now wondered whether they had been friends at all. She lived with an aunt who was retired, and her parents gave her a little money to live on. She could not imagine being rehired after this extended hiatus from law and employment. There was a nagging feeling in my mind, and in hers, she implied, that the accident had almost provided a cover for an anticipated implosion. If it had not been the accident, it would have been something else. I wondered about substance use but she denied current use.

When we discussed her goals, Jen said quickly that she needed to get back on her feet. She realized this would be difficult, but she had been in therapy with a senior, well-known clinician while in college, and he had helped her tremendously through the right mixture of advice and insight. She thought therapy would help again. I gently suggested that the responsibility was on her to take charge and get back to work, even though it would be difficult. I could not tell yet whether an affective connection (bond) would develop; I was alarmed at her inactivity and what I imagined was her magical expectation that I would help her and give her direction.

I just stuck to my tasks: ask questions, try hard to understand, be open-minded, and not inject my values and opinions. She seemed to perform her tasks as well: she was talkative, self-revealing, and expressed a striking degree of self-awareness. She knew she should get back to work, but she was not going to accept just any job she was offered; it had to be pretty good. She felt that she got along well with people, but did not suffer fools gladly, and she tended to get

annoyed and critical if she felt others were not intelligent or reasonable. She was a high-performance sports car; give her the right fuel
and the right conditions, and she was terrific. But if she was not
treated well, then she could not work.

The first meeting was an extended evaluation, and after an hour
and fifteen minutes, she looked at me at said, "Well, I've decided
you seem honest and also smart, so I might as well tell you the rest.
I don't want you to jump to a judgment about this, and you might,
but you seem like the kind of person who might not." It turned
out, that the crucial additional piece of history was that during her
convalescence, while feeling ill, taking painkillers and sedatives, she
had stolen jewelry from her aunt, sold it for a substantial sum, and
had found a way to cover her tracks.

Jen had decided to perform the task of the patient—honest
revelation about one's history and the details of one's life, including those elements that are shameful, embarrassing, and painful.
Of course, this revelation further increased my alarm about her
problems, her capacity for destructive behavior, and her substance
use.

This example illustrates the evolution of a commitment to the task
component of the therapeutic alliance, albeit in a patient who shows
some antisocial features from the beginning of treatment. The previous
example demonstrated the development of shared goals. What about the
bond component of the therapeutic alliance? In our experience, trainees learning psychotherapy tend to focus more on the bond component,
especially in the beginning. They want the patient to feel good about
them, and they are especially concerned about whether they "like" the
patient, and the patient "likes" them. Perhaps this reflects the universal
wish to be liked and loved. They tend to be enthusiastic about patients
with whom there is a good bond and report that "things are going really
well." But how should the bond feel for the therapist?

There is a particular quality of feeling that one has toward a patient
when the therapeutic alliance, and the bond in particular, is strong. One
feels very involved with the patient and cares greatly about what happens
to him or her. There is a feeling of affection and respect for patients, for
their strengths, their ability to withstand and adapt to travail, and for
their talents. The patient's weaknesses, frailties, limitations, and annoying habits are there, but they do not bother the therapist. One can easily
imagine how others experience the person, for example, their relationships with friends, family, or spouses. Yet the therapist does not really
want to talk with the person outside the office and would not particu-

larly look forward to seeing the inside of the patient's home and would not really choose to be at a family wedding.

It is the very separateness of the therapeutic relationship, the one-sidedness of it, that allows the therapist to feel so close and so positive. If it were a real relationship outside the office, the therapist would have his or her own needs to contend with. The patient's limitations would be frustrating, or her strengths might bring up competitive feelings. One of the most wonderful things about being a therapist is that you have the opportunity to get to know many people, often so different from those you would meet in the course of everyday life. You get to know them so well in a particular way that allows you to see them at their best, and from a vantage point that allows you to relate to them at your best.

How does this bond develop? It requires more than just the passage of time. It is based on the patient's capacity for trusting relationships and the therapist's capacity for warmth and affection. The bond grows stronger when both are effectively performing tasks and working together on goals. Positive feelings toward patients tends to be a taboo topic, of course, because affection can lead to boundary violation, and this is the all too frequent and destructive. But warm and affectionate interest in someone else, and the acceptance and empathy that come with it, is the sine qua non of the bond from the therapist's perspective.

THE THERAPEUTIC ALLIANCE AND PSYCHODYNAMIC PSYCHOTHERAPY

So far, the discussion has been about developing an alliance with patients, without specific reference to psychodynamic psychotherapy. Bordin's ideas, although based on psychoanalytic concepts, were designed to have broader application. The examples given were from the first few sessions, rather than later in a longer treatment. What additional components, both theoretical and conceptual, are specific to psychodynamic therapy?

Greenson (1967) distinguishes three dimensions of the patient's relationship with the therapist: the therapeutic alliance, transference, and real relationship. The therapeutic alliance component is what we have been discussing all along in this chapter. The transference refers to the feelings, thoughts, perceptions, and fantasies the patient has about the therapist based on earlier life experiences, especially those experiences with primary caretakers during childhood. Understanding the transference is a gold mine in dynamic therapy, because it allows the patient and therapist to see and experience old reactions right in front of them in the office. The therapeutic alliance is a construction in the here and now by patient and therapist, and it rests on an adult collaboration on goals, tasks, and bond. The transference is not current and not realistic; it is based on relationships in the past.

Last in Greenson's scheme is the real relationship. This refers to the particulars of this therapist and this patient, and their actual interaction, not necessarily in relation to the therapeutic task. An example of the real relationship would be the fact that a therapist speaks accented English, and the patient does too. This may contribute to the therapeutic alliance (or impede it), and it may help to shape the transference reaction, but it is not essentially part of either. Other examples would be the therapist's work or vacation schedule, the proximity between the therapist's office (or home) and the patient's home, or the actual fact of time spent between patient and therapist. The real relationship obviously exists, it is fodder for the development of the therapeutic alliance, and it certainly contributes to the transference. It is of great concern to beginning therapists who may be anxious about what to do if they meet a patient in the elevator, at a restaurant, or as it happened to one of us, in a dorm room in a youth hostel in a foreign land! Not much can be done about it, either to help or hinder the therapy.

There are forces that work against the development of the therapeutic alliance. The patient's drive to repeat and reenact experiences from earlier in life will conflict with the development of the therapeutic alliance. This conflict gives rise to the concept of resistance. This term is unfortunate because it implies that the patient has a conscious negative stance toward the treatment, when, in fact, it is largely unconscious. The patient may be truly attempting to build a therapeutic alliance with the therapist. But at the same time, there are feelings, perceptions, and thoughts based on past experiences that impede the alliance. For example, a patient may experience the therapist as intrusive, demanding, and self-centered from the beginning, when the clinician has actually been empathic and respectful. For this patient, the experience of being asked questions by another person stimulates such powerful feelings of intrusion that a basic element of the therapeutic alliance is hard to accept.

In the early phase of treatment, the therapeutic alliance needs the attention. Later, when it is solidly in place, the field is set for exploration of the transference. We observe that some trainees make the mistake of commenting on the transference too early, before an adequate therapeutic alliance has been built. This contributes to early dropout. On the other hand, many trainees are reluctant to point out the transference for fear that the patients will think they are self-centered and egotistical.

As you can see, the concept of resistance is just another way of thinking about transference, because they are both manifestations of conflict in the therapeutic relationship. The term *resistance* emphasizes the way that old conflicts prevent open discussion of the problems the patient came to address in treatment. *Transference,* which refers to the replay of feelings, thoughts, and perceptions about early relationships with the therapist, refers to the same problem, but refers to the replaying of old relationships.

The therapeutic alliance and the transference will always coexist. The effective therapist keeps a finger on the pulse of both, looking for manifestations of each. In the example of Beth, who had been abducted by her father, the therapeutic alliance developed slowly but surely in the first few months of treatment. She collaborated well with the therapist until the moment when she became suspicious of him after he discouraged her from returning to her boyfriend. At this point, it was clear that she had a negative transference reaction based on her relationship with her father. Prior to this point, there may have been an unrecognized positive transference reflecting whatever trustworthy relationships she had as a child, perhaps with her mother. The assumption that resistance and transference inexorably arise in the treatment relationship is a distinguishing feature of dynamic psychotherapy and becomes a tool for helping the patient understand herself.

The concept of enactment, which refers to the replaying of (reenacting) earlier experiences in the therapeutic relationship, was introduced to help detect subtle but important manifestations of transference and countertransference. Whereas transference refers to what the patient feels and does in response to old relationships and experiences, countertransference reflects the therapist's engagement with this old script. Sometimes the unspoken assumptions and unconscious reactions of both the patient and therapist come together to produce a way of relating to each other which is not readily observable to either. Examples of enactments could include a feeling that the therapist is an inquisitor and the patient is the victim, or the patient is special and deserving and the therapist is the admirer. The transference and countertransference become evident in the playing out of roles. Thinking about what kind of enactment might be going on is a particularly useful approach to help answer a therapist's inner question of why he feels a certain way in a session, or why he relates in an uncomfortable or unusual way with a patient. The concept of enactment reminds us that we do not simply react based on what is going on with the patient, but we also bring subtle and even not so subtle reactions and feelings of our own. What happens in the relationship arises out of an interlocking of both of these feelings, and has a life of its own. Psychotherapy is an encounter between two people and all of their baggage.

An example will help to tease out the aspects of therapeutic alliance and the transference (including resistance and enactment). Distinguishing between the alliance and the transference is cleaner conceptually than practically, but it is essential to try to catch the unfolding of each in the therapeutic relationship.

Ed was a pleasant and likeable young surgeon who came for consultation because he was trying to repair his marriage after having been caught in an extramarital liaison. His other problem was that he was very anxious that his patients might suffer complications of the procedures he performed.

Ed was the middle of three sons of a warm and engaging father and an intense, ambitious mother. His childhood experience was complicated—there was much love and support, but he always had the feeling that his position in the family was insecure. He felt he had to compete hard for acceptance and attention, especially from his mother. He was an excellent athlete and he remembered wanting to win so badly in Little League that he publicly embarrassed himself with aggressive and unsportsmanlike behavior.

This young physician had always valued his attractiveness to women, and had numerous affectionate and sexual relationships. Women found him very desirable, and he often felt that he fell into relationships as though he had little choice about it. He married an accomplished woman, but several years into the marriage he became infatuated with a female colleague who was rather needy and demanding. He could not say no, and they had a brief affair. He ended the relationship, but the scorned lover told his wife what had happened. Ed's wife loved him and wanted to try to repair the marriage, as did he.

The focus of Ed's therapy was on understanding what drove him to the affair, as well as working on his anxiety about his patients' developing a surgical complication. In his practice, he frequently became intensely worried and guilty and assumed he had made careless errors or was just plain incompetent. He was sure he would be sued, found guilty, and would be embarrassed in front of colleagues and the other patients in his practice. His rumination about this could be all-consuming. Ed wanted to be respected and popular.

In the evaluation and subsequent therapy Ed was talkative, cooperative, motivated, and interested in feedback and observations. He was always more comfortable talking about what he was afraid of (being sued or getting in trouble) than what his urges were (success, victory, admiration). There was no conflict or misunderstanding between us, and he seemed to view me as positive, helpful, and kind. The therapy seemed easy and productive. But I had the nagging feeling that nothing ever goes entirely smoothly, and if it does, there is probably a reason.

Ed's core problem was low self-esteem, and two interconnected themes emerged in the therapy. Ed needed to be loved and tried hard in each and every situation to elicit affection and interest from others, especially women. This came out in his romantic relationships, relationships with women at work, and, of course, his mother. He was also intensely competitive and wanted to do better than other men, while feeling at times that he did not measure up. He was afraid that he would be found out to be inadequate, and would be cast out and punished for his attempts to be a man. Both his affair and his professional ambition had roots in his need to prove how loveable and valuable he was. Ed felt guilty about the intensity of his wishes (for both romantic and career success) and worried that he had hurt someone else because of them (wife, lover, and patients).

Ed formed an effective therapeutic alliance—he was a regular and steady participant in the therapy, committed to goals, performing his tasks well, and there was a strong bond with the therapist. He knew he wanted to be loved and admired—by mother, wife, girlfriend, father, colleagues, and therapist. But the competitive theme of his relationships with men was subtly present as well. Ed's demeanor constituted a resistance in therapy because it impeded direct discussion of some of his major conflicts; he spoke easily of his fears, but tended to hide his competitive feelings. It was also a transference because it involved themes in his relationship with his father (avoidance of conflict). He never competed with the therapist directly, but there was a certain amount of excessive respect, and less collaborative give and take than with many patients. This was the enactment. When the therapist realized it and pointed it out to Ed, he realized he wanted to see himself as a faithful student of the therapist. He also acknowledged that occasionally he felt competitive and wanted to be seen as better than the therapist, like he wanted to be better than his colleagues. His loyal and pleasing demeanor was his technique for dealing with the conflict between his competitive feelings and his need to be liked—if he was likeable, then he would not be seen as aggressive, and if he was not aggressive, he would be loved and admired.

It is important to recognize that resistance, enactment, and transference exist alongside the patient's many strengths. Alongside the conflict is a healthy, mature adult with a realistic and contemporary focus. That is, Ed also had an accurate mode of perception and good problem-solving skills.

POSITIVE AND NEGATIVE EMOTION

Positive and negative emotions meet in psychotherapy in the therapeutic alliance. Essentially, the alliance is a new kind of relationship where old, painful emotions coexist with new, positive ones. The alliance reflects respect, affection, and interest from the therapist and engenders these feelings in the patient toward himself. The field of positive psychology, which emerged in the late 1990s, makes positive emotions a direct subject of inquiry. Fredrickson's (2001) broaden-and-build theory locates the value of positive emotions in an evolutionary context. She attempts to explain why there are positive emotions and what survival value they may have. If anxiety promotes vigilance and survival and depression reflects loss and attachment, then what is the purpose of happiness and joy? Fredrickson's theory is that positive emotions build relationships and the capacity for resilience and problem solving. More specifically, Fredrickson shows that positive emotion is valuable because positive affective states promote improved capacity for problem solving; prior positive emotional experiences increase resilience when there is a new current problem to solve; and positive emotional experiences that increase interpersonal connections increase social resources. Thus positive emotion causes a broadening of coping strategies and a larger repertoire of potential solutions to a problem (Fredrickson, 2001).

We suggest that an essential part of the bond in the therapeutic alliance involves experiencing positive emotion at the same time as the negative emotions associated with the patient's problems. It may be this admixture of the negative and positive that is an essential element in the therapeutic relationship, which makes it so different from other relationships. This new relationship, like all attachments, must involve something positive. The broaden-and-build theory gives a conceptual framework for understanding this clearly felt but little-discussed aspect of the therapeutic alliance.

In the traditional psychodynamic literature, supportive interventions were contrasted with exploratory ones. Comments that support, validate, and encourage were seen as useful but antithetical to exploration and deeper understanding. We suggest, however, that positive, encouraging comments, shared humor, direct praise, recognition of patient strengths, and expressions of optimism serve to elicit positive emotions in the patient. These positive emotions do not suppress negative emotions and make it harder to explore areas of conflict. Rather, the positive emotions exist alongside the negative emotions that have brought the patient to treatment, and indeed there is evidence to support the notion that positive and negative emotions are not highly correlated (Watson, Clark, & Tellegan, 1988). We believe that positive emotional experiences enhance the therapeutic alliance and thereby increase the patient's problem-solving capacity the way Fredrickson's broaden-and-build theory suggests. With more positive emotion, a patient will have a greater ability to separate himself from painful feelings and reflect on them and deal with them more creatively. When such successful experiences of self-reflection are repeated, there is greater resilience in the therapeutic relationship, which only serves to embolden the patient further to talk about upsetting and difficult things.

THERAPEUTIC ALLIANCE SKILL DEVELOPMENT

How does one facilitate the development of a therapeutic alliance, and how should we teach others about this? There are scant important data about this topic (see Summers & Barber, 2003, for a review). Patient qualities, therapist qualities, and therapist "technical activity" are the broad categories of factors that are thought to affect the development of the therapeutic alliance. Moras and Strupp (1982) noted that 25% of the variance in a patient's collaborative participation in therapy is linked to qualities of the patient, such as the nature and quality of the patient's other interpersonal relationships. In support of this, Satterfield and Lyddon (1995) found that therapists' prior dependent relationships predict a negative view of the therapeutic relationship.

Patients' expectations of improvement predicted a better therapeutic alliance early in therapy, and previous hostility in relationships predicted a poorer alliance (Connolly-Gibbons, et al., 2003). Not surprisingly, the same is true of the therapist. Dunkle and Friedlander (1996) found that less self-directed hostility in the therapist, more perceived social support, and comfort with closeness led to a stronger bond component of the therapeutic alliance.

The therapist "technical activity," that is, what the therapist does, represents perhaps the most teachable component of the therapeutic alliance. Grace, Kivlighan, and Kunce (1995) demonstrated that counselor trainees who were taught to explicitly discuss patient nonverbal communication had improved therapeutic alliance scores compared with trainees who simply expressed empathy. Weiden and Havens (1994) identified specific behavioral techniques for improving the therapeutic relationship with severely disturbed patients. Crits-Christoph, Barber, and Kurcias (1993) reported that accurately interpreting patients' core conflicts early in treatment results in increased therapeutic alliance later on in treatment. Safran, Crocker, McMain, & Murray (1990) noted that the ability to repair the inevitable ruptures is essential for strengthening the therapeutic relationship.

Therapeutic alliance skills may also develop with clinical experience and duration of training. Mallinckrodt and Nelson (1991) looked at the relationship between training and measurable therapeutic alliance in the Bordin model. They found that greater experience is associated with higher goal scores, less powerfully with improvement in task scores, and is not correlated with bond scores. Dunkle and Friedlander (1996) found that training experiences did not predict increased goal and task scores. Davenport and Ratliff's (2001) study of family therapy trainees found that therapeutic alliance was correlated with cumulative number of patient hours. More recently, Crits-Christoph et al. (2006) trained a small group of relatively naïve therapists in what they called alliance-fostering therapy, a 16-session treatment for major depressive disorder that combines interpersonal–psychodynamic interventions with techniques for enhancing the alliance based on Bordin's model of the alliance. They were able to show at least moderate effect size change in the patients' rating of the therapeutic alliance with the training.

Kurcias's (2000) qualitative study of psychology trainees and their supervisors' conceptualization and implementation of the therapeutic alliance suggested an evolution in the trainees' work. Trainees showed increased sophistication, complexity, and focus in their conceptualization of the patient and of the alliance, greater comfort in discussing patient–therapist relationship issues, greater patience with the slow pace of change, and increased recognition and more skillful management of relationship ruptures over the course of their training.

In our review of teaching about the therapeutic alliance (Summers & Barber, 2003), we urged more focused didactic opportunities, increased attention to this area in supervision, and the use of therapeutic alliance rating scales to help trainees learn more about their patients' perceptions of them in this area.

STRATEGIES FOR FACILITATING THE THERAPEUTIC ALLIANCE

This chapter has outlined the concept of the therapeutic alliance and its key components. Each component was illustrated with examples, and we reviewed many issues involved in learning how to develop a good therapeutic alliance. Now here are some practical tips on how to facilitate it.

1. Give a brief explanation of the procedure of psychotherapy. An example is: "We will meet weekly to talk about what you are feeling and what you are struggling with, so that you can understand it better. The better you can understand what is going on, the better you will be able to figure out what part of it is from baggage from your past, and what part is really a problem in the present. This will allow you to see things as clearly as possible and then decide how you would like to manage and deal with them."

2. Maintain your curiosity and self-awareness in the relationship. Your ability to try to see your blind spots and your patient's, or at least your attempt to do so, will embolden the patient to do the same.

3. Have faith that if you inject warmth, enthusiasm, support, and empathic skepticism about the patient's coping strategies, he will become interested and focus on problems and patterns. If the patient becomes focused and interested, you have truly developed an effective therapeutic alliance.

4. Find those qualities that are likable in your patient rather than ones that are not, and periodically acknowledge them. Enough people in the patient's life have found him or her unlikable.

5. Keep a continuing focus on your own feelings, using them to understand potential countertransference reactions and emerging enactments. Use whatever degree of genuine warmth and interest you feel to facilitate the bond. It is an essential part of the therapeutic relationship to develop some kind of positive emotional experience between therapist and patient. You must be an active participant in this. Positive emotion will augment the empathy you offer, and this will strengthen the patient–therapist bond.

6. Stick to your essential tasks: listening, understanding, reflecting, empathizing. Gently educate the patient about what his tasks in the therapy are: honesty, verbalizing what is on his mind, sticking to it when he feels upset and anxious, coming to appointments, and valuing curiosity. Encourage and counsel patience.

7. Try to understand the patient's goals, implicit and explicit, and develop a clear understanding of what you and he will be working on (discussed further in Chapter 8).

8. In your conceptualization of your developing relationship with the patient, distinguish between those aspects of the relationship that reflect the therapeutic alliance and those involving transference and resistance. Resistance and transference are inevitable, and your attitude toward them should be curiosity and interest, not judgment and criticism.

9. Every comment about resistance should be preceded by an empathic comment implying your understanding that the patient is in pain. For example, "When you talk about the arguments with your husband, you seem to focus on all of the ways that he has hurt you and how angry you are. That is really understandable, as it has been devastating, but doing so seems to prevent you from stepping back and trying to understand how you are reacting and relating to him."

10. Watch for too much pleasure or too much anxiety on your part. These are clues to an enactment that you must understand in order to help the patient reflect on himself and his impact on others.

11. Note the inevitable disruptions in the therapeutic alliance (Muran & Safran, 2002). When it happens, ask the patient about it, validate it, try to understand what happened, and do not be afraid to apologize. Connect this understanding and the disruptive event to the emerging picture of their core problems and conflicts.

12. See the best in human nature, having empathy for the patient's unique trials and tribulations, but do not let him off the hook in being accountable for how he affects others. Your patient needs to deal with reality, and he knows it. He will look to you to judiciously remind him of it.

13. Tips about your manner and approach to the patient:

- In your overall demeanor and manner, behave toward the patient like he is someone sitting next to you at a pleasant dinner party.
- Keep an eye on the anxiety thermometer; too little makes for pleasant conversation but not much therapy, too much creates excessive discomfort for the patient.

- Understand what the patient is looking for emotionally in each session, and make sure he gets a little bit of it.
- Ally with the healthy side of the patient, that is, the part that is distressed by what he or she is doing, feeling, and experiencing.
- Maintain a reasonable degree of focus, enough so that the anxious patient feels he is taking something specific from the sessions, but loose enough to shake off the prearranged agendas.
- Do not work too hard in the session, or remain passive and do too little.
- Do not encourage the patient to like you, but to respect you.

The application of these strategies helps the therapist build the therapeutic alliance while observing the unfolding relationship. Core problems, conflicts, resistance, enactment, and transference are expressed from the beginning and all through the treatment. Learning how to be a psychodynamic therapist involves a high-wire balance of working with these conflicts while attending to and cementing the healthy aspects of the therapeutic relationship at the same time.

SUMMARY

The therapeutic alliance is essential to effective psychotherapy. The three components of the alliance—goal, task, and bond—each require attention and focus by the therapist. Potential ruptures in the alliance are inevitable but important to repair. Empathy, attunement, education, early identification of the patient's core problem, and professional demeanor on the part of the therapist help to build the alliance, and there are a host of specific techniques and tips that will strengthen it.

CHAPTER 5

Core Psychodynamic Problems, Part I

In preparing for battle I have always found that plans
are useless, but planning is indispensable.
—DWIGHT D. EISENHOWER

An energetic woman in her early 50s with closely cropped dark hair
and alert eyes quickly took in the office surroundings. Her husband
had announced that he was thinking of leaving her. This shocked
her; she was completely taken by surprise. She felt scared, ashamed,
guilty, and angry. She said, "I just want him back, I'll do anything."
Quickly, she described her relationship with her husband, and all
that she did for him and their family. She described her concerns
about him, and about herself and their children. She talked about
typical family arguments, issues about money, and one child's health
problems. Her worries were specific and unique to her.

Are there hundreds or thousands of different human problems, each
distinct from one another? Or is there a finite number of problems that
have individual variations? To practice therapy effectively you need to be
able to pay exquisite attention to each person and empathize with each
experience discussed. But you must also look for essential patterns, and
not reinvent the wheel with each treatment. The patient who says to his
therapist, "I'm sure you have heard this sort of thing before, it must be
boring," is wrong, because no one has ever felt and seen the world like
him before, and because it is almost always interesting to listen to people
talking honestly about themselves. But he is also right in the sense that
his problem is probably a version of something common, and recognizing common problems helps therapists understand and anticipate.

There is uncertainty about the type of patient who is best treated in psychodynamic psychotherapy. Students sense that for dynamic therapists, all problems are psychodynamic, and all psychodynamic conflicts are problem filled. If that is true, then what are the boundaries and limits of the treatment, and what problems is it best for? Which diagnoses, personality types, symptoms, and contexts do well with this treatment? All too often, practitioners throw a wide net of inclusiveness around potential patients, finding evidence of emotional conflict or unconscious meaning a justification for therapeutic exploration. Against the indiscriminate view that all problems would benefit from insight and the defeatist view that there are a few "introspective worried well" for whom dynamic psychotherapy is a just dessert, we suggest that the core psychodynamic problems are finite and definable, prevalent and important.

We contend that six problems (Table 5.1)—depression, obsessionality, fear of abandonment, low self-esteem, panic anxiety, and trauma—account for 80 to 90% of those who are appropriately treated with psychodynamic psychotherapy. These common psychodynamic problems have either clear empirical data (depression, panic anxiety, fear of abandonment) or clinical experience to support responsiveness to psychodynamic treatment. Our brief list clarifies what to look for and treat and helps to distinguish between problems that will yield to treatment and those less likely to. Certainly these are not the only problems that respond to dynamic treatment, but they are the most common ones. We are not suggesting that dynamic therapy is the best or most effective treatment for these conditions, as we recognize that other treatments such as CBT or medication may be at least as effective. Although the efficacy of dynamic therapy is a function of the patient's diagnosis, it also requires that the patients possess general qualities that predict psychotherapy response, like motivation and psychological-mindedness (these factors are discussed later in Chapter 8).

TABLE 5.1. Core Psychodynamic Problems

- Depression
- Obsessionality
- Fear of abandonment
- Low self-esteem
- Panic anxiety
- Trauma

Although it is easy to concisely describe a list of problems, the process of searching for and recognizing these problems in actual therapy may be much more difficult. Some patients easily fit the profile of one problem well, and some may have features of more than one.

Each of these core problems contains characteristic patterns and manifests in typical ways. Although there are DSM-IV-TR diagnoses that map well onto some of these problems, we organize and describe the problems by both their surface manifestations and their deeper characteristics.

It has been said that psychoanalysis is in dire need of a "theorectomy," a surgical removal of unused and incorrect aspects of its theory. With more than 100 years of development, the proliferation of theories has resulted in multiple, overlapping ideas, with older theories littering the landscape along with coexisting more recent ones. Nowhere is this more true than in talking about diagnosis and disorders. Among therapists, patients' problems are described in different ways, using different diagnostic terms, employing theoretical models that are numerous and confusing. Because there are so many ideas, and so many are difficult to disprove, there has been little systematic elimination of the less useful terms and theories. For example, the word *narcissism* is used colloquially to refer to selfishness, diagnostically to refer to an abnormal vulnerability in self-esteem, theoretically to refer to a normal and universal aspect of human life, and developmentally to define an aspect of the self that changes throughout the life cycle (Pulver, 1970).

A century of theoretical and conceptual work on diagnoses, usually done with an impulse to split rather than lump, certainly leads us to feel humble in defining a list of core problems. We firmly side with the lumpers, and our menu of problems is relatively simple and coherent. Our scheme could be attacked from all sides by those who support alternative classifications, undoubtedly with some merit, but we maintain that the ability to learn psychodynamic psychotherapy has been hampered more by the sheer volume and variety of schemes than it has by attempts to simplify and clarify, which lack subtlety.

We use the term "psychodynamic problem" to denote problems with common underlying patterns. Historically, psychoanalysts have spoken of psychoanalytic diagnoses—for example, obsessional neurosis, hysterical character, and phobic neurosis, among others. These were relatively well-defined entities, with characteristic symptoms, identifiable (although inferred) dynamics, and hypothesized etiologies. But the psychoanalytic diagnostic system was unreliable and difficult to apply clinically because of its reliance on a high degree of inference. One man's obsession was another man's phobia.

Some of the classical psychoanalytic diagnoses are useful, intuitive, and fairly easily observable, but they also carry theoretical assumptions that may not be true and unnecessarily complex. For example, the cause of the classical neurosis is developmental fixation, that is, trauma during a particular developmental phase. Supposedly, this defining event and the phase when it occurred determines the subsequent type of neurotic symptomatology. But did all patients with obsessions have anal-phase trauma, and did all eating disorders result from early feeding problems? Although theoretically elegant and certainly intuitive, there are few data to support this radical privileging of early developmental experience over genetic vulnerabilities, subsequent environmental factors, and later life experiences. In summary, the classical psychoanalytic approach to diagnosis, which was based on inferred dynamics and a deterministic view of early relationships, has suffered because it does not fit the data and is rigid and laden with excess assumptions.

DSM-III was the first psychiatric nosology that was organized around observable (relatively) symptoms and signs and that attempted to be free of theoretical bias about the causes of disorders. DSM-IV continued in this vein, tweaking the descriptions, and rearranging the diagnoses. The weaknesses of this system have been extensively discussed in the mental health literature (see, e.g., Sadler, 2002), and include the grouping of problems by phenomenological features rather than by underlying entities or diseases, and an implicit bias toward equating symptoms with illnesses and treatments with symptom reduction. The *Psychodynamic Diagnostic Manual* (PDM Task Force, 2006) and the *Operationalized Psychodynamic Diagnosis* (OPD Task Force, 2008) are recently proposed psychodynamic systems; it is not clear yet how widely they will be accepted and tested.

The six problems we are highlighting and embracing are psychodynamic (and psychoanalytic) in format, and they provide a helpful narrative understanding of a person's condition. We regard these as organizing explanations that make up in therapeutic narrative value what they lack in empirical rigor. A useful list of psychodynamic problems that helps the practitioner understand and practically treat patients should have neither the excessive conviction of classical psychoanalytic theory nor the surface orientation of DSM diagnoses.

Instead, we use a heuristic approach to categorization, aiming for what is clinically useful. The six problems are characterized by their key psychodynamic conflicts, historical conceptualizations, and the psychoanalytic model most useful for understanding them, as well as the character strengths that are most affected in those suffering from the problem, and the usual treatment goals. They are recognizable by therapist and patient alike. These are problems that can be understood and worked with therapeutically, not necessarily genuine disease entities with the theoretical baggage of etiology, structure, course, and so forth. In the actual clinical world, these real problems can present singly or in combination, and a particular problem can dominate the patient's life (and therapy) at one point in time and may be replaced subsequently by another. The student of psychotherapy would be well served by developing an intellectual and "gut" understanding of these essential problems. During the early stages of learning, pattern search and recognition is a deliberate, effortful, conscious, and rational process that later becomes rapid and intuitive with experience.

References to relevant literature are included in our descriptions, but we cannot possibly do justice to the rich psychoanalytic and empirical literature, which includes a tremendous breadth of descriptive, theoretical, and clinical writing about these problems. We also make no claims of originality in our description of these problems, but rely heavily on classical and recent conceptualizations that we have found useful.

Gender, race, and ethnicity (as well as history) shape individuals' problems and how they are perceived. Some problems seem to be found more among one sex, or perhaps among specific subpopulations. We recognize, for example, that fear of abandonment may be seen relatively more often in women than men, and recognize that this may reflect social expectations about relationships, as well as social definitions of what constitutes a problem and typical pathways for coming to treatment. Thus we do not pretend that this categorization sits outside the current social context. Instead, we assume that it may reflect social norms and biases as it tries to describe what therapists and patients see. There is a danger that it could reinforce stereotypes, and therefore it may need to be revised and amended as times change.

Strengths coexist with problems. The traditional psychodynamic approach attends greatly to problems and their resolution and trusts that well-being will follow. We suggest that a well-rounded view of our patients includes taking into consideration both pathology and strengths, because treatment may need to build strengths while it diminishes problems.

Assessing patient strengths is an important part of therapy, and we observe that problems typically sap individuals of their strengths. Peterson and Seligman (2004) have enumerated character strengths and virtues, attempting to develop an "un-DSM" that describes strengths, instead of illnesses, that are present across time and across cultures. Their taxonomy, summarized in Table 5.2, has generated significant

TABLE 5.2. Virtues and Character Strengths

Virtues	Character strengths
Wisdom and knowledge	Creativity, curiosity, open-mindedness, love of learning, perspective
Courage	Bravery, persistence, integrity, vitality
Humanity	Love, kindness, social intelligence
Justice	Citizenship, fairness, leadership
Temperance	Forgiveness, humility, prudence, self-regulation
Transcendence	Appreciation of beauty and excellence, gratitude, hope, humor, spirituality

Note. From Peterson and Seligman (2004). Copyright 2004 by Oxford University Press. Reprinted by permission.

interest in empirical research on personality strengths (Seligman, Steen, Park, & Peterson, 2005). They define virtues as overarching categories, each composed of three to five character strengths. We see character strengths as important in therapy in the following areas: development of the therapeutic alliance, the personal narrative, processes of change, and degree of resilience after treatment is over. We discuss these issues in the chapters dealing with these topics. Here we comment on the core psychodynamic problems and their relationship to character strengths and make some suggestions about building character strengths in psychotherapy.

Which character strengths become diminished in illness probably depends on what kind of problem the patient is struggling with. For example, depression seems to sap one's courage, humanity, and capacity for transcendent experiences, and obsessionality undermines one's wisdom and humanity. The question of which strengths are compromised by which particular problems is only beginning to receive empirical study, and our comments are based on clinical experience rather than evidence.

WHICH PROBLEM DOES THE PATIENT HAVE?

Table 5.3 summarizes the psychodynamic problems and describes them in detail. This includes the key conflicts, associated DSM-IV diagnoses,

TABLE 5.3. Core Psychodynamic Problems and Their Treatment

	Depression (Peter)	Obsessionality (Ben)	Abandonment fear (Sarah)	Low self-esteem (Stan)	Panic anxiety (Alice)	Trauma (Ellen)
Essential problem						
	Loss and self-criticism	Rumination and resentment	Attachment and abandonment	Self-esteem and protection	Acute paroxysms of anxiety	Safety
Key conflicts and problems						
	Abandonment, attachment, conflict over aggression	Autonomy, fear of loss of control, conflict over aggression	Abandonment, attachment, primitive defenses	Self-esteem, abandonment	Separation, repressed anger	Fear of loss of bodily integrity, attachment and abandonment
Predominant psychodynamic model used for formulation						
	Ego psychology	Ego psychology	Object relations	Self psychology	Ego psychology	Object relations
Typical CCRT						
	Wish to be loved; rejected by others; feel depressed, angry	Wish to be in control of emotions and impulses; others are controlling me; feel angry, anxious	Wish to merge/be close; people are abandoning me; feel abandoned, angry	Wish to be taken care of, loved, respected or admired; not given enough respect, love, or admiration; feel empty and not admired	Wish to be close and loved; people leave me; feel loss, fear, anger	Want to trust and be safe; others violate my trust; feel afraid and not trusting
Most associated DSM-IV diagnoses						
	Major depression, dysthymia	Obsessive–compulsive personality disorder,	Atypical depression, Cluster B personality disorder,	Narcissistic personality disorder, dysthymia	Panic disorder with or without agoraphobia	PTSD, Cluster B personality disorder, atypical depression,

Disorder	Psychodynamic treatment goals	Character strengths affected	Therapeutic alliance issues
somatization disorder, some eating disorders	Increased sense of security and empowerment, increased healthy trust in relationships	Courage, humanity	Clearly spelled out boundaries and expectations, mutual respect, attention to fact and reality
	Increased independence and ability to be assertive without overwhelming anxiety and anger	Courage, transcendence	More frequent sessions, empathic attention to episodes of panic, close exploration of precipitants, psychoeducation about panic, ability to tolerate the patient's necessary discomfort
	More accurate and positive self-image, increased ability to tolerate vulnerability	Wisdom and knowledge, humanity, temperance	Attention to empathic bond
somatization disorder, some eating disorders	More stable image of self and other, decreased mood reactivity, increased stability of relationships	Justice, temperance	Empathy, development of contractual relationship leading to relationship development
subclinical obsessive–compulsive disorder	Decreased guilt, increased tolerance of affective experience	Wisdom and knowledge, humanity, transcendence	Psychoeducation about therapy and importance of affects, elicitation of feelings
	Decreased vulnerability to abandonment, decreased self-punishment	Courage, humanity, transcendence	Empathy, encouragement, instillation of hope, education about depression

(cont.)

97

TABLE 5.3. (cont.)

	Depression (Peter)	Obsessionality (Ben)	Abandonment fear (Sarah)	Low self-esteem (Stan)	Panic anxiety (Alice)	Trauma (Ellen)
Typical resistances						
	Overwhelming affects, hopelessness, passivity	Characteristic obsessional defenses (intellectualization, isolation of affect, reaction formation, etc.), overvaluing of thought over feeling	Fear of abandonment, premature ending of therapy	Inevitable ruptures in empathy	Dependency, avoidance	Fear leading to reenactment of traumatic situation
Technique issues						
	Initial phase of empathy, support, encouragement of function, second phase of identification of key themes of abandonment/loss, and conflict over resentment about losses, maintenance	Active listening, focus on feelings, gentle but firm confrontation, attention to anger and guilt, some directiveness, use patient's cognitive skills to help identify patterns	Concept of containment, appropriate management strategies, mixing of supportive and exploratory interventions, progression from relationship development to	Consistent emphasis on ruptures in empathy, repair and recognition of this continuing vulnerability	Identify precipitants, challenge avoidance; interpret conflict associated with panic, focusing primarily on precipitants but connecting to historical antecedents and transference; encourage widened	Collaborative, flexible attitude, focus on empowerment and realistic perceptions, truth-telling, respect for boundaries

	Typical transferences	Typical countertransferences
phase related to early recognition of increased conflict and planning for effective solutions	Abandonment, dependency, idealization, anger	Rescue fantasies, feeling incompetent, sucked dry
working through dependency to true working alliance	Controlling, passive-aggressiveness, "resistant," anger and hostility, anxiety about being controlled, struggle for freedom and autonomy	Frustration, feeling of being controlled, retaliatory fantasies, boredom, distance, futility
	Mirroring, idealizing, twinship	Rescue fantasy, grandiosity, anger at feeling defeated, boredom
scope of behavior; tolerate resurgence of separation reaction at termination	Separation, loss, abandonment; anger about loss; fear of further loss or retribution because of anger	Maternal, rescue and caretaking; frustration with dependency and rejection
	Lack of trust, fear and vigilance, rage at lack of help, need to control therapist, reenactment of trauma	Identification with victim, helplessness, identification with perpetrator, bystander/witness guilt, secondary PTSD, confusion

treatment goals, character strengths affected, psychodynamic model that best explicates the problem, typical resistances, transferences, counter-transferences, CCRT themes, and techniques. Our subsequent discussion of each problem outlines the evidence base for the treatment of each.

We encourage clinicians to think about which core psychodynamic problem best characterizes the patient. Our students like the clarity of the six psychodynamic problems, and they rapidly recognize their patients in the descriptions. They find it helpful to be able to quickly recognize the core issues. When they begin to employ the conceptualizations with ease, the user-friendliness of this scheme leads to an interesting clinical problem. How do you determine which problem best fits an individual patient? Sometimes they are able to build a case for several problems for a given patient. The considerations in making this choice are:

- What is the dominant painful affect or symptom the patient is struggling with (e.g., does the patient complain of depression, frequent losses, panic attacks, or insecurity)?
- Do the problem and the associated dynamics help explain essential history, current problems, and the patient's troubling emotions? Is it the clearest, simplest, and most comprehensive explanation of the six problems?
- Does the patient have some degree of recognition of this psychodynamic problem? Can he or she see it in when discussed?

Some problems are at a deeper level of inference, such as obsessionality and trauma. Patients are less likely to self-report these problems and less likely initially to recognize them in themselves. But initial patient acceptance is not the only consideration, and accuracy and thoroughness are ultimately more important.

The era of one-size-fits-all psychodynamic psychotherapy has been fading since the development of DSM-III and the recognition that the empirical study of psychopathology trumps theory as the driver of new ideas about treatment. We regard PPP as "problem-specific" and see tailoring the treatment to the problem as just as important a step in improving psychodynamic psychotherapy as it is in other treatments. Specific problems are best treated with specific treatments. Although the descriptive and very specific diagnoses used in DSM-IV are essential for overall treatment planning and perhaps for guiding the timing and type of psychotherapy, we suggest that the "diagnoses" that are most relevant for planning and carrying out psychodynamic psychotherapy are the six psychodynamic problems.

Our view of each problem reflects a synthesis of the literature and our clinical experience. We do not propose a novel treatment model for each of the six problems. Rather, we have integrated the work of many clinicians and researchers in our recommendations and reference the major influences on our thinking. Trainees will need to supplement our brief discussion of each problem with further readings of the literature to treat these problems most effectively. This chapter discusses depression and obsessionality, and Chapter 6 covers fear of abandonment, low self-esteem, panic anxiety, and trauma.

DEPRESSION: LOSS AND SELF-ESTEEM

> I am in that temper that if I were under water
> I would scarcely kick to come to the top.
> —JOHN KEATS

Past losses make people sensitive to new losses, and depression is the most common problem that brings people to therapy. Under its broad tent coexist sadness, loss, melancholy, boredom, frustration, irritability, fear, abandonment, and hopelessness. Although these feelings are ubiquitous and present transiently for most everyone, when they persist they often start a vicious cycle of negativity—sadness, loss, withdrawal, demoralization, and increased self-criticism, leading to further withdrawal and negative outlook. Subjectively, depression involves prominent persisting feelings of self-criticism, negativity, and loss. From a symptom perspective, depression is often associated with the typical somatic symptoms, including changes in sleep, appetite, and energy, along with problems in focus and concentration and the ability to enjoy oneself. Suicidal thinking and urges may creep in, and there may be loss of sexual interest.

> Youthful and intense, Peter walked into the office for his first appointment. It was late in the first semester of his freshman year of college. His steady gaze was framed by long, dark hair and punctuated by gold wire-rimmed glasses. He started right in with an exceptionally articulate description of his inner pain—he was anxious, self-critical, afraid, and certain that he would not succeed socially or academically. His suffering was intense and palpable.
>
> He was the eldest of three children, the only son, born to a quiet engineering professor and his wife. Peter was quick to express his frustration with his mother, who talked excessively and seemed to take everything about their relationship too seriously, includ-

ing telling him about her disappointments with his father. He was close to her but angry about her neediness. His father was kind but remarkably aloof, almost a caricature of an engineer; he was stuck in his "left brain."

Peter had intense crushes on several girls at college; he was fascinated and preoccupied with each. But he was so focused on being accepted and loved that it was hard for him to think about how he really felt about them. He was easily wounded and angry when he was hurt. He ruminated about what the girls thought and felt and what move he should make next. He had some male friends, but they were not nearly as important to him as satisfying his intense need for a romantic relationship. He felt very lonely and insecure.

Peter had difficulty sleeping, constant sadness and anxiety, trouble concentrating, loss of the ability to enjoy himself, and he often thought of suicide. Prior to coming for treatment, he had considered purchasing a gun to shoot himself in the head. It was just too painful to live this way, and when he felt rejection by a girl or a slight from a friend, he was catapulted into intense hurt, anger, and hopelessness.

Peter was very smart and thought about things carefully—he organized a high school initiative for environmental awareness when this was barely beginning to be popular and had creative and interesting ideas for his coursework. But he regularly became bogged down while working on projects and was filled with self-doubt, self-criticism, and fear that he would be seen as mediocre and unimportant. His procrastination caused him tremendous anxiety, and he had to take a semester's leave because of poor academic performance.

Psychodynamic Conceptualization

Freud's profoundly original conceptualization of depression in *Mourning and Melancholia* (1917b) emphasized the importance of loss of close relationships as the cause of depression. Contrasting the self-limited sadness of grieving with the self-critical despair of depression, he hypothesized that those we lose (referred to as the lost "object," in psychoanalytic parlance) are internalized, taken into our minds, and identified with—they become part of us. Anger at the lost object becomes directed to where the object now lives, in the self. This leads to the criticism and anger directed toward the self that is so characteristic of depression, for example, self-doubt, self-criticism, and guilt. It was hard to miss from Peter's history that his problems became full-blown when he left home for college. He loved his parents and sisters and was usually annoyed and disappointed with them, but they were his closest relationships; although he was thrilled to leave the demands of his family behind, going to college was a big loss.

Melanie Klein (Mitchell, 1986) put forward a similarly brilliant but also somewhat tortuous theoretical conceptualization of depression. She held that early infantile experiences of love and hatred (based on frustration) are managed by projecting such feelings onto the mother and then introjecting them (a primitive form of internalizing) back into the self. Like mother birds who predigest food for their young, human mothers must be present and close enough to their very young children to allow them to engage in this projection and introjection, allowing the children's anger to be detoxified. Klein defined the stage dominated by this feeling about the mother as the schizoid position because the love and hate are so split apart. The next stage is called the depressive position; here the child brings together the feelings of love and anger, recognizing their coexistence, and tolerates the depressing feeling of hating the very same person she loves. Klein's contribution to theoretical thinking about depression emphasizes the struggle between loving and angry feelings and the experience of depression as fundamentally tied to the difficulty in attachment to early caretakers and the subsequent stand-ins for these important relationships. Peter was seething with conflict about his love and hate—his mother was his closest confidant, and he disliked both himself and his mother for this. He got very attached to potential girlfriends, but he was more often angry and frustrated with them than loving toward them.

Edward Bibring (1953), a European psychoanalyst émigré who settled in Boston, developed a theory that is easier to understand. Relying on the concept of the ego ideal as the part of the mind that contains the hopes and dreams about what kind of person one wants to be, Bibring hypothesized that good self-esteem depends on how close your perception of yourself is to your ego ideal. Live up to your dreams and you will be free of depression. Be the kind of person you really are, and if it is far from what your ego ideal, you will be depressed. Bibring's view illuminated part of Peter's depression. He was in great pain at the difference between who he wanted to be—loved, handsome, smart, successful—and who he felt at times he really was—insecure, unattractive, deficient, unlovable.

Heinz Kohut (1971), the father of self psychology (discussed in Chapter 3) took the study of narcissism and narcissistic personality as his starting point. He noticed that there was a subgroup of patients who found the rigors of classical psychoanalysis especially difficult, feeling ashamed, self-protective, and constantly hurt by the distant analyst and lonely couch. He distinguished a particular type of depressive feeling in those who feel chronically insecure, unloved, and susceptible to searing feelings of loss, abandonment, and shame (he called these patients narcissistic). He saw the Freudian and Kleinian depressions as arising from internally conflicted anger and love and related to these drives and how they are managed. By contrast, he was interested in the effect of a lack of closeness, reciprocity, empathy, and affirmation in relationships. He saw these compromised attachments as frequent and debilitating and a cause of a new type of depression. Thus the Kohutian depression is one of limited attachment as well as chronic subacute disappointment and abandonment. Indeed, Peter felt lonely, detached, and dangerously thin-skinned when it came to relationships. His strong feelings of shame and low self-esteem were matched only by the intensity of his self-criticism and self-flagellation.

Though there are many other thoughtful and penetrating writers about depression, Busch, Ruden, and Shapiro's (2004) monograph on the psychodynamic treatment of depression provides a very useful synthesis of the main ideas. They bring together the Freudian and Kleinian attempts to understand aggression in depression, as well as the Kohutian focus on self-esteem and intimacy. Their formulation is: Frustration with early attachment leads to anger and guilt; this anger is turned back on the self in the form of self-criticism. The patient with depression then attempts to salvage a sense of self-esteem and well-being by trying to connect to others, idealizing them and hoping to rescue self-esteem through the love of a new, loving parent. This is doomed to disappointment because of the depressed person's high and unrealistic expectations. The latter part of this dynamic, the self-esteem salvage operation, makes use of Bibring and Kohut's thinking about the importance of the patient's low self-esteem and the use of relationships to heal and save.

Busch et al.'s cogent formulation provides a structure for organizing Peter's symptoms, history, and dynamics. His relationships with his needy mother and distant father resulted in intense feelings of loss, frustration, and anger. The anger made for a powerful superego with resulting intense self-criticism. These attachment difficulties also led to an uncertain sense of self and fragile self-esteem. Peter sought out new relationships with girls to salve his sense of loneliness and emptiness; these girls were idealized, and thus the fantasy of being with them made him feel loved and whole. But he was constantly disappointed because his hopes were unrealistically high. These rejections fueled his anger and frustration, some of which was turned onto himself with self-criticism and occasional self-destructive behavior. The twin themes of self-esteem fragility with cycles of hope and disappointment and of frustration leading to angry self-criticism reinforced each other. When the therapist first met Peter, he was terribly insecure and angry at himself. With time, he came to understand that he was also very angry with both his mother and father, the former for being excessively indulgent and the latter for being too distant. Peter's wobbly self-esteem rose and fell in response to how others felt about him; this preoccupation with how the others responded to him made it hard to go through the day, do his schoolwork, and socialize with friends.

Needless to say, the psychodynamic conceptions of depression do not preclude the importance of genetic and biologic vulnerability, but they do help to understand the mental processes as they are, and they propose a developmental narrative of how the characteristic feelings come into being.

Strengths

Awareness of Peter's strengths balances the discussion of his problems. Depression seems to take a particular toll on the strengths of courage, humanity, and transcendence, and these are the areas that may need special tending in the treatment. Indeed, Peter had a natural courage, sense of conviction, and independence, yet this was particularly challenged by his concern about what others would think of him and the terrible upset he felt when he was rejected by girls. His frequent inhibition, ambivalence, and uncertainty seemed to reflect his illness and the struggle with it. His humanity, characterized by love, kindness, and social intelligence, was an area in which he was especially well endowed. Although not surprising, it was striking to note that when not depressed, his function in each of these areas was so much better and deeper, and so much more limited when he was.

It is hard to be loving, compassionate, and perceptive when one is desperately preoccupied with keeping one's emotional head above water. It is hard to be kind when one feels angry about being rejected. Likewise, with his strengths in the area of transcendence—Peter was a talented writer, and he had strong moral convictions and a belief that society could be better. When depressed, he procrastinated terribly in attending to his work, and he lost interest in thinking about his larger community and its problems.

There are two different perspectives on the relationship between pathology and strengths. They may be opposite sides of the same coin, and the presence of strengths means the relative absence of illness, and vice versa. An alternative perspective is that pathology exists alongside strengths, and there is some degree of reciprocal causality. That is, perhaps depression causes decreased courage and humanity, or more courage and humanity diminishes depression. These two different perspectives suggest theoretical and empirical questions that need to be studied. At this point, we take a pragmatic approach and observe that a continuing focus on patient strengths helps patients find in themselves qualities they respect and feel proud of. For depressed patients this means helping them see their courage in their struggle with depression, or appreciating that they will feel more loving when they feel better. It means encouraging attention to those moments of transcendent experience—appreciation of something beautiful, or laughing at comedy routine—that can remind patients that those parts of themselves are still present.

Goals of Treatment

The goals of the psychodynamic treatment of depression are to decrease the patient's vulnerability to abandonment and decrease the tendency for harsh self-criticism. Although this seems simplistic, it helps the therapist keep an eye on the future of the relationship, what to look for to assess whether there is progress, and the combination of openness and curiosity and a guiding hand on the tiller that makes for good therapy. The goals for Peter were to develop the ability to ride out the expected bumps in friendships and close relationships by tolerating and surmounting the inevitable feelings of abandonment he will experience, and have a healthier and more positive sense of self that will be more immune to self-criticism when he is angry and hurt. He will look more to himself to feel good, and less to others, and set himself up less for hurt and disappointment.

The psychodynamic treatment of depression combines a detailed exploration of how the patient reacts to the present as though it were the past, with support for behavioral change. Our treatment discussion is also primarily informed by Busch et al.'s monograph on psychodynamic psychotherapy of depression (2004). An important caveat is that depression is a heterogeneous problem, and we assume here that appropriate diagnosis and treatment selection have already taken place. This means that the patient has been screened for possible medical disorders (e.g., hypothyroidism), and what appears to be depression is not actually something else, such as acute grieving, substance abuse, or a psychotic disorder. A clinical history with emphasis on neurovegetative signs and symptoms, other active psychiatric symptoms, and a screening for medical symptoms will provide the data needed to clarify the diagnosis.

> Through therapy, Peter achieved both symptomatic improvement and a change in his sense of himself and the strength of his relationships. He will probably always have a vulnerability to rejection and loss, but it is now muted, more expected, and predictable. He is quite good at recognizing when he is overreacting to the present based on his sensitivities and when he is looking to a relationship to provide salvation. He makes better decisions about his relationships. His mood is more stable, and he tends to "go with the flow" more. He chose a career path and is pleased with it despite how hard he has to work. He is dating and deals with the uncertainties and opportunities in his relationships with far more equanimity than in the past. In the past, he was terribly anxious about his relationships, always concerned about whether he was liked and loved, and had difficulty enjoying being in the moment. Now he is more able to appreciate people for who they are, and more open to spontaneity.

This is the hoped-for outcome of psychotherapy for depression. The patient no longer has specific symptoms of depression, and has not had them for several years. But the change is deeper than this, as his experience of himself, his relationships, and his work is also different. He is not desperate, and he can enjoy himself, follow his interests, deepen his talents, and appreciate others for who they are. He is probably less vulnerable to relapse as well, and this is reflected in the fact that he has not been depressed for about 5 years.

Developing a Therapeutic Alliance

The therapeutic alliance with patients with depression develops rapidly when the patient is scared and suffering. Dependency in the patient, when the therapist is supplying all of the energy, hope, and constructive attention, will certainly make for a quick, powerful attachment. But developing a good alliance requires more than the patient liking the therapist. It also requires the patient to perform the necessary tasks of self-reflection and trying new things. The therapist must take a practical perspective and push the patient to be as active as possible, both in the hard work of therapy and in the engagement with the world.

Some patients who are quite depressed and hopeless may have little interest in developing a new relationship. Why would therapy work when they have so little to live for? So an essential aspect of treating depression is helping to rekindle hope in the patient. This is done directly through encouragement, as well as through education about depression and how treatable it is. The hopeless patient needs some time to have small successes or moments of satisfaction. It may be hard to avoid overidentifying with the patient and begin to feel hopeless, too. There can be a very powerful pull in this direction. You may need to step back from the patient's own experience of her situation and consider it from the outside; is the degree of pessimism warranted? Might some people find a way of adapting and working through the problems?

We may alternate between excessive ambition for our patients and hopelessness and detachment. Both of these positions involve some avoidance of feeling what the patient is feeling—misery and hopelessness. The empathic link is so uncomfortable the therapist can become desperate to change the patient or detach from even trying. This alternation can reach an extreme in dealing with the severely depressed or suicidal patients. Because it is so painful to be with patients who are in acute anguish and who are also very angry about their losses, therapists tend to detach without realizing it. Similarly, depressed patients' significant others respond to their depression by distancing themselves (e.g., Coyne, 1976). Therapists do this, too, to manage helplessness or anger at patients for making them feel so powerless (this dynamic is described well in Maltsberger & Buie, 1974). But despite this description of the dynamics encountered in developing a therapeutic alliance, most depressed patients step into their role in therapy and develop a good alliance.

Technique

The initial phase of therapy involves promoting a supportive environment and providing education about depression. The education is rather straightforward. The syndrome of depression means that upset feelings, typically about loss, have taken on a life of their own, and the patient is preoccupied with negative, hopeless thoughts, and neurovegetative symptoms. There is usually a mix of genetic vulnerability and life stressors that precipitate and maintain the depression. Patients need to be told about the diagnosis and encouraged that this problem will get better from a variety of treatments. They may need to be informed that they will be vulnerable to depression in the future.

Sometimes just starting therapy results in the patient becoming more active, but often it is helpful for the therapist to specifically encourage activity and engagement in the areas the patient identifies as important and rewarding. Doing things and engaging in physical activity usually makes people feel better. Encouraging activity does not limit the potential for learning from the transference in therapy, and it is certainly required in many situations. There is often an improvement in mood and function during the first phase, and these gains ideally will be maintained through the second phase.

The second phase of therapy focuses on identifying the key themes of (1) abandonment and loss, and (2) resentment about the loss and subsequent conflict over this resentment.

> First, Peter worked hard on recognizing the typical sequence of feelings he struggled with in his social life—rejection sensitivity, resentment about feeling so hurt, guilt and worry about his anger. He experienced this repeatedly in the therapy, feeling it deeply, then looking at it and discussing it. The therapist asked about his feelings and perceptions of the situations where he felt rejection and loss. Over time he began to feel that his reactions were excessive and that the degree of anger and worry about his anger was misplaced. He did want to make friends, and be close to others, but he began to feel that his reactions were out of proportion to the situations he was really in. He became able to connect his intense responses to friends with old feelings about his parents, and he could see how much his current feelings about loss and rejection were really the reactivation of old feelings about his parents in childhood.
>
> With this increasing awareness, Peter could more flexibly consider his friends and what they were like, and whom he really liked and didn't like. He could see them more for who they were, rather than as a reflection of his feelings and needs. He saw his tendency to idealize others, especially women, and how this set him up for disappointment. With this recognition, his dating pattern began to change. He was able to chase women less intensely and wait to see whether they were genuinely interested in him. He worked harder at being active and outgoing, knowing that this increased his social circle, even when he felt discouraged, breaking an old pattern of retreating when he felt hurt.

The techniques we described for increasing self-awareness, changing perceptions, and trying new behaviors are the main focus of this phase of treatment. Some patients become increasingly upset as they explore current and old feelings of loss, and sometimes they feel worse during this phase. These bursts of intense pain are usually accompanied by a return to an even mood. That is, the patient becomes more resilient and gains confidence that when he is upset he will be able to figure it out and feel better.

The third phase of the psychodynamic psychotherapy of depression, which could be seen as more of a maintenance phase of treatment, focuses on consolidation of the understanding achieved in the second phase and a deepening and working through of these feelings. The attention here is on early recognition of situations that bring up conflicts and recognition of the differences between old and current feelings. The patient works consciously to plan for solutions to these problems. Late in Peter's treatment, he could analyze situations himself and report on them in the next therapy session.

Some patients do not linger in the maintenance phase, and move on quickly to termination. Not surprisingly, this last phase of treatment can be especially potent because patients with depression may reexperience their earlier losses with the loss of the therapist. They may also be afraid of a recurrence of depression, as the natural history of depression often involves relapses. The general issues of termination are discussed in more detail in Chapter 15, but our experience is that this phase of the treatment of depression involves a genuine sense of loss, both reexperienced via the transference, but also of the realistic aspects of the treatment relationship. The relationship with the therapist is a deep one, and there is an aura of sadness that both therapist and patient will likely feel. It is important to accept this and let the patient grieve in a healthy way. You should caution the patient (and yourself) that a future relapse does not mean the treatment has not been effective, as even the best therapy may leave the patient vulnerable to future depression.

Transference and Countertransference

The most frequent transference reaction of the depressed patient is a feeling of abandonment and hunger for a closer connection. This transference is typical of patients who have a more anaclitic, or abandonment-related, depression. It is frequently associated with a dependency reaction, where the patient regards the therapist as an essential helper. He feels he cannot function on his own and regressively expects and hopes the therapist will take care of him. Some patients idealize their therapists, seeing them as the bountiful source of emotional supplies they need to survive. The other side of this dependent transference reaction is the angry transference, where the patient is filled with a sense of rejection and disappointment. Early losses are replayed with the therapist in the role of the absent or hurtful parent. Patients with introjective, or guilty, depression tend to experience the therapist as critical and rejecting.

It is the therapist's task to note these transference reactions and see them as a reflection of the typical dynamics of depression. Patients are expected to have transference reactions and become able to identify and understand them, but this takes time. Therapists are expected to have countertransference reactions, but when they rise to the level of dominating our feelings and affecting our actions in any tangible way, there is a problem.

A common therapist response is the rescue fantasy, a countertransference reaction in which you feel you personally can make the patient better. You feel you can help him become healthy and whole through a close relationship with you, and you feel that your interest and warmth will make the patient feel that life is worth living. Some patients feel so deprived, and are so pleased with the therapist's attention, that they treat us and make us feel like we are wonderful rescuers. Of course, this is too much of a good thing. There is a big difference between being a good therapist trying to help, and feeling that you are going to rescue the patient. In a healthy therapeutic relationship the patient is expected to take responsibility and do work on his own, and use you as well as others for help.

Frequently therapists react to sad and hopeless patients by feeling incompetent and like they are unable to do anything right. This often occurs in response to patients' transference reactions of anger and disappointment. Connected to this response, but a little different, is the countertransference feeling of being sucked dry. Here the therapist has tried to help, but empathy, support, suggestions, and interpretations all feel like they have not had much effect. The patient is still suffering and not much has changed. This is very frustrating and can lead to resentment and detachment on the part of the therapist. Of course, these are the therapist's feelings and not necessarily an accurate representation of reality. We discuss the therapist's strengths and capacities that will help you manage these experiences in Chapter 12.

Therapists conducting dynamic therapy must be aware of and monitor these countertransference reactions, connecting them to the patient's transference reactions. Your goal is to be able to distinguish—and help the patient distinguish—between what is current and realistic, and what is old and transferential.

Evidence Base

Increasingly, psychotherapy outcome studies of major depressive disorder have shown equivalent effectiveness for psychodynamic and cognitive therapy. Leichsenring (2001) published a meta-analysis comparing brief dynamic therapy to CBT and found almost no difference in outcome. In that meta-analysis, Leichsenring, like Crits-Christoph (1992), included interpersonal psychotherapy as a form of dynamic therapy. There is a controversy, which we will not try to resolve here, about whether interpersonal psychotherapy is a psychodynamic treatment. Interpersonal psychotherapy is similar because it focuses on repetitive scenarios involving loss and transition and uses empathy, exploration of painful affects, and occasionally transference. Of course, it is different in that it is highly focused and includes a major educational component. Without making a judgment about whether interpersonal psychotherapy should be included, both meta-analyses reported that their main results were not changed if interpersonal psychotherapy was excluded.

More recently, Leichsenring et al. (2004) identified 17 well-conducted studies of short-term psychodynamic psychotherapy published after 1970 and found that these short-term psychodynamic psychotherapies yielded large pretreatment–posttreatment effect sizes for target problems (1.39), general psychiatric symptoms (0.90), and social functioning (0.80). According to Leichsenring et al., the effect sizes of this treatment significantly exceeded those of waiting-list controls and treatments as usual. No differences were found between short-term psychodynamic psychotherapy and other forms of psychotherapy. The meta-analysis clearly shows that further research on dynamic psychotherapy in specific psychiatric disorders is needed.

Although meta-analyses are powerful because they allow us to review a large number of studies and average effect sizes across different studies, they also have the weakness in that they rely on the quality of the studies that they include. Meta-analyses by Leichensenring and Crits-Christoph included several types of psychodynamic therapies—interpersonal psychodynamic therapy (not interpersonal psychotherapy), time-limited psychodynamic (including supportive–expressive) therapy, and supportive dynamic therapy. All the studies involving a dynamic therapy comparison with some other treatment were included in at least one of the four meta-analyses examining the efficacy of time-limited dynamic therapy published since 1991 (Svartberg & Stiles, 1991; Crits-Christoph, 1992; Anderson & Lambert, 1995; Leichsenring et al., 2004). Overall, the very few studies examining the efficacy of dynamic therapy for depression indicate that dynamic therapy is no less effective than other established treatments (Hersen, Bellack, Himmelhoch, & Thase, 1984; McLean & Hakstian, 1979; Gallagher & Thomson, 1982; Thompson, Gallagher-Thompson, & Steinmetz Breckenridge, 1987). Nevertheless, the scarcity of studies using manualized modern forms of dynamic therapy (besides interpersonal psychotherapy) with reasonably experienced therapists examining depressed patients in a range of ages is notable, given its popularity.

In summary, depression is described here as a core psychodynamic problem that is frequently conceptualized using the ego psychology model. Old experiences of loss lead to anger and frustration that becomes internalized and leads to ill-fated attempts to restore self-esteem, which only lead to further disappointment. We have described typical goals for the psychodynamic treatment of depression, as well as expected resistances, transferences, countertransferences, and essential techniques. This discussion establishes the format for our discussion of the other five core psychodynamic problems.

OBSESSIONALITY: CONTROLLING FEELINGS

> BAILEY: I happen to have a human thing called
> an adrenaline.
>
> SPOCK: That sounds most inconvenient. Have
> you considered having it removed?
> —*Star Trek*

Ben, a well-dressed, successful attorney, spoke elegantly and at length about his frustrations with work. He polished his rimless glasses carefully several times each session. He acknowledged the absurdly long work hours he kept and spoke of the inevitable disappointments of his work, the ungrateful clients, demanding partners, and unsatisfactory support staff. With crisp sentences and well-formed paragraphs he maintained a pleasant and slightly abstracted expression on his face while describing incredible frustration. He complained about the burdens and obligations he felt, but then explained them away as understandable, reasonable, and a consequence of fate. I listened with a sense of detachment (he described everything as though it was happening to someone else). But at the same time, I felt strongly that his burdens were my burdens and I wanted to break free from it all.

Ben had trouble getting to the point. If I did not interrupt to ask a question, inquire about a feeling, or clarify, Ben would speak through much of the session without interruption. All the while, he maintained rapt attention to my face, as though scanning for reactions. He did not invite me to respond or ask questions.

Ben was involved in the expansion of his law firm and was in charge of delicate negotiations. But he had so much difficulty asking others to help with preparing and conducting the negotiations that he had made several potential crucial errors on staffing and financial commitments. He was scared and deeply disappointed with himself. On the personal side, his wife was pregnant with their first child after a long course of fertility interventions. The future baby

seemed like an obligation rather than a source of joy and excitement. This likeable but somewhat distant man came for treatment
because he felt anxious, depressed, and demoralized about his life
and the future.

Caricatured in the role of Mr. Spock, the Vulcan on *Star Trek*, the
patient with obsessions is preoccupied with rules, ideas, and procedures,
and is distant from feelings or emotion. It is not that such patients do not
have feelings—they do have very strong emotions. It is that they regard
the emotions as an "inconvenience," and a threat to well-being.

Shapiro's (1965) discussion of obsessionality begins by noting
Wilhelm Reich's apt description of an obsessional patient as a "living
machine." The style of thinking is rigid and hard to influence, and Shapiro observes that the patient is dominated by the feeling of having no
autonomy. He feels "I should" instead of "I want," and maintains an
iron discipline in hewing to the line in doing what "should" be done.
These patients experience a subjective sense of loss of autonomy because
they have difficulty making decisions. Shapiro claims that these patients
are indecisive because the emotions involved in decision making are not
given much free play. Finally, he notes that obsessional patients constantly doubt because they lack a deep personal sense of conviction and
instead follow their sense of what should be done (1965). Ben speaks of
responsibilities and requirements rather than emotions and needs. He is
in charge, yet he does not feel he has choices.

The core psychodynamic problem of obsessionality does not map
cleanly onto the DSM-IV system. DSM-IV distinguishes between two
forms of obsessionality. Obsessive–compulsive disorder is a genetically
loaded and self-perpetuating illness that involves irresistible repetitive,
intrusive thoughts or powerful urges to repeat irrational ritualistic behavior like cleaning or checking. Obsessive–compulsive personality disorder
is a lifelong disorder involving preoccupation with details, interpersonal
aloofness, interest in form over substance, and tight control over emotions and relationships. Both disorders can be characterized by similar
psychodynamic patterns, which we describe below.

Dynamic therapy is probably indicated only for obsessive–
compulsive personality disorder (Barber et al., 1997), the aloof, inhibited version of the problem, and for milder and subsyndromal forms of
obsessive–compulsive disorder, the highly ego-dystonic variant. It has
not been shown to help the full-blown syndrome of obsessive–compulsive
disorder. Hence, we use the term "obsessionality" for the core psychodynamic problem that is similar in both of these conditions, and which

is amenable to psychodynamic therapy. From a DSM-IV perspective, Ben has obsessive–compulsive personality disorder, with characteristic attention to rules and procedures, perfectionism that results in difficulty completing tasks, excessive devotion to work at the expense of leisure and personal relationships, inability to delegate, and rigidity.

Psychodynamic Conceptualization

The main theme in the psychoanalytic literature on obsessionality is the conflict over aggression and the use of specific defenses. The initial psychoanalytic interest in obsessionality focused on the concept of anality and the developmental issues of autonomy and control. Abraham (1923) described the anal triad—cleanliness, orderliness, and parsimony. Psychoanalytic writers connected these characteristic anal preoccupations with the way that obsessional neurotics seem to value order, ritual, and thought over emotion, and proposed that obsessionality had its origin in anal phase developmental problems (Freud, 1908). There are few data to support this notion.

Subsequent thinking, primarily from the ego psychology school of psychoanalysis, emphasized the obsessional patient's feeling that anger is bad; it is to be gotten rid of, controlled, and disarmed (A. Freud, 1966). This relieves the patient of guilt, leaving a feeling of goodness and cleanliness. The patient accomplishes this by using characteristic defenses, each of which operates unconsciously and results in the patient feeling less conflict, especially less anxiety about anger.

There are five characteristic defenses. *Intellectualization* is the focus on complex cognitive processes rather than gut feelings. *Isolation of affect* is the separation of thoughts from feelings. *Reaction formation* involves substituting a positive feeling for a negative one. *Displacement* means shifting the feelings and conflicts from one situation onto another that is unrelated, like road rage after a family argument. *Doing and undoing* refers, like it sounds, to the tendency to express something (verbally or through behavior) and then undo it by expressing the opposite. Making a humorous critical comment followed by the smiling aside, "Just kidding," is an example of this. Ben had many typical obsessional characteristics—his seamless exterior, careful control, interpersonal distance, disavowal of anger, and difficulty tolerating and expressing his feelings illustrate the core psychodynamic problem well.

Salzman (1968) extended the central formulation of obsessionality: conflict over aggression resulting in prominent guilt. He observed that patients with obsessional problems maintain, and feel a need to maintain, strict control over their emotions. They need to control others so that their own feelings do not get too stirred up. Ben was chronically angry about the burdens and obligations he lived with and had impulses to tell off his clients, partners, and family, but was so anxious and guilty about these angry thoughts that he had to manage them with the usual obsessional defenses. He needed to control himself lest he felt angry, guilty, and then anxious. He rarely let the therapist speak because he was so intent on keeping his conflicts under control. If the therapist spoke, Ben was afraid he would get too stirred up.

As society has become more complex, with technology and bureaucratic procedures involved in every facet of life—work, government, household management, and even leisure—the obsessional patient's qualities have more adaptive value. Our veneration of and ambivalence about coolness and rationality, sticking to procedures, and "machine-like" functioning are epitomized in the social role of the nerd. In popular culture, the nerd is glorified but also an object of ridicule.

Strengths

Although they possess much rational knowledge, obsessional patients seem to have less of the personality strengths of wisdom and knowledge (this requires judgment and conviction, seeing the forest for the trees) and instead show doubt or rigidity. Although they are very decent people, such patients do not strongly manifest humanity, as they tend not to have much access to their feelings of love, empathy, and altruism. The personality strength of transcendence, which calls for the ability to experience inchoate emotions like beauty, gratitude, hope, and humor, is difficult because it requires flexibility and irrationality, and the obsessional patient must maintain control. The goals of treatment, discussed below, involve a decrease in the degree of conflict, but also an attempt to help patients deepen their capacity for flexible thinking and deeper feeling.

Goals of Treatment

The treatment goals for obsessionality reflect the psychodynamic theories for understanding it. The chief aims are (1) helping the patient experience a wider range of emotions, (2) increasing tolerance and acceptance of negative and positive emotions, and (3) decreasing the degree of guilt that drives the defenses and the need for self-punishment.

For Ben, this meant exploring his anger, which turned out to be about early losses related to his father's distance and criticism, competition with many younger siblings, some oedipal frustrations vis-à-vis his mother, his father's untimely death, and the obligations placed on him by his family after his father's death. Ben had had a contentious although loving relationship with his father, and his sudden death and the requirement that he help to support the family unroofed his previously buried anger. Ben was very anxious about his anger, fearing it would be dangerous, and his personality style was an attempt to contain this. His angry and competitive fantasies about his father were only thoughts, but the interpretation was made that unconsciously he feared they had slipped out and resulted in his father's death.

The therapy helped Ben name these feelings, stick with them, and find a greater acceptance and tolerance for his emotions. Accepting his anger and frustration allowed him to examine these feelings, and this led to a decrease in guilt and less need for punishment. He let himself feel his sad feelings more, which allowed him to grieve and move on. Freeing up these painful negative emotions resulted in his feeling freer to experience positive feelings, and Ben was able to feel and act closer to his wife and child.

The heart of the problem in working with obsessional patients is their difficulty in tolerating and experiencing emotions, especially painful emotions. Anger is the most difficult emotion, and obsessional people worry about being destructive. This often leads them to feel out of control and worry about retaliation by others. The goal for obsessional patients is to help them experience more pleasure, spontaneity, emotion, and autonomy and decrease the burdensome sense of pressure, guilt, anger, and fear. This happens through experiencing and reexperiencing anger and loss in the treatment relationship without the feared consequences.

Developing a Therapeutic Alliance

Obsessional patients are so concerned that their feelings are bad that interpretations about using the defenses of intellectualization and isolation of affect can easily feel like criticism. Therefore the therapist needs to be sensitive to possible ruptures in the alliance and must confront obsessional individuals carefully. One of the ways to increase the alliance is by encouraging patients to conceptualize their problem. This helps to give them a sense of control and mastery as they proceed and promotes the alliance as long as the therapist does not get seduced into too much theoretical back and forth. Some intellectualization can help to promote the therapeutic alliance.

Interpretations (in general, not just with obsessional patients) should start with empathy, move on to observations about the patterns, and conclude again with empathy. An example of this would be: "You feel so much responsibility it is crushing for you. I think that maybe you are also feeling angry about how much responsibility you have, but you feel very guilty and afraid of the angry feeling. This guilt is so powerful, and you are so afraid of what you might do if you really got angry, that you need to make sure you control this, and so you are good and responsible and nice."

Technique

All psychotherapy patients may benefit from psychoeducation, an explanation of the treatment and how it will help with the problem. Obsessional patients are particularly interested in this preparation for therapy because of their love of rules, procedures, and ideas. A good, simple explanation of what psychotherapy is, how it is done, and how change occurs is in order. The patient's main responsibilities—to talk about what is going on in his mind and what he is feeling—are emphasized as a simple prescriptive.

You must look for affects and elicit them carefully with obsessional patients. You cannot simply listen, support, and vaguely evoke feelings. Directly inquire, observe body posture, and explore the subjective experience of each type of feeling and each experience. In other words, you need to help the patient recognize the affect that is being avoided, for example, "When you came home to an empty house last night, what did it feel like?" or "When she said that, what was that like for you?" You may point out common reactions to situations the patient is in and ask the patient whether he is having those reactions. You might need to keep the questions open-ended but not give up on getting an answer when the patient demurs. You may need to return to important questions.

Later on you can focus more on the anger and ask what it feels like, for example, "What are you afraid of when you are feeling his way?" Emotional experiences must be clarified and named. Mirroring, empathizing, and active expressions of acceptance of feelings are helpful, as obsessional patients have strict superegos, with harsh self-criticism and shame. Remember, these patients are focused on what they *should* feel, trying to avoid the upset of what they *do* feel.

More than any of the other psychodynamic problems, treating obsessionality requires persistence and an active stance. Patients may debate a course of action over weeks. Action should be encouraged, and then later the results can be examined and dissected. The obsessional patient's tendency to ruminate rather than act needs to be met with a firm guiding hand, encouraging practice, trying new behaviors, experimenting. Of course, there is a danger of enacting a control battle in the name of good therapeutic intentions, and therapists should try to find a way to guide and encourage with a light touch, avoiding a potential counterproductive control struggle. Even when guiding and directing, the emphasis is always on the emerging affects.

Harold, a likeable, polite, and kind man in his 40s used to leave the house to go running several evenings per week just around the time that his young children needed to go to bed. It was a typically chaotic moment in the house, and his wife was frazzled and the kids were demanding. Harold felt angry at his wife for her insistence on help from him and her frequent criticism of him. He revealed his habit of escaping into a run with some embarrassment, but discussed it as though he simply needed to leave because it was so loud in the house.

It was clear to me that Harold could not stand the conflict and emotionality of the household at that time of day. Everyone was tired, worn down, and vulnerable to erupt. So was he. When probed gently for what he felt, Harold insisted that he just wanted to be somewhere quiet and by himself. He did not know why. As he spoke about this again, I detected a moment when he seemed annoyed with his wife, and I asked him more about that. After a few questions along these lines, he finally acknowledged that he did not like the way she treated him when they were getting the children ready for bed, and he wanted to get away. But he was not sure why he needed to leave and appeared more ashamed of this than before.

Several weeks later the same topic came up, and we got a little further. Harold was talking about his wife and her strong personality, and how this was tiring at times, and irritating. He was able to express, with much empathizing and support from me, that he got angry at her often, and did not know what to do. He felt guilty because she is a good person, and a good wife and mother. I connected this with his nightly escapes and wondered whether he left because he was angry with her and did not like the feeling. Perhaps it scared him? This time, he was aware of feeling angry and having the urge to escape. But it was followed quickly by feeling embarrassed. I commented that he seemed ashamed, which was understandable when looking at it from a contemporary adult perspective, but that maybe there were some deeper emotions and fears that were not so rational.

Slowly, and in fits and starts, Harold began to see his pervasive pattern of anger and his fear that the anger would go to generate terrible conflict. This was triggered especially when he felt a sense of rejection or loss. He was afraid that others (his wife, colleagues at work, children) would get angry with him and reject him. There often seemed to be a greater intellectual awareness of this pattern than an emotional familiarity, and we returned to it over and over again.

It was hard at times because we seemed to go over the same ground repeatedly, but usually I was aware that it did not feel like the same ground to him. Each time was a little more revelation, with a little more emotion. The dilemma was to keep it fresh and not sink into intellectual repetition, and to keep the focus on the emotions he was experiencing—naming them, helping him to see the pattern, empathizing with his struggle, and encouraging new solutions to the emotional conflict.

Transference and Countertransference

Typical transference reactions for obsessional patients include the need to control the therapy and the therapist. This is usually a desperate attempt to manage the possible emergence of bad and dangerous feelings. It accounts for the sometimes dry and distant feeling of the sessions with these patients, who may struggle for control to preserve their freedom and autonomy, and thus may frequently regard you as controlling. They will rebel or avoid you as though you were an implacable force set on stamping out their autonomy. They may test you and your tendency to want them to be a certain way or make certain decisions. There may be overt feelings or indirect expressions of anger and hostility. This type of transference reaction may be more evident in patients who are less compensated and adapted to their obsessional conflict, or as the treatment progresses and the patient becomes more able to tolerate his anger.

Common countertransference reactions are frustration and the feeling that the patient is deflecting and not engaging with the therapist. In the example of Harold, it required patience to stay with the slower pace of understanding and analyzing the troublesome repeated scenario. The therapist could feel angry and have the urge to push through the patient's carefully constructed defenses, or could feel boredom and distance. Sometimes the game of cat and mouse feels futile and pointless.

One may also find oneself responding to the patient's underlying anger, which is repressed or suppressed so carefully.

Evidence Base

Barber et al. (1997) studied the efficacy of moderate-length (52 sessions) supportive–expressive therapy (Luborsky, 1984; Barber & Crits-Christoph, 1995) in patients with avoidant or obsessive–compulsive personality disorders. By the end of treatment, 39% of the avoidant personality disorder patients still met diagnostic criteria for their disorder, while only 15% of obsessive–compulsive personality disorders retained their diagnosis at the end of treatment. These data, although tentative, suggest that supportive–expressive therapy was quite effective at helping patients with a diagnosis of obsessive–compulsive personality disorder. Other studies have looked at patients with personality disorders treated with dynamic therapy, but most of them did not break out their results for obsessive–compulsive personality disorder.

SUMMARY

A clear definition of the six core psychodynamic problems allows the clinician to rapidly recognize typical patterns, bring to bear useful psychodynamic conceptualizations, anticipate challenges in building the therapeutic alliance, employ effective problem-specific therapy techniques, and be aware of likely transference and countertransference reactions. The first two psychodynamic problems, depression and obsessionality, were discussed in this chapter, and the remaining four are the subject of Chapter 6.

Core Psychodynamic Problems, Part II

You will find yourself running through the six core problems in your mind as you interview patients, trying to decide which one fits best. If the patient seems to have more than one problem, which problem seems to capture the patient's current experience and includes the data you have gathered? Which problem would the patient find most useful to work on initially? In this chapter we review the remaining four problems: fear of abandonment, low self-esteem, panic anxiety, and trauma.

FEAR OF ABANDONMENT

> We long for an affection altogether ignorant of our faults. Heaven has accorded this to us in the uncritical canine attachment.
> —GEORGE ELIOT

Unfortunately, the completely secure and uncritical attachment Eliot speaks of does not come through our relationships with other humans. Of course, some people are much more sensitive to loss and abandonment than others. Fear of abandonment as a psychodynamic problem shows itself in insecure attachment to others, with a persisting feeling of vulnerability to separation and abandonment. Patients with fear of abandonment use desperate strategies to stay connected with others; they try to tolerate painful feelings of loss and loneliness. If you constantly feel alone and are scared of losing what little you have, you may appear chaotic and unstable to others because of the strategies you employ to stay secure.

There is a spectrum of fear of abandonment, ranging from very symptomatic and dysfunctional to reasonably functional with uncomfortable inner experiences. Kernberg's (1975) and Gunderson's (2000) studies of borderline personality disorder describe typical characteristics of patients with severe attachment problems: intense feelings of abandonment, chronic anger, multiple physical and psychiatric symptoms, alternating good and bad internal representations of self and others, absence of good sublimations (engaging and successful activities), frequent feelings of emptiness, impulsivity, use of the characteristic defenses of splitting and projective identification, and a tendency to briefly lose touch with reality in intense interpersonal situations. Other patients have significant problems with separation and abandonment, which manifests in relationship instability with dependency and anxiety. These more functional patients have fear of abandonment, but they struggle with less intense loneliness and emptiness. Their use of splitting is less severe and less pervasive, they are less prone to projective identification, and they are more able to use higher level defenses like sublimation and humor.

Psychodynamic Conceptualization

The traditional psychodynamic and psychoanalytic literature discusses abandonment fears in terms of the diagnosis of borderline personality disorder. The term "borderline" itself has a pejorative connotation in the mental health arena. It came about innocently, used to describe people who seemed, from the perspective of 1950s psychoanalysis, to be on the borderline of psychosis. But the word contributes to stigma, alienation, and objectification that is painful and destructive for patients and brings out less attractive responses in therapists as well. There is not a better formal diagnostic term used in the literature for patients with serious abandonment reactions, but the attachment paradigm developed by John Bowlby (1958) provides a broader context for understanding this problem and a useful construct for understanding and treating patients.

Perhaps more than anyone in the 20th-century psychoanalytic movement, John Bowlby (1958) established a connection between theory and observable behavior. He took an ethological—that is to say, he observed behavior—approach to understanding the problem of attachment, and the simplicity of his framework provides a remarkably useful, experience-near account of abandonment and its vicissitudes. Bowlby observed toddlers in the process of separating from and returning to their mothers. He studied this process in detail, observing their behavior and emotional expression, and described four types of attachment: (1) *secure attachment*, in which the toddler is able to leave the mother and feel good alone and upon reunion with the mother; (2) *anxious attachment*, where the toddler responds to separation with apparent anxiety and clinging when the mother returns; and (3) *avoidant attachment*, when the child stays away from the mother upon reunion, as though fearful of feeling connected and then abandoned again. He later added the notion of (4) *disorganized attachment*, which occurs in those who manifest chaotic and poorly organized responses to separation.

Bowlby observed the relationship between children and their caregivers and focused on the nature of the attachment, its security, and the child's responses to its disruption. Subsequent psychoanalytic literature on attachment had more of an intrapsychic focus. The traditional psychoanalytic perspective on the genesis of borderline personality disorder came from the work of Margaret Mahler (1972), who described a critical period of development in the attachment of the toddler and mother (caretaker). Following the normal symbiotic exclusive relationship between mother and baby comes a period of separation, individuation, and rapprochement (the normal alternation between closeness and separation), which ideally results in a secure sense of self and confidence in the presence of the mother. Mahler's theory located the source of the difficulty for borderline patients in the rapprochement phase, concluding that they were not able to successfully try out independence, reconnect and refuel with the mother, and then separate again. Her theory was not based on longitudinal developmental data, but rather on the similarity between observations of this childhood phase and patterns that theorists infer in the minds of patients with fear of abandonment.

Otto Kernberg's (1975) dense and brilliant writings attempt to systematically combine these descriptive characteristics and the language of object relations to describe the inner world of borderline patients. Kernberg was highly influential in his emphasis on the aggression and rage these patients experience. He posited a constitutional excess of aggression that was intensified and accelerated during the rigors of the separation process. This is a controversial proposition, and some would suggest that Kernberg's emphasis on aggression is excessive. Kernberg's recommendation to confront the rage directly, especially in the transference, is one of the hallmarks of his treatment approach. Most recently, his work has evolved into a manualized treatment for these patients, transference-focused psychotherapy (Kernberg et al., 1989; Clarkin, Yeomans, & Kernberg, 1999).

Sarah was a scared social work student who tended to get overly attached to potential boyfriends, and whose mood fluctuated with each phone call, casual meeting, or date. A small woman with blond curly hair and a pixie-ish demeanor, she was very smart and successful at her academic work. She felt desperately alone in the middle of a busy academic program with many like-minded peers. She had an intact family that included her father, mother, and a younger brother. But no one seemed trustworthy, and unless they pledged endless loyalty, she mistrusted and constantly tested those she hoped to count on. Her mistrust led her to use poor judgment. When she dated another student, she "Googled" him and his family members, and then sent him an e-mail using someone else's address to ask whether he was dating anyone.

Sarah's obsession with relationships showed itself in the therapy as well; she strolled by my office when she did not have an appointment, looking to see who was in the waiting room. She saw the office door open, and looked in, staring intently. It was a chilling experience—as though she was intensely connected way beyond what seemed to be the reality of our relationship after 10 weeks of treatment, and I felt anxious, guilty, and a little violated. She found my home address in a directory and mentioned it one day when she was feeling particularly upset.

Her fear of abandonment was so clear. She made occasional suicidal threats, frequent veiled references to desperation, and developed an insistent focus on me. She needed to be and stay intensely connected to me. Nothing mattered as much as the feeling of being loved; it was not an erotic, sexual love, but rather a parent–child, caretaking, enveloping love that she seemed to want so badly. Everything that happened with me, or with her friends and family, meant either that she was loved and cared for, or it confirmed her feeling of loss and abandonment. She had to lasso others into a safe and unbreakable bond.

The chaos that may surround abandonment-sensitive patients results from their chief technique for dealing with their overwhelming insecurity—they try to control relationships and feelings, both in the external world and inside themselves. They prevent the experience of abandonment by keeping others bound to them. Sarah's attempts (often so unsuccessful) to achieve security with boyfriends, and her therapist, were the external manifestation of this painful endeavor. She demanded so much of others that they often rejected her and kept their distance.

Inside, Sarah experienced the split sense of self so characteristic of this problem, and did everything she could to keep current the positive valued self-image (Kernberg, 1975). In childhood, Sarah developed two distinct images of herself and of those around her. Her good self was the loving, helpful, interested, competent, lovable self she both was and wanted to be entirely, but alongside of this, there was a dark side. She was angry, frustrated, destructive, and convinced of her unlovability. This was especially painful because it made her feel that all of her misery was her own fault; maybe her loneliness was because she was so unlikable and bad. This duality extended to her view of others. People were loving, maternal, nurturing, rescuing, and ideal, or disappointing, inconstant, selfish, rejecting, and unavailable. Ambivalence is a ubiquitous experience, and involves feeling both good and bad, while splitting is different because the patient feels either good or bad.

Splitting causes confusion and dismay in those around a patient with fear of abandonment, but it also helps the patient maintain a beacon of love and hope inside. It allows for a positive sense of self and a positive feeling about others, untainted by anger and hatred. Splitting maintains that sense of goodness and allows for something inside that the patient can count on. But, of course, this defensive operation causes a tremendous amount of collateral damage.

Many of the other core features of attachment problems follow from this understanding. Sarah had difficulty finding activities to invest in (although she had her academics) because they seemed unimportant compared with her emotional need for attachment. She was impulsive about expressing her positive and negative feelings in relationships, depending on what was most prominent at the moment. Sometimes she felt empty, sensing that there was nothing inside her that was stable and truly *her*; she was just the sum of her fears and insecurities. Her occasional loss of reality-testing occurred when she was in the thrall of her negative and bad views of others. She could only see the other person as a bad object, and not a fully developed person with good and not-so-good qualities.

Many abandonment-sensitive patients have less severe symptomatology; they use more developed and mature defenses and may not significantly employ splitting. Bowlby's concepts of clinging attachment and avoidant attachment are helpful explanations. These patients tend to manifest their abandonment fears more directly in their significant relationships and experience insecurity and fearfulness about any perturbation or change in those they rely on. This milder version of fear of abandonment appears as a proneness to dependency. Some people have overt clinging type behavior in relationships, while others hold themselves apart or reject others before they are rejected, to manage their experience of abandonment.

Strengths

What positive character strengths are challenged and compromised in the face of these chronic fears of loss and abandonment? Humanity—the ability to feel love, altruism, and empathy—is weakened because both sides of the split representations of self and others are inaccurate and wrong. The patient is neither as good nor as bad as the self-representations portray, and others are neither so lovable nor as evil as they seem. A strong sense of humanity requires the ability to manage and experience ambivalence. Justice, which includes citizenship, fairness, and leadership, is compromised as well. When one is fighting for one's life, it is easy to lose sight of others and their needs. Because the urge for secure attachment is paramount, and justice essentially requires an ability to step outside oneself and see oneself in a larger context, this is particularly difficult.

Much of the traditional psychoanalytic literature on fear of abandonment emphasizes the patient's anger and pathological defenses, and deals extensively with the countertransference dilemmas stirred up by splitting. Identifying strengths and supporting them are essential tasks for the therapist of patients with fear of abandonment, and we discuss the importance of coaching more fully in the section on treatment.

Treatment Goals

The treatment goals for fear of abandonment include a more stable and integrated (good and bad) image of self and other, decreased emotional reactivity, and more stable relationships (see Gunderson, 2000). The therapeutic challenge is to help these patients contain their destructive emotions, develop an increased ability to be effective and active in the world outside treatment, and increase their ability to reflect and "mentalize" (Bateman & Fonagy, 2008) or understand needs and feelings. The goal is to help Sarah feel she is loveable, neither perfect nor awful. She should be able to count on loyalty from others, but accept that they have their own needs and cannot always do what she wants. For those patients with more mild abandonment issues, the goal is a more secure attachment in Bowlby's sense, and an ability to weather the inevitable sense of threat they feel in close relationships.

Building a Therapeutic Alliance

What distinguishes the patient whose core problem is fear of abandonment from patients with other core problems that also involve experiences of abandonment such depression, panic, and trauma? The centrality of loss in the patient's current experience, and the use of defenses to manage it, are the main features of this problem. Not surprisingly, these defensive strategies for dealing with abandonment are rapidly enacted in the relationship with the therapist.

The therapeutic alliance is built under the sway of the patient's intense need to connect, and his or her fear of separation and loss. Confidence in the therapist can go from zero to 60 miles per hour in a single session, with the patient concluding that the therapist is the best ever, with absolute confidence that the relationship will be sustaining and productive. Or the therapist is seen as cold, rigid, and uncaring because of the seemingly short duration of the session, or the fee, or something in the interaction. The relationship may begin one way and change by the next session, and then change back. Therefore calmness, patience, and unflappability on the part of the therapist are a must.

A strong alliance is more likely to develop through repeated experiences of containment and coaching. Understanding the patient's vulnerability to abandonment and proneness to split will give you some detachment as well as fortitude when it inevitably occurs. The goal is for the patient to be aware of both sides of the split, because this makes the self-experience more stable, perceptions of others more accurate, and it leads to better adaptation to the stresses of relationships. This will take quite a while, but early empathy for the difficulty of extreme mood and perceptual oscillations, frequent educational remarks about how this is a consequence of feeling abandoned, and understanding for how it helps to protect but also causes new problems will help to build the alliance.

Technique

Gunderson's (2000) description of the stages of treatment of borderline personality disorder is clear and practical, and the stages are appropriate for the broader group of patients with fear of abandonment. The initial phase is devoted to developing the treatment contract; fleshing out this understanding usually involves some testing of the therapist. Next is the phase of relational development, which means the patient and therapist begin to engage on a deeper, more emotional level. Transferences and countertransferences are noted but are not the focus of treatment. The phase of positive dependency is next; here the patient begins to use his other relationships to try out new self-perceptions and perceptions of others. He practices the ability to be connected and close to someone else, vulnerable to hurt and loss, but able to avoid using splitting to the same previous pathological degree. The last phase is called the working alliance. This term is used somewhat differently from our usual discussions of the therapeutic alliance. Gunderson refers to it as a hard-won achievement and a state of the treatment relationship in which the patient can begin to do traditional psychodynamic work—insight-oriented attention to the past, present, and transference, with the use of interpretations, as opposed to the degree of coaching and support that has been present up until now.

Gunderson suggests that it takes almost 6 years to be able work through these stages in the typical treatment of borderline patients. This time frame seems reasonable for patients with more severe fear of abandonment, but many with less serious attachment problems achieve important gains in much shorter periods of time. Often those patients with more severe fear of abandonment move from one therapist to another, and different parts of the work may be accomplished with different therapists. Although some time-limited treatments for borderline personality disorder, like dialectical behavior therapy (Linehan, 1993) and transference-focused psychotherapy (e.g., Kernberg et al., 1989), describe much shorter time duration, we could not find controlled data to support the notion that there is a meaningful reduction in the fear of abandonment during the 1 or 2 years of treatment they provide. Gunderson's stages are still relevant for patients with less severe abandonment fears, but the time frame is shorter, especially for the earlier stages.

For the abandonment-sensitive patient, verbalizing feelings of loss and anger is important. But putting these deep feelings into words is only the beginning, and sometimes it makes the patient feel worse. Encouraging behaviors that help the patient self-soothe may be necessary— exercise, rituals, meditation, religious observance, music, or television. The notion of containment refers to helping patients tolerate extreme negative affects, such as rage or despair, without resorting to parasuicidal or suicidal behavior. Dialectical behavior therapy is particularly useful for these patients with persisting acute symptomatology.

In the earlier phases of treatment of fear of abandonment, coaching and support are essential. With Sarah, this meant pointing out her social awareness and good judgment when she was not upset. It also meant emphasizing her considerable academic talents and encouraging her persistence and ambition. Coaching is different from support because it means discussing very specific problems the patient is facing, and encouraging their solution through the application of strengths. Coaching helps create success experiences for the patient that will promote growth. For example, after Sarah e-mailed her date under an alias, the therapist encouraged her to think about whether this approach was likely to help her feel good about herself (although it would reassure her about her fears). The discussion was about what behaviors could help her feel strong, confident, and how she could improve her ability to assess a date's interest.

For patients who struggle with intense and overwhelming feelings, it is important to have a treatment contract that spells out what behavior is acceptable in session, the limits for behavior outside sessions, and the patient's responsibility for potentially self-injurious behavior. There also must be a clear plan for the therapist's role in crisis stabilization and management of self-injurious behavior. A typical contract is discussed and negotiated with the patient early on. It takes the form of the therapist offering to work closely with the patient if the patient is able to follow the terms of the contract, and an understanding of the contingencies if the patient is not. This might mean transfer to another therapist, fewer sessions, hospitalization, and so forth. Kernberg and his colleagues' discussions of the treatment contract (Selzer, Koenigsberg, & Kernberg, 1987) and Gunderson's (2000) description of working with borderline patients in the earlier phases of treatment may be helpful. Linehan's dialectical behavior therapy (1993) involves the extensive use of patient self-soothing skills, which is a very valuable tool for patients with more severe fear of abandonment.

Because one of the goals is to increase the patient's strengths, it is important not to facilitate a regressive dependent relationship in which the patient develops excessive reliance on the therapist and calls too frequently outside of appointments. Flexibility, availability, and responsiveness are necessary because the core problem is, after all, fear of abandonment. Reasonable limits are helpful because they encourage the patient to contain emotions and at times actually try to repress them.

Sarah continued in psychotherapy for almost 2 years. The first year or so included frequent testing of the strength and the limits of the therapeutic relationship. She called the emergency number one night after an apparent breakup with her boyfriend, sobbing and overwhelmed, after having taken a few pills from his medicine cabinet.

She felt bereft, alone, scared, and desperate, and she took pills to get away from these overwhelming feelings. She also seemed to want to be taken care of. A few months later, after my 2-week vacation, she did not show up for two appointments and needed two phone calls to convince her to return. She was detached and angry and decided to cut off the relationship with me because I was so cold and uncaring. During this brief hiatus in treatment, Sarah hooked up with a male student whom she would subsequently have to see regularly in her classes.

I met her impulsive behavior with empathy for her sense of loss and abandonment. I suggested that she was trying to detach from me to handle her anger and hurt and encouraged her to consider more adaptive ways of managing these powerful feelings. I offered regular guidance and coaching (much more than with a less chaotic patient) about her academic work, dealing with a professor she had conflict with, whether she should continue the relationship with the fellow student, and about a problem with her apartment that caused her to argue with her landlord. Each of these discussions included some observations about her emotional vulnerability to loss and her tendency to manage her emotionality in a dysfunctional fashion. But I pointed out her healthier wishes and the strengths she was using and encouraged her in her healthy assertiveness.

We suspect that the mechanism of therapeutic change in patients with fear of abandonment relies more heavily than the other psychodynamic problems on the new experiences inside and outside the therapeutic relationship. The accumulation of positive life experiences—of safety and security in relationships, effective function in work and life, or the ability to manage stormy emotions—provides the patient a more balanced experience of himself and the world.

Transference and Countertransference

Patients with fear of abandonment often see the therapist as all-good, helpful, and the longed-for loved parental figure, or as selfish, evil, dishonest, and frightening. These alternative and alternating reactions reflect internal splitting. Patients on the less severe end of the abandonment spectrum tend to feel powerful dependency. Countertransference reactions are profound and are more often the cause of the demise of psychotherapy than the patient's transference reactions or the acting out. The aphorism, "If you don't make it worse, it will get better," captures the therapist's task well.

The therapist can use several techniques to cope with these emotional patients. Focus some of your attention to the patient's positive qualities and the positive feelings about the patient that you naturally have, and give frequent voice to these feelings. Stay aware of the extent and depth of the patient's struggles, remembering that behind every difficult behavior is pain and fear of abandonment, and any aggressiveness or manipulativeness is an attempt to stave off these painful feelings. Find ways to step back from the experience of being rejected or criticized by the patient. As painful and immediate as it is to be criticized, this is a reflection of the patient's anger and it is not about you. Be respectful of how resourceful these patients can be.

It is the therapist's job to manage the powerful countertransference reactions, chiefly the feelings of helplessness, of being abused, or anger and hostility, and of careless detachment. It is easy to see how these feelings are stirred up in the therapist by the patient's struggle with powerful alternating split-off experiences of merger and abandonment. It is not easy to keep a healthy distance and not act out oneself. There is a tradition of blaming these patients for their interpersonal difficulties, and it is surprising how frequently trainees and faculty make derogatory jokes about these difficult patients, creating distance and blaming the victim. Vaillant (1992) notes that the term borderline personality disorder is used as an epithet and often reflects unrecognized countertransference.

Evidence Base

There is some recent evidence to support the use of dynamic techniques for patients with fear of abandonment. Transference-focused therapy (Clarkin et al., 1999), a manualized therapy developed by Kernberg and colleagues for borderline patients, focuses intensively on the transference. This treatment emphasizes recognition and interpretation of the transference and promotes reflective functioning and narrative coherence (Levy et al., 2006). Some data suggest that the extent of attention to the transference is correlated with the degree of positive change in patients' experience of relationships (Gabbard et al., 1994; Høglend et al., 2006, 2008). Furthermore, Crits-Christoph, Cooper, and Luborsky (1988) showed that accurate interpretation of the patient's core conflict was associated with good outcome. Mentalization-based therapy (Bateman & Fonagy, 2008) relies on the notion that highly abandonment-vulnerable patients lack the capacity for mentalization, that is, the ability to self-reflect and conceptualize their own mental states.

LOW SELF-ESTEEM

Trust yourself, then you will know how to live.
—JOHANN WOLFGANG VON GOETHE

Stan was a remarkably talented and very likeable pharmaceutical company executive who came for treatment shortly before his 45th birthday, depressed and ruminative. He had a fleeting broad smile that lit up the room when he spoke of some of his past accomplishments, but he was generally dejected. His clothes were rumpled and his shirttail was out.

Stan had been summarily rejected by a younger woman with whom he was having an affair. She broke off the relationship, concluding that he wanted more from her than she wanted to give. Stan felt she also did not need him any longer, as she had already gained access to his valuable business contacts. Stan was disenchanted with his long-suffering wife, and he was despondent that a long hoped-for promotion had not materialized.

Stan was brilliant and was an accomplished pianist and tennis player, yet he alternated between recognizing and reveling in his accomplishments, and experiencing a terrible feeling of aloneness, smallness, and loss. He was either elated and excited about the future, or hopeless and negative. His ambition was "the sky is the limit," and he believed he could do and be whatever he wanted. Yet he was terribly envious and competitive and paid a lot of attention to others' money, status, and opinions of him.

Stan came for treatment because he felt depressed and demoralized. In advance of the first appointment, he asked if he could forward a series of e-mails from the girlfriend so that I could see what had happened. I agreed, thinking this might help in developing the therapeutic alliance. In the initial meeting, he asked for help because he felt so bad and wanted assistance in figuring out what was really going on with the girlfriend and why she had broken up with him. He was confused, stunned, broken, and beaten. I empathized with his pain and rejection and commented that the girlfriend seemed rather manipulative.

The beloved only child of upwardly striving working-class parents, Stan felt that his mother had focused all her hopes on him. His father had worked hard as a subway operator and was out of the house for very long hours. Sadly, he developed lung cancer and died when Stan was 16 years old. He felt his mother was overly dependent on him; when he was a child she needed strength and emotional support, and when he was an adult, she frequently asked him for money.

Stan's focus in the therapy was mostly on himself, how he felt, and what would help him to feel better, more successful, and more secure. Despite his descriptions of success and talent (and he really was talented), it quickly became clear that inside he felt helpless in a world in which others took advantage of him.

He despaired about the end of his affair, and the break-up made him feel unattractive and unlovable. He missed the relationship and the feeling of closeness, but the acute pain was about how badly he felt about himself. He fantasized about being back with the girlfriend, and this made him feel healthy, strong, and appealing.

Psychodynamic Conceptualization

Freud was very interested in those who struggle with low self-esteem and noted that their problems caused them to tend to focus on themselves. Characteristically, Freud (1914) looked to development to understand the roots of this problem. His formulation was that infants and very young children are normally focused entirely on themselves. This state of "primary narcissism" involves intense impulses for food, holding, warmth, and bodily relief; the needs are all-consuming and the infant cries out and waits for satisfaction. Maturation and development lead to the awareness of others and their needs, and compromises must be made between impulses and the needs and the constraints of the environment. Thus "secondary narcissism" occurs when there is a developmental interruption—a crisis in which there is too much loss or too much anxiety—and a return to this earlier narcissistic state. A sick person who cannot focus on anything but his aches, pains, and bodily ills, or a grieving person who withdraws from the outside world thinking only of the terrible loss are examples of Freud's concept of secondary narcissism.

When this self-focus is persistent it insulates the individual from feelings about others. There is an avoidance of the painful feelings of rejection that inevitably come from involvement in close relationships or meaningful work. The core psychodynamic problem of low self-esteem involves an inner experience of insecurity and loneliness that is managed through self-preoccupation and self-oriented gratification. In our work, we do not use the term narcissism because that refers to the compensatory strategy these patients use, rather than the problem itself, and it tends to make patients feel criticized and ashamed, rather than understood and supported.

Kernberg (1975) distinguished between those who are narcissistic and borderline by calling attention to the grandiose, entitled, excited, and ambitious attitudes that narcissistic patients have. Different from the borderline good and bad self, the narcissist has a hugely exciting and magnificent self, and a sad, small, depleted, shameful self. Kernberg posited severe frustration in early parenting as a cause, and noted that narcissism often helps people become successful in the earlier part of their lives, but becomes a problem in midlife. High self-regard, competition, and a drive to master can lead to early success, but in midlife, satisfaction, love, and close relationships become more valuable than fame, wealth, and competition. Gore Vidal quipped that "a narcissist is someone better looking than you are," calling attention to the intense feelings of envy that are also part of the picture. Others seem to the have the love, beauty, strength, wealth, or position that those with low self-esteem covet.

Kohut (1971, 1977, 1984) changed the field of psychoanalysis with his sensitive awareness that many patients, including those Freud would have described as being in a state of secondary narcissism, are so filled with shame, inferiority, embarrassment, and low self-esteem that virtually everything they think, feel, do, and say is directed at trying to feel better about themselves. He acknowledged Freud's description of entitlement and megalomania, but his contribution was to explore and articulate its painful underbelly. Entitlement is a reaction to feelings of powerlessness, loneliness, and fear.

Kohut defined a normal part of parenting as providing a "selfobject" for growing children. This merger of child and caretaker, with optimal empathy, validation, and protection of the budding self in the child, is necessary for the development of healthy self-esteem. Neither too protected nor too exposed to frustration and hardship, the child who is part of a selfobject develops self-love, vitality, creativity, and assertiveness, as well as healthy love and empathy with others. In his later work, Kohut went on to suggest that narcissism had its own distinct developmental progression, which was necessary alongside of other developmental achievements like cognition, psychosexual, and physical.

Kohut's emphasis on anger and entitlement as secondary to hurt differed deeply from Kernberg's view. Kohut and the self psychologists see these classic narcissistic symptoms as a reaction to the environment, perhaps the unhealthy environment, rather than an irreducible drive. Kohut used the term "vertical split" to refer to sectors of the personality dominated by differing self-images, both grandiose and inferior.

From Kernberg's perspective, Stan is an angry, frustrated man whose splitting and grandiosity help to maintain the sense of a loving self and a loving object in a world of anger. Kohut's Stan is a sad, scared, lonely, and vulnerable man whose elation and entitlement is a last-ditch effort at security, and who only gets angry when he feels deeply rejected. In our work with low self-esteem we emphasize the Kohutian view, as it rests more squarely on the substantial empirical evidence for the importance of the therapeutic alliance in treatment outcome.

Strengths

Stan's innate strengths were compromised by his problems; excessive focus on the self made it difficult for him to love, and his social intelligence had blinders at times because of his concern about being manipulated and taken advantage of. Stan's exquisite sensitivity to humiliation and shame rendered temperance and the strengths of forgiveness, humility, prudence and self-regulation in short supply. Humility is confused with inferiority, and prudence hardens to defensive manipulation in a dangerous and uncertain world. Self-regulation is difficult when you are starved.

Treatment Goals

The treatment goals for those with low self-esteem are a more accurate and positive self-image and a greater ability to tolerate vulnerability in relationships. Helping Stan to reconcile his disparate views of himself and understand how they came about, along with helping him build new, healthier relationship experiences, will decrease the painful, shameful inferiority as well the counterproductive grandiosity. He will be able to approach the second half of life and its challenges with a greater opportunity to have support from family and friends.

Patients who feel insecure, ashamed, defective, or unlovable tend to be skeptical about treatment. Initially, the positive regard for the therapist, or the fantasy of magical transformation, is sustaining. But soon enough, the old feelings return and the patient usually feels that talking about feeling bad just does not help. The therapeutic relationship is fundamental to bringing about change here, perhaps even more than with the other psychodynamic problems. The patient must feel known, admired, and supported. The narrative, although important, is in some ways less complicated, more conscious, and less powerfully mutative than for other problems.

Building a Therapeutic Alliance

Self psychology regards anger as the result of frustration and the failure of empathy in childhood and adult relationships. In Stan's treatment, the therapist met his anger at his girlfriend and wife (and, occasionally, at the therapist) with empathy and an attempt to restore the empathic bond. Indeed, the development and maintenance of the therapeutic relationship seems central to the psychodynamic treatment of this problem, because it restores the selfobject function for someone who has lost it.

The essential technique is to support and empathize, watching for and dealing actively with the patient's inevitable disappointment, hurt, and anger in the therapeutic relationship. There is an extensive literature on ruptures in the therapeutic alliance (e.g., Muran & Safran, 2002), concluding that this is a ubiquitous phenomenon in psychotherapy, but it may be most problematic in patients with fragile self-esteem. If you feel insecure, you will be especially sensitive to criticism and rejection by your therapist. Ruptures and their recognition are seen as essential to maintenance of the alliance. Each rupture, the precipitants, the feelings stirred up, and the repair, are like a "teachable moment," where another building block of security and self-esteem are added.

Stan successfully negotiated a business deal that involved making a contact, Al, who subsequently offered him a very lucrative position in his company. Stan reported on the contract negotiations in some detail. Al was friendly and seemingly generous, but as the dialogue proceeded, Stan felt that Al was not giving enough and did not recognize his potential contribution to the new company. Al began to seem disrespectful and devaluing. It was not overt, but Stan sensed it, and felt a tone was being set for the future. He became quite angry. In several sessions he railed against Al and the new company, accusing them of manipulation and arrogance; he was clearly afraid Al was going to take advantage of him.

It was hard to fully appreciate both sides of the situation. Stan's perceptions almost always had an accurate core, but the weight of his past experiences of exploitation and insensitivity probably also distorted his perceptions in that direction. I commented that he had a particularly acute sense of when he was being taken advantage of, because he felt he needed to do what his mother wanted or else she would be unhappy and disappointed with him. I told him it did seem like he might be in some jeopardy, but the intensity of his feelings was probably greater than was justified by the real current situation. He was interested in this clarification, agreed, and discussed this at some length. Shortly, he became angry, critical, and self-justifying about Al again. This interaction continued over several appointments, as the job offer seemed to be foundering. I sensed that the new company was getting tired of Stan's aggressiveness and souring on the relationship.

While remaining polite, Stan was clearly increasingly angry with me. I was pointing out his "flawed" reactions repeatedly. To him, I was taking their side, as though I was like his mother, not seeing his feelings, perceptions, and needs. He missed an appointment. When I realized what was going on, I tried to repair the rupture in our relationship. This involved a number of genuine expressions of concern, validation of his perceptions of Al (who had now withdrawn the offer), and empathy for his feeling that I did not understand him. It did not matter that my comments might have been useful insight and advice. This content had to go by the wayside in the face of Stan's feeling of being criticized. We could, and did, come back to Stan's contribution to the conflict with Al later.

Technique

Early-career therapists find this kind of shifting position uncomfortable, and they can get caught up in the question of who and what is right. It is an easy trap to fall into. As therapists, our role is often to "suspend judgment." We may focus on the ideas discussed rather than what is happening in the relationship, and what needs to happen—empathy, a concern for reality and the need to deal with it, and then empathy again about how this is difficult. This is the essential "selfobject" function that Kohut talks about. Putting this into action over and over again in the treatment seems to be the essence of what helps.

Another way to conceptualize this central element in the psychotherapy of low self-esteem is that you are helping patients understand and try new skills in interpersonal relationships. You are reminding them of their impact on others, something that they are not aware of because of their low self-esteem. You are trying to help them increase their social intelligence by helping them see what is really happening in an interaction from both sides, and supporting them in their side and their needs.

The psychotherapy of low self-esteem is rarely short, because it depends so heavily on the relationship itself. There are no quick insight fixes. Sometimes these patients come to treatment for a while, discontinue, and come back when they have been hurt and disappointed again in their lives, and then repeat this cycle. The traditional psychoanalytic view is that this represents the acting out of negative transference, usually the feeling of being criticized and envious. This may well be true, but it may also turn out to be a reenactment of the healthy separation process, depending on the parents, being with them, leaving, and then depending on them again. The development of a healthy selfobject function requires that the object be there when needed and not have overwhelming personal needs.

This process may also be conceptualized as the development of strengths in context of a therapeutic relationship. For example, the strengths grouped under the rubric of wisdom and knowledge are increased with the insight and perspective provided by the therapist. Humanity is increased by the repeated attention to understanding what others feel and need, and temperance grows in response to the therapist's support for containing painful feelings and limiting dysfunctional interpersonal behavior.

Transference and Countertransference

Kohut's work (1971) laid out the common reactions of the patient with unstable self-esteem to the therapist and suggested that these transferences are ways to recognize and diagnose the problem. Mirroring, Kohut's term for the intense need for admiration and empathy, is a replay of old needs that went unfulfilled, and may have an insistent quality because painful feelings of shame and unlovability are always just around the corner. Idealization of the therapist soothes the patient because it restores the feeling of being close to someone so special, loving, and wonderful. Even though these reactions may be excessive in relation to adult needs, they are often desirable for the therapy and therefore should not be challenged initially. The therapist's job is to support these feelings, allowing them to take root, and help the relationship withstand the inevitable threats that make patients feel hurt, rejected, and misunderstood. Like the parent who must gradually but decisively expose a child to reality, protecting and then challenging, the therapist gradually tempers these perceptions with more realistic ones. The patient's rigid requirement for constant mirroring becomes a need that can be fulfilled more easily and more flexibly. Idealization is gently challenged and reality is tested, and over time the patient does not need it as much.

The philosophy of this approach is that what the patient needs must be fulfilled by the therapist (or the parent), and that this fulfillment slowly results in developmental change. Thus the common countertransference reactions include a rescue fantasy that the therapist will be the first really good person in the patient's life and will provide the love and kindness that will make everything better. Other reactions include enjoyment of the idealization without gently pointing out its unrealistic nature, boredom with repeated vignettes with the same themes, and resentment about feeling defeated or controlled by the patient's great focus on him- or herself. If the transference and countertransference are clear to the therapist and the gradual process of working out ruptures and misunderstandings takes place, these patients can greatly benefit from the treatment.

Evidence Base

In their review of the literature on personality disorders, Crits-Christoph and Barber (2007) did not find any study that examined the efficacy of dynamic therapy for patients with narcissistic personality disorder, the descriptive diagnosis closest to low self-esteem. We see this as a fertile field for further study.

PANIC ANXIETY

> A wave of panic passed over the vessel, and these rough and hardy men, who feared no mortal foe, shook with terror at the shadows of their own minds.
> —ARTHUR CONAN DOYLE, SR.

Panic attacks are acute paroxysms of anxiety that appear to arise spontaneously. Profound somatic symptoms such as shortness of breath, palpitations, sweating, and trembling are often accompanied by feelings of overwhelming fear, dying for air, or feeling of imminent doom. People who experience panic attacks may become sensitized to locations where the attacks occurred, and agoraphobia results when there is a constriction in the radius of activity and the places that feel safe from panic.

Alice was a 28-year-old lab technician with brightly dyed hair, dark makeup, and artistic garb who reported at the beginning of her first appointment that she felt "just fine." Yes, she had been experiencing disabling panic attacks, but she could handle them. Approximately two to three times daily she felt acute anxiety with typical somatic symptoms, and the attacks seemed to flow from one into the next over the course of the day.

Her first panic occurred when she was 6 years old. The attacks became full-blown in her teens. Alice's coping strategy was to "take ownership of my mind and body." She forced herself to continue with what she was doing and make sure she could function. She was the eldest of four children, and the only one from her mother's first marriage. Her mother had an extended period of depression when she was young and had abused substances to blunt her emotional pain. During this period of her childhood, Alice acted upbeat and tried to cheer her mother up with jokes and distraction. As a girl she had felt "alone, in a bubble," and remembered that she tried to be cool and in control like Mr. Spock and not let herself be disturbed by the intense sad and fearful feelings inside.

Alice had a boyfriend with whom she was quite enmeshed at the beginning of treatment. Although she saw him all the time, she hung on his phone calls and contact, feeling alternately pleased and gratified when he contacted her, and anxious and abandoned when he did not. She helped nurse his emotional wounds when he was in trouble, but felt taken for granted. The usual precipitants to her panic attacks were anticipating or experiencing rejection by the boyfriend, or feelings of fear of failure when she had to speak up at lab meetings in front of her colleagues.

Alice was smart, verbal, insightful, energetic, creative, and intense; she was like a coiled spring. Her distinct pattern in each session was to express her sadness, anger, or disappointment, and then immediately take it back reassuring me that none of this bothered her.

Psychodynamic Conceptualization

Early psychoanalysis was founded on the study of anxiety and anxiety symptoms in young women like Alice. More recently, panic disorder became a favorite problem for cognitive-behavioral therapists and psychopharmacologists to treat. In behavioral and medication treatment, the panic symptom is regarded as the illness, while from the psychodynamic perspective the panic is seen as a symptom of underlying conflicts that need to be addressed.

Freud's first conceptualization of panic was that it was an "actual neurosis," that is, the result of an "actual" traumatic experience. His later formulation of anxiety neuroses (1926) posited that unconscious conflicts produce signal anxiety, that is, small, tolerable amounts of anxiety that serve as a signal or stimulus to the ego to develop defensive reactions and protect the person from the greater anxiety connected with the repressed material. This signal anxiety is conscious, and the only aspect of repressed conflict the patient is aware of. Neurotic symptoms develop when this smoothly functioning system involving conflict, signal anxiety, and defense is interrupted by a powerful stressor, or when the defenses no longer hold. Thus from the psychodynamic perspective, panic is the breakout of symptomatic anxiety in response to underlying conflict.

As you read about the various psychodynamic problems in this chapter, you have probably noted that the characteristic conflicts associated with each problem seem to have similarities. But why is the symptomatic presentation different for each core problem, while the underlying conflicts are not as distinct? Why a particular symptom develops is known as the problem of "neurosogenesis" in the psychoanalytic literature. Is there a one-to-one correspondence between the nature of the underlying conflict and the type of symptoms that result? We think the connection is fuzzy, and in keeping with our pragmatic perspective, we regard this as a conceptual problem, but not a major practical and therapeutic one. Remember, the core psychodynamic problems are attempts to build a coherent and useful framework for understanding the problems; they are useful heuristics.

Over our careers, each of us has struggled with this paradox. We have a complex and interesting explanatory theory, but it does not really determine specific symptoms. Is it really a scientific theory, then? One of us (RFS) felt deeply convinced of the psychodynamic thinking early on in training and practice and has had several periods of skepticism and cynicism since. During those phases, psychodynamic theory seemed to explain such a small part of motivation and ignored so many other important, practical factors. But then, after a powerful experience working with a patient who changed more than expected, or after hearing a brilliant and incisive case discussion, what had seemed like limitations in the psychodynamic model seemed more like personal limitations in applying the ideas. With more conviction, more sensitivity, and less personal baggage, maybe more therapy experiences could be this powerful.

Yes, depression, obsessionality, and panic all seem to involve anger toward others, and defenses against anger. Fear of abandonment and low self-esteem are characterized by attachment problems, as is panic. We do not know why one person's attachment problem emerges as low self-esteem and another's as abandonment sensitivity. Nor do we understand why anger results in either depression or obsessionality. We do know, however, that from the patient's perspective it feels very different to be depressed than obsessional, and each has a distinct narrative that helps a patient understand him- or herself. The core problems satisfy the subjective need of patients (and therapists) despite their unclear epistemological status.

Milrod et al. (1997) performed systematic psychoanalytic interviews of patients with panic symptoms, attempting to define their essential conflicts with the goal of developing a focused psychodynamic psychotherapy. They reviewed the psychoanalytic literature, including Freud

(1895); Andrews, Stewart, Morris-Yates, Holt, and Henderson (1990); and Tyrer, Seivewright, Ferguson, and Tyrer (1992); as well as the psychiatric literature. Milrod's group developed a formulation for panic disorder that integrates neurobiological vulnerability with experiences of separation, anger, fear of expression of anger, specific child–parent interactions, and current stressors. She notes that the central conflicts in panic patients involve separation and loss, inhibited aggression, and sometimes anxiety about sexual excitement. Panic anxiety is an especially interesting symptom because the "fight or flight" response has deep roots in our evolutionary heritage. The neurobiological literature on anxiety (LeDoux, 1996) suggests explanations for panic anxiety, but they do not satisfy the need to connect panic symptoms with precipitants and maintaining factors in the patient's life.

Neurobiologically vulnerable children, such as those with behavioral inhibition or shyness, may be sensitive to the normal separation experiences of childhood. They tend to experience anger and frustration, and they become conflicted about this. They fear that their anger will hurt the relationships with caretakers and that it must be inhibited. This results in separation sensitivity, dependency, and inhibited anger, and out of this brew comes a readiness to develop panic in the face of losses or increases in demands by others in relationships or at work. The panic expresses the loss and fear, defensively hides the anger, and maintains a position of dependency. Those who are not shy or behaviorally inhibited (panic symptoms without the neurobiological vulnerability) usually have a history of more overtly conflicted relationships with parents, with significant losses or abandonments, and real compromise in their close relationships when anger was expressed. Shear, Cooper, Klerman, Busch, and Shapiro (1993) observed that dependency in panic patients manifests in a "separation-sensitive" presentation with excessive reliance on others, and a "suffocation-sensitive" type in which patients are uncomfortable with their dependency needs.

Alice probably did not have the neurobiological vulnerability to panic; she was not a behaviorally inhibited child. But her early losses, including her parents' divorce and her father's departure from their life, and her mother's subsequent depressions and addiction, likely contributed to the development of her panic. Indeed, her symptoms started at age 6 after the parents split and while her mother was ill. The later exacerbation of her panic symptoms came during periods of loss and separation along with the development of other defensive strategies. For example, during adolescence she had eating disorder symptoms, and in her early 20s after leaving college, she engaged in recurrent self-cutting.

This ended about 2 years before she came to treatment for her panic. When she was engaged in cutting, Alice had minimal panic symptoms, and when she was able to stop cutting, her panic recurred. This illustrates the notion that an underlying separation conflict can manifest in a variety of symptoms and suggests that a purely symptom-focused treatment might not have helped this patient get better.

Alice struggled with her feelings of dependency and attachment. Her panic attacks worsened when she moved away from the city in which she had grown up, and she dealt with this by forming the enmeshed relationship with her boyfriend that was an initial focus of treatment. She panicked when she was afraid he would not call her or see her. She was angry with him but had great difficulty expressing this. Instead, it came out through panic. Her other precipitant for panic was speaking up in her classes. She discussed this at length, and it became clear that she was worried that shining in class would alienate her from her classmates and expose her to the possibility of being the teacher's favorite—she might not be able to live up to that, and then she would lose the special relationship with him.

Strengths

Patients with panic symptoms also have strengths. But fear and anxiety make it difficult to feel courageous and behave courageously. The immediate sense of danger and worry that these patients feel makes it difficult to let themselves go enough to engage the personality strengths of transcendence. Appreciation of beauty, awe, spirituality, and humor occur when the person has a basic degree of security. We comment in the technique section below on the specific approaches for addressing courage and transcendence.

Treatment Goals

The goal of psychodynamic treatment for panic is to help the patient understand the conflicted feelings of dependency and anger that have been outside of awareness and allow him or her manage relationships and activities in a more adaptive way. These patients need to develop a more realistic and contemporary view of how much closeness and intimacy they really require. Increased assertiveness and the capacity for independence will render the panic dynamics less relevant and lessen the intensity and frequency of symptoms.

Developing a Therapeutic Alliance

The development of the therapeutic alliance is intertwined with the patients' struggle with their symptoms—that is, the new relationship may provide an opportunity for support and increased confidence and a buffer for their marked sensitivity to separation and loss. For Alice, there was a rapid attachment to the therapist and a quick reduction in symptoms. Although this is sometimes called a "flight into health," we see it as an opportunity, as it buys time to work on, and through, the conflicts.

Patients who use avoidance to deal with their symptoms—either through rigid control over their attention, or their activities, or in frank agoraphobia—tend to have a more difficult time developing an alliance. They may protect themselves from the therapist because they are concerned that the new and potentially challenging relationship will destabilize them and expose them to frightening feelings of loss or anger. They fear the therapy might precipitate panic. These patients are actually correct, as effective therapy for avoidant patients does encourage them to come into close contact with upsetting feelings, which may increase panic.

There are several techniques for facilitating the development of a strong therapeutic alliance. Frequent sessions promote security and consistency. This makes sense because these patients are so sensitive to separation and aloneness. Careful empathic attention to panic attacks and close exploration of the precipitants to panic help the patient reflect on the symptom and provides some distance from it. Education about the psychodynamic model of panic gives the patient perspective and a rationale for therapy—early loss, anger, and somatic vulnerability can allow a person to avoid feeling frightening emotions, maintain repression, and struggle with panic symptoms rather than with the underlying upsetting feelings. The panic attacks are terrible, and patients will do practically anything to prevent them, but they are only subjectively uncomfortable, and in fact, the patient is physically and mentally safe. From the therapist's perspective, it is important not to overidentify with the patient and these symptoms. If you cannot tolerate your patient panicking, you will not be able to help the patient tolerate the painful feelings that need to be uncovered over the course of treatment.

The typical resistances in psychotherapy for panic reflect the challenges in developing a therapeutic alliance with these patients. The most common resistance is excessive dependency. Patients feel you can solve their problems and guarantee their security. They want you to take care of them and prevent them from feeling alone. Other panic patients come for treatment because they know they need it, or they have been pushed into it, but they do not really want to feel anything uncomfortable. Avoidance as a resistance can be internal (use of repression, suppression, disavowal) or external (proscribed behaviors, agoraphobia, use of phobic companions to allow engagement in anxiety-producing behaviors). Patients often try to control the interaction in the therapy to maintain their avoidant stance.

Technique

The course of treatment has been clearly described by Milrod et al. (1997), and our comments are based on their work. With the goal in mind of decreased symptoms, increasing independence, and the ability to be assertive, the initial phase of treatment is characterized by the development of a therapeutic alliance and exploration of the panic history. The detailed exploration of panic attacks, especially looking at the precipitants to panic, both historical and current, sets the stage for the treatment. Often patients are unaware of the psychological meaning of the events that trigger panic and feel the attacks come on entirely unconnected to these events. It is striking how often one can construct a meaningful narrative about the events that precede panic. Usually it comes back to loss or separation in some form, or the fear of anger and losing one's temper destructively about a loss or rejection. But the first phase is collecting the information and developing a good database of panic attacks and their surrounding context.

In those patients who are not actively panicking, but who have this as an important part of their history, or those whose lives are organized around phobic avoidance of the panic, the treatment will stall if the patient feels no anxiety and simply continues the avoidant behavior. One patient kept her husband with her for most of her errands; she also cleverly but unconsciously changed the subject over and over again in sessions. Confrontation of the avoidance in external behavior and in the relationship with the therapist is a staple of treatment for patients in this phase. The confrontation takes the form of pointing out the avoidance, not telling the patient how to behave. Typically, avoidant patients need this interpretation a number of times before they can begin to take conscious responsibility for pushing themselves.

Next, interpretation of current panic allows the patient to begin to see the repetitive pattern. This takes the form of connecting the precipitating event and the experience of separation, or anger about separation, and the panic attack itself. This must be repeated numerous times ("worked through") with different experiences of panic or limited-symptom panic attacks. The work is bolstered by historical interpretations about the same dynamic in the patient's early relationships, and it will certainly manifest itself in the transference and countertransference as well. One hopes to ultimately be able to make an interpretation that ties together the repetitive pattern in the past, present, and transference. An example of this kind of interpretation is:

Your drive on the turnpike, where the infrequent exits make you feel trapped on the road, brought up a frightening feeling of being alone and unable to control your environment. This triggers an old feeling of separation and aloneness, like when your parents were fighting, leading them not pay attention to you and your needs. Back then, you were afraid you would entirely lose your base of security at home, and this was terrifying. This is also like the feeling you had when I told you I would be on vacation next week, leaving you to deal with your panic "by yourself." You were also angry at your parents, and maybe at me, too, about this separation. Each of these situations triggers a feeling of loss that leads to panic and fear of more panic. This comes out as a panic attack, which prevents you from feeling the feelings directly, and you are left with a confusing but terrible symptom.

The work on panic implicitly encourages patients to widen their scope of behavior, including those situations that expose them to separation triggers. The new awareness that panic is related to old historical danger situations, rather than elevators, shopping malls, and enclosed spaces, for example, emboldens most patients to want to try to expand their sphere of activity.

Recognizing that the separation fears are old fears, with the accompanying decrease in panic anxiety, gives panic patients increased confidence in their ability to withstand stressful and upsetting life experiences. This increases their resilience and courage to take on new challenges. It can be helpful to explicitly recognize and validate this when patients begin to change their behavior and expand their sphere of activity. The strengths grouped under the rubric of transcendence (appreciation of beauty and excellence, gratitude, hope, humor, spirituality) seem to naturally reawaken with decreasing panic symptoms. These qualities emerge spontaneously with reduced anxiety.

Transference and Countertransference

The typical panic transferences involve separation and loss and the patient's various reactions to these. Feelings of closeness and separation are prominent early in the treatment. But rescheduled appointments, lateness, and vacations are felt keenly as separation, and they stimulate earlier feelings of loss and aloneness, and sometimes panic itself. One patient had her first panic attack in months the evening after a therapy appointment when ending treatment was first tentatively discussed.

The patients will experience you as the person who abandoned them—whether this experience is rooted in a frank abandonment or the kind of temperamental mismatch that leaves a child feeling misunderstood, unvalidated, and scarily alone. Typically, these patients experience separation as overwhelming and inchoate—their world will come to an end, or they will not be able to take care of themselves. It is hard to describe in words. But the quality of the feeling is such that they do not feel the feeling of aloneness clearly; instead it is felt in the body as an intense and frightening physical sensation, the panic attack. There can be covert anger at the therapist because of the separation, which may trigger feelings of fear and guilt, as the patients usually feel that their anger is part of the reason that parental figures abandoned them. In addition to these dynamics, there is anticipatory anxiety about having another panic attack.

Typical countertransference reactions include feeling a maternal caretaking urge. This maternal reaction denies the separations and losses the patient may be experiencing and allows us to avoid painful feelings about our own separations and losses. But frustration with the patient's dependency may also surface, with a need to reject the patient, pushing him out of the nest, and freeing the therapist from the incessant demands for closeness. Both of these reactions are natural counterparts to the patient's own dependency struggle and represent our difficulties in confronting and interpreting these problems for our patients because the treatment is painful for them.

As the treatment draws to a close, it is no surprise that transferential feelings of separation and loss come to the fore, and there is a potential for resurgence of panic symptoms. Because of the work done on this already, it should be possible to connect these feelings to the recurring interpretations about separation and panic.

Evidence Base

Panic-focused psychodynamic psychotherapy (Milrod et al., 1997) was compared with applied relaxation training in a pilot randomized controlled trial (Milrod, Leon, Busch, et al., 2007), and a large effect size improvement was noted. In a follow-up analysis, Milrod, Leon, Barber, et al. (2007) reported even greater superiority for this dynamic treatment among panic disorder patients with a comorbid personality disorder. A randomized controlled trial is currently in progress comparing the efficacy of panic-focused psychodynamic psychotherapy with CBT and applied relaxation training.

TRAUMA

Pain is inevitable. Suffering is optional.
—DALAI LAMA

Traumatized people have experienced something outside the realm of normal that threatens their sense of safety and well-being. They have had real-life tangible experiences that are more than just psychologically threatening. The human organism has been shaped by evolution to respond adaptively to dangerous events, and while sometimes trauma leads to illness, we are far more often resilient to external threats than we are made ill by them (Konner, 2007).

Traumatized patients have reliving experiences, including flashbacks, dreams, and other forms of reexperiencing. They experience ongoing mistrust of others, difficulty in close relationships, and problems in self-esteem, identity, and a sense of autonomy and competence. They do not feel powerful. There is invariably avoidance of stimuli reminiscent of the trauma, and it is striking how a traumatized person can become acutely agitated and distressed when triggered by something reminiscent of his traumatic experience. Avoidance can also be manifested in a kind of global numbing of feeling. Vigilance and hyperarousal, a tendency to dissociate and detach from everyday experience, vulnerability to a wide range of physical symptoms in multiple organ systems, and secrecy are all part of the picture. Often these patients have not had predictably good responses to psychotherapy or psychopharmacology, and there may have been boundary problems in the treatments and intense countertransference reactions by the therapist. Those who do not naturally recover from the impact of trauma have a persisting sense of distress and an oscillating clinical state. Trauma survivors are often intensely reactive, with rapid decompensation and recovery. Just as quickly as they get worse, they rapidly get so much better. In summary, the fear and intensity of the original traumatic experiences lives on in the minds of victims and is palpably present in the experiences they have with others.

Psychodynamic Conceptualization

The history of psychoanalytic thinking on trauma is checkered, with important insights and missed opportunities. Although early psychoanalysis helped to understand the extent and impact of childhood sexual and violent trauma, subsequent thinking was dominated by excessive attention to the intrapsychic meaning of trauma. This turned attention away from the need to recognize, address, and deal with the impact of bad external events. All too often, the attention was on how a patient might have been ambivalent or even gratified by the traumatic experience. Rather than review the very extensive literature on this debate (Herman, 1997), we present a contemporary perspective on trauma arising from biology, cognitive processing, and psychotherapeutic findings.

A trauma is an overwhelming event that threatens the health, safety, and security of the individual and cannot be emotionally and cognitively processed. Preexisting conflicts are stirred up, and the emotions of shock, fear, and danger that are generated by the trauma are too much for the person to tolerate and to relate to other usual life experiences. For example, how could it be that the perpetrator of the trauma is someone who otherwise seemed safe, or upon whom the victim is dependent. The bubble of safety in which we live is invaded and something inconceivable has occurred. Previously trusted people may turn out to be untrustworthy, or situations previously innocent are now revealed to be dangerous. Detachment from reality, dissociation, and the development of a split in the personality result when the experiences associated with the trauma are not integrated with the dominant associational network of memories. Inevitably, the dissociated part of the self leaks back into awareness, leading to reliving experiences; meanwhile, avoidance of stimuli reminiscent of the trauma helps maintain the split in memories and feelings.

> Ellen was an intelligent, compassionate, warm, and caring woman with a very strong sense of values and ethics. She was deeply committed to her family and was a sensitive and thoughtful wife and mother. Her middle-class upbringing was normal in many ways, but her brothers engaged in inappropriate and demeaning sex play with her as an early adolescent. During this time, a boy from school sexually harassed her regularly on her walk home from school. As an adolescent she was raped on a date with a man who was a number of years older than she. Anxious, guilty, and insecure, she could not tell her parents about any of this.

Her marriage to a kind, strong, loyal man helped her launch an adult life with children, religious observance, and altruistic activity in her community. Several years before she came for treatment, she was approached by a friend of her husband's, a predatory man, who convinced, manipulated, and cajoled her into an affair. He threatened her to try to prevent her from exposing the relationship, and Ellen had the awful feeling she could not escape. She had been depressed before this, but now her terrible feelings of shame and guilt tortured her to the point of suicidality.

Initially, Ellen was acutely agitated, focused only on how unforgivable her behavior was. She remained quite functional and was generally able to take care of her children and husband. Sometimes she took to bed when her children went off to school and got up shortly before they came home. But she had periods of detachment, drinking binges, and sudden intense self-critical episodes. She avoided men, including her brothers. She could almost hear a man's voice in her mind criticizing and demeaning her, but she knew it was her own thoughts heard aloud. Over the course of her treatment, she often felt rapidly worse and then better, and struggled with terrible feelings of mistrust toward her parents and siblings.

Ellen's prior traumatic experiences predisposed her to the advances of this manipulative man because she relived the experiences of her childhood, feeling helpless and powerless and under the influence of males who were aggressive and selfish. Despite her values and current emotional connections, she experienced this new trauma according to the same template as the old ones—fear, powerlessness, and passivity. The problem with un-worked-through trauma is that that the thoughts and feelings related to the traumatic experience are generalized to many subsequent adult experiences (Charney, 2004). It was Ellen's shame and distress about what she had done, and her confusion about how it was so different from the person she thought she was, that brought her to treatment.

Common secondary effects of trauma include a disturbance of identity, which Ellen had—although she had a sense of herself as intact, compassionate, and helpful, there was a persisting feeling of being ugly and bad. Her secrecy and avoidance of her brothers and the man with whom she had the affair, along with feelings of isolation, anger, fear, sadness, and loss of hope are characteristic, too. Common adaptations include perfectionism, avoidance, repetition of the traumatic situation, and dissociation. Sometimes there is a counterphobic reaction in which the trauma victim becomes very aggressive, fearless, and almost the mirror opposite of the usual fearful avoidance. Some traumatized people develop "street smarts" that allow them to become exquisitely sensitive at seeing the potential for evil and danger. Others develop a strong capacity for dealing with pain. Most gain a gritty realism from their suffering.

Strengths

Ellen was a woman with quiet natural courage and a powerfully nurturing, loving nature. This was evident even in the midst of her worst suffering. But when she was most ill, these qualities were sorely compromised. Indeed, the character strengths of courage and humanity can be worn away by traumatic experiences, and trauma victims learn that courage can sometimes result in worse harm. Faith in humanity—their own and others'—is shaken and tested by the awareness of what others can do to them. In the case of natural and environmental trauma, the veil of safety provided by close relationships is revealed to be thin indeed. Working through the trauma and restoring empowerment and accurate perception will help to restore these character strengths.

Treatment Goals

The treatment goals for traumatized patients are focused on empowerment and an increased sense of safety and security. Knowing the difference between trustworthy relationships and those that are unhealthy leads to increased trust and a greater ability to feel close and safe. It is necessary to reexperience old traumatic experiences, seeing them as unavoidable consequences of being in a dangerous situation. Reexperiencing takes the form of telling the story and feeling what it really felt like. This helps patients decrease the many negative conclusions and attributions they make: it's their fault, they deserved the pain and suffering, it will happen again, they cannot and should not try to protect themselves, and so on.

The treatment of trauma restores the sense of empowerment and reality to the patient, reconnecting split-off and overwhelmed feelings with the main experience of life and dismantling past useful responses that are no longer necessary. This discussion of treatment generally follows the work of Judith Herman (1997). The goal is an accurate narrative of the past, an increased sense of security and empowerment, and increased healthy trust in relationships. Our definition of this problem refers primarily to those with a history of trauma perpetrated by others, whether it is physical, sexual, or mental, and is less immediately relevant to those with traumas from natural disasters.

Building a Therapeutic Alliance

Traumatized people often do not trust others to maintain healthy boundaries and engage in a mutually respectful relationship. This is especially true if the trauma has involved violence or sexual abuse. Thus the task of building and strengthening the therapeutic alliance is carried on continuously during the entire treatment. It will take time for the patient to develop trust that the therapist will follow the appropriate tasks and have the appropriate goals.

Because the trauma has often been denied or ignored, or at least downplayed by others, these patients are especially focused on the question of what is real, and what really happened. Did they exaggerate, did they make up their memories? Are they complaining excessively? Are their memory and judgment intact? Accepting and believing that what happened really happened, and that it had a huge impact, is a painful but essential element of trauma treatment. The resistance of not knowing, or not really believing, is very common. In working through trauma, there are frequent cycles of feeling it and believing it, and then denying it.

This uncertainty manifests itself in the treatment relationship as well. The patient is often very concerned with what is really going on in the treatment relationship—what you are really thinking or feeling, or why you responded in a certain way. There is, early on especially, difficulty in looking at these feelings as transferential. The patient wants to know what is real and is made more anxious by attempts to explore fantasies or feelings about the therapist. The patient may have experienced psychological manipulation in the past, or the uncertainty itself may provoke anxiety. Thus, the therapist must commit to genuineness in the relationship, and not hide behind therapeutic neutrality, even if this is well-intentioned.

Clarity, honesty, and transparency are necessary. You will continually have to prove that you are not an abuser. This requires confidence in yourself when you are accused or regarded with suspicion. You will have to focus your attention so that you do not inadvertently do the things the patient is frightened of such as minor expressions of anger, retaliation for the patient's difficult behavior, or overly personal expressions of affection. But even if you do all this, a patient with a history of physical abuse may worry that the therapist will get angry and attack. It might take repeated calm expressions of interest and positive regard, and several months of therapy, before the patient can settle down enough to be able to begin see these fears as self-generated and transferential, as opposed to a result of a real danger situation.

The resistances manifested in the treatment of trauma are the patient's attempt to manage feelings of fear or contain anger. Trauma results in the splitting off of traumatic memories and responses, and this dissociation then shows itself in the treatment. There are periods of time when the patient does not seem to have much to work on, and other periods when the patient is so overwhelmed by emotion that they do not feel they can leave the office and reenter the world. The therapeutic alliance will strengthen if the therapist encourages discussion of the traumatic memories, feelings, and reactions, but leaves enough time at the end of appointments for the patient to reconstitute and return to the contemporary reality. Patients may dissociate in session under the sway of these memories and feelings, and you will need to help them find a safe place to be after sessions, and find techniques for soothing themselves when they are distressed outside the session.

Technique

The road map for treatment starts with education about the arc of psychotherapy for trauma—empowerment, exploration and evaluation of memories, and use of that knowledge to inform current relationships and decisions. The initial phase of treatment involves a cautious exploration of the present and past, with support, empathy, and the maintenance of a clear perspective. That is, the therapist expresses the conviction that the bad things that happened were wrong, they should not have occurred, and they produced possibly lasting effects. But the trauma is in the past, and in the present the patient will be able to develop techniques for managing the emotional sequellae and be in charge of current perceptions and decision making. The painful memories and emotions need to be contained in the therapy, using support, appropriate availability outside the appointments, and clarifications about the reality of the therapeutic relationship.

The next phase, working through, involves repeated discussion of the traumatic memories, but also the many current life situations and how the traumatic experiences may be distorting current perceptions. The patient recovers a sense of control, mastery, and confidence by taking charge of how he sees things in the present and makes new decisions more free from repeating aspects of the old traumatic scenarios. For example, the patient does not have to shrink back from situations that are not really dangerous but are reminiscent of the trauma, nor does he have to counterphobically prove himself to be safe. He does not have to doubt his perceptions, which will sometimes include skepticism or criticism of others' behavior, and does not have to second-guess his perceptions and decisions in the same way.

The working-through phase will, to some degree, involve a deeper experience and exploration of the traumatic transferences (and, for you, the countertransferences), and a deeper kind of trust will enter the therapeutic relationship. Treatment will draw to a close when the old traumatic feelings and perceptions are relatively less powerful and the patient has a renewed sense of self-efficacy and mastery.

Transference and Countertransference

Traumatic transferences are often quite specific. That is, the patient feels things about the therapist that are replays of traumatic experiences in earlier relationships. For example, a male patient who had been sexually abused in childhood by an older woman felt the female therapist was dangerously seductive when she smiled because his abuser had smiled at him in a particular way. A female patient had difficulty looking at the therapist because the male therapist's eye contact reminded her of a manipulative man with an aggressive stare who had once threatened her. For another patient, the long hallway outside the therapist's office often triggered memories and feelings related to the hallway in her childhood home where abuse took place.

Frequently the patient regards the therapist as a potential abuser of some kind and brings to the relationship a lack of trust. It is often incomprehensible to a traumatized patient how the therapist could only have the agenda of listening, helping, and trying to understand, and not have more selfish motivations that will lead to dangerous behavior. The patient is afraid of the therapist and feels that the only way to protect himself is to maintain constant vigilance. It is important to be on guard, not reveal too much that might make one vulnerable, and never relax too much, or something dangerous could suddenly occur.

The rage trauma victims feel toward those who hurt them is often reawakened in the transference, accompanied by guilt or fear that the abuser (therapist) will retaliate in some way. This reflects the bind they felt as helpless victims. Another variant of this problem is when the transference is based on those who were bystanders and did not help. Other family members who did not come to the rescue, or who helped to maintain secrets, were a focus of anger and mistrust, and the therapist can be seen in this light. Here the anger is about the bystander's betrayal, passivity, or cowardice. It is important to distinguish between these two reactions, both based on anger—anger at being hurt and anger at not being protected—because they each reflect an important aspect of the legacy of trauma and its effect on subsequent relationships.

Traumatized patients present many challenges to the therapist, although ultimately it can be a deeply satisfying experience if one is able to help them regain a sense of control and mastery over themselves and their lives. Countertransference reactions tend to be strong, like the transference reactions. There are six common countertransference reactions. First, one may identify particularly strongly with the patient's suffering and the overwhelming sense of hurt, fear, and rage. As always, empathic identification helps one understand what the patient is feeling and struggling with, but it can cause difficulty because it is harder for the therapist to take a dispassionate view and push the patient to help him move forward. The identification can turn into overidentification and downright passivity, hopelessness, and loss of the helping role.

Second, you may downplay the seriousness of the trauma. A therapist is especially vulnerable to this when the patient is minimizing or in denial of the significance of the abuse. Therapists deny abuse because it is so awful to consider, and empathizing with the abuse leads to painful emotions—fear, anger, vulnerability, hopelessness.

Third, the therapist may identify with the perpetrator. In this case, the therapist feels angry or controlling feelings toward the patient, subtly slipping into regarding the patient's needs and feelings with disrespect, like he is not quite equal. When there is a traumatic reenactment going on—the patient is feeling that the therapist is abusive—even the therapist may experience himself that way. This is often accompanied by feeling guilty and bad. Sometimes, the therapist treating a traumatized patient just feels bad and guilty, even if there does not seem to be anything realistic to base it on.

Fourth, you may feel helpless. In response to the patient's passive bystander transference, you can feel like you are just not doing enough. You are witnessing a person in extraordinary pain, and you are just standing by doing nothing. In reality, talking, reflecting, and problem solving are the very things the patient does need, but sometimes it feels like the therapist's work is so ethereal or so minor, it is practically trivial. This is the countertransference guilt of being the bystander.

Fifth, you may feel overwhelmed with feeling. Hearing about trauma, especially when there are repeated instances, becomes overwhelming at some point. Patients need to be able to talk about their experiences as much as they want, and they will need to repeat their stories numerous times. Indeed, in prolonged exposure, the efficacious structured behavioral treatment for PTSD developed by Edna Foa and colleagues, patients verbalize their major traumatic experiences many times (e.g., Foa, Hembree, & Rothbaum, 2007).

Hearing over and over again about trauma can lead to a subtle form of posttraumatic stress disorder, with avoidance, anxiety, and reliving experiences. The best approach to dealing with these feelings in yourself is supervision and discussion with peers. You need some support and guidance in processing your own powerful responses to hearing about the trauma, in a fashion parallel to the patient's therapy. It might be important to limit the number of seriously traumatized patients you treat at any one point in time.

Last, there is a particular type of confusion you may experience that is actually a form of countertransference. You may forget parts of the patient's history, or what was discussed at the previous session, or you may find yourself not being able to synthesize your understanding of what the patient is talking about. Your thoughts and feelings may swirl, or you may retreat into a state of anxious confusion. This is often the kind of feeling the patient had in response to the trauma. It is the subjective state of being so overwhelmed that the usual cognitive functions are interrupted. It may help you understand how the patient felt or feels sometimes now in dealing with the traumatic memories.

We have described the issues involved in developing a therapeutic alliance and the usual transferences and countertransferences with trauma patients at somewhat greater length than with the other psychodynamic problems because they are so powerful that the treatment will likely become derailed if they are not recognized and attended to.

Evidence Base

There is not a single modern randomized controlled trial comparing dynamic therapy to CBT for PTSD. Brom, Kleber, and Defares (1989) compared a short-term psychodynamic treatment based on Horowitz's form of time-limited dynamic therapy (Horowitz, 1976) to systematic desensitization and hypnotherapy. They found that 60% of patients in each group improved. In addition, they reported that psychodynamic psychotherapy resulted in greater reduction of avoidance symptoms, while systematic desensitization and hypnotherapy resulted in greater reduction of intrusion symptoms. Despite these positive results, we are not aware of any studies continuing this promising line of research. This is surprising because many interpersonal, developmental, and personality aspects of PTSD suggest that dynamic psychotherapy should be considered for this population (for an excellent review of this literature, see Schottenbauer, Glass, Arnkoff, & Gray, 2008).

SUMMARY

This review of the six core psychodynamic problems—depression, obsessionality, fear of abandonment, low self-esteem, panic anxiety, and trauma—helps the therapist recognize and anticipate the unfolding of each type of patient's psychotherapy. Having identified the core problem and begun to develop the therapeutic alliance, your next task is to develop a comprehensive formulation with the historical and personal data you have gathered.

CHAPTER 7

Psychodynamic Formulation

The formulation of a problem is often
more essential than its solution.
—ALBERT EINSTEIN

When we were in training, those teachers who could listen to a case presentation and instantly grasp the patient's essential problem had a luminous quality for us. They perceived the patients' key conflicts and used them to explain everything important in their lives. This almost magic ability seemed unattainable, and we saw it as the ultimate skill in our new field. Now we know that what appeared to be magic is actually the learned ability to formulate a case rapidly.

Perry et al. (1987) make the important point that writing out a formulation is not just an educational exercise; rather, it is an important and concrete way of making sure you commit yourself to a way of thinking about the patient. They quote E. M. Forster's alleged comment, "I never know what I think until I read what I write." Although open-mindedness and an ability to be flexible and change set are essential skills for the therapist, vagueness and ambiguity have too often allowed us to hide our confusion and muddy thinking, and a thoughtful formulation is an attempt to move past that.

Any reasonable reader at this point will likely be reacting with alarm. How does one integrate all of the material about the patient's life

---

Much of the material of this chapter has been adapted from Summers (2002). Used with permission of the Association for the Advancement of Psychotherapy.

with the core psychodynamic problem, illustrating the central conflicts and discussing neurobiological factors that are important but which we can only guess at? Like any complex new mental task, writing a formulation is best accomplished by breaking it down into its parts, focusing on the completion of each component and waiting for the moment when it all comes together. Our trainees feel overwhelmed with the first formulation they attempt, but it gets easier with experience. By their third attempt, they are writing successful formulations and are struggling instead with a deeper understanding of the patient, realizing that the formulation writing is a worthwhile tool for pushing them to clarify their clinical thinking.

Here is a formulation for Peter, the young man with depression discussed in Chapter 5. We have learned from our students that it is helpful to read through an entire formulation first before discussing the structure and the components. Each component of the formulation is labeled for easier reference.

Part 1: Summarizing Statement

Peter is a 19-year-old man in his freshman year of college with chronic low-grade depression, social anxiety, disappointments in love, and high academic achievement. He describes feelings of extreme loneliness, anxiety, and constant suicidal preoccupation. He experiences a great longing for intimacy, both in a romantic relationship with a woman and in friendships with men, and feels constantly disappointed. He has difficulty completing his work and meeting deadlines. The most intense periods of depression, anxiety, and suicidality follow social disappointments. He had marked childhood shyness, depressive symptoms beginning in the preteen years, and a family history of depression and schizophrenia.

Part 2: Description of Nondynamic Factors

Peter meets the diagnostic criteria for major depressive disorder. His paternal grandmother had paranoid schizophrenia, and his father, an esteemed academician, is described as emotionally aloof, overly rational, and inhibited. His mother suffers from chronic low-grade depression, and she is emotional and often needy for his attention. Peter was an anxious and chronically shy child with behavioral inhibition. He had prepubertal onset of intense social anxiety and a markedly fluctuating mood with low self-esteem. Prior traumatic experiences included frequent teasing and humiliation by other boys during the teenage years, and rejection and public humiliation by his first girlfriend. He found prior psychotherapy helpful and responded fairly well to prior treatment with serotonin reuptake inhibitor antidepressants with reduced interpersonal sensitivity and less catastrophic responses to disappointment.

Part 3: Psychodynamic Explanation of Central Conflicts

Peter's core psychodynamic problem is depression. The main conflicts involve his early sense of loss, with anger, guilt, and a tendency to idealize others and be disappointed by them [*statement of core psychodynamic problem and essential conflicts*].

Peter recalls many memories of his mother confiding in him about her frustrations and loneliness in her marriage, and complaining about his father's lack of warmth. She made a big point of thanking Peter for touching her shoulder at her father's funeral. These experiences, and her special singling out of him for companionship, made him feel very close to his mother but overwhelmed by her neediness. He felt that she did not adequately support his needs for independence and vigor. Instead, she seemed to want a companion who would be tied to her. His father was hyperintellectual, and Peter never felt comfortable with him, and longed to feel more masculine. In childhood, the attachment problems with both parents resulted in a feeling of loneliness with much anger at both parents, and intense guilt about this [*childhood experience*].

Peter became increasingly depressed and struggled with angry and suicidal feelings over the recent semester. He felt lonely and was rejected by several girls. He experienced intense rejection, feeling that everyone but he was paired off with a member of the opposite sex. This made him feel more suicidal, but also very angry at the girls who rejected him. He yearns for closeness with men—other students and professors—wanting to be guided and protected. He responds to this need for others and his fears of not measuring up with self-defeating behavior, such as turning in work late, keeping others waiting, and confessing excessively about his history of depression. After a recent disappointment by a girl whom he wished to date, he cut himself superficially on the thigh. This expressed his hurt, self-directed anger, and yearning for understanding [*recent experience*]. The CCRT for Peter would be: a wish to be close and idealize others, a response that others are disappointing and rejecting, and a response of self of disappointment, anger, and guilt.

These issues are also reflected in his pattern of difficulty completing college courses, meeting work deadlines, and being consistent about extracurricular activities. He expresses his anger at impending rejection, yet brings it about at the same time. Sometimes he manages his neediness through aggressive and even argumentative behavior. In high school, he initiated a one-person environmental campaign, writing articles about environmental threats in the school paper and organizing meetings. Yet he did not reach out to include others in his protest [life events].

Striking intelligence, articulateness, and a kind of dogged persistence helped him deal with all of this travail. Peter was a "fighter" [*strengths*].

Peter's neurobiological vulnerability to social anxiety and shyness, as well as his predisposition to depression, probably contributed to proneness to rejection as a child and intensified his experiences of disappointment and anger. This likely made him even more dependent on his mother, and more sensitive to the disappointments in his relationship with his father. His schizotypal vulnerability (grandmother with schizophrenia, father with some schizotypal traits) may cause his reaction to these losses and frustrations to be more chaotic and disorganized that otherwise expected [*biology affecting psychodynamics*].

On the other hand, Peter's fear of rejection, and the self-defeating behavior that has become associated with it, tend to perpetuate the recurrent depression and social anxiety. His sensitivity to rejection is a trigger to episodes of illness. Thus his depressive psychodynamics likely reinforced his biological vulnerabilities, resulting in the acute symptom picture he presents in coming for treatment [*dynamics stimulating biological vulnerability*].

Part 4: Predicting Responses to the Therapeutic Situation

Peter has many positive prognostic features, including a high level of academic function; consistent and stable, if conflicted, relationships with parents; and a history of prior participation in therapy. His intelligence, verbal facility, and persistence will be very helpful and probably critical to weathering the transference storms.

Following the development of an initial positive transference attitude, Peter's angry and competitive feelings associated with his father and the conflicted dependent feelings related to his mother may begin to develop toward the therapist. Thus he might feel disappointed and rejected, and it is possible that there could be self-destructive behavior or an angry counterdependent reaction. Peter's attitude toward psychopharmacology may follow the same pattern, with a wish for help but ambivalence when it is received.

What were your reactions to reading this formulation? We hope it conveys this patient's themes of hurt, anger, and self-defeating behavior and traces them from early origins to current presentation. It also attempts to demonstrate the relationship between those dynamics and the biological vulnerability. Although a comprehensive formulation can provide a rich picture of the interweaving strands of experience and vulnerability, it often raises as many questions as it answers.

As you can see, a formulation is not a history. It is a pithy summary condensed around one core psychodynamic problem. It organizes the patient's symptoms, experiences, important relationships, and seminal life events into a focused and coherent whole. There is always a tension between waiting for an understanding of the patient to "bubble up" through extended exploration and discussion, and reaching a judgment about what the core problems are. If we rush the process, our conclusion will be formed too early in the treatment based on incomplete data and understanding. But caution has its costs as well. The conservative stance, waiting until all things are clear and the patient herself arrives at a concise picture herself, is often slow and unrealistic. It exposes the patient to too much uncertainty and anxiety and the feeling of floundering. This is one reason patients complain their therapists are not "doing anything" for them.

The formulation enables you to apply your understanding of the six core psychodynamic problems, generic as they are, to the unique patient in front of you. It also helps you define appropriate treatment goals and anticipate the unfolding of the therapeutic relationship. Most forms of therapy emphasize the need to derive a formulation to guide the goals of treatment and to decide on the best interventions (for a comprehensive overview of formulations from a different perspective, see Eells, 2006). The formulation approach we describe here is comprehensive, meaning it includes the neurobiological, social, and systems aspects of the patient's problem, as well as the psychodynamic aspect. This approach requires you to judge the relative importance of psychodynamic factors compared with other factors in the development and maintenance of the patient's condition.

The example of Peter illustrates the structure and content of a formulation. In this chapter we describe its evolution as a clinical tool and the data you need to gather to derive it. We conclude with some of the practical pitfalls and problems you may confront in generating formulations.

THE TRADITION
OF PSYCHODYNAMIC FORMULATION

Freud made succinct conceptualizations of his patients without using the term formulation—for example, in the famous case of Dora (Freud, 1905), he pinpointed the patient's conflicts with her father and other

men. Much subsequent interest in the structure and format of psychodynamic formulation came from educational rather than clinical settings.
Formulation was seen as a good way of helping junior clinicians sharpen
and clarify their thinking about patients and a stimulus for good discussion with teachers and supervisors (MacKinnon & Michels, 1971;
MacKinnon & Yudofsky, 1991; McWilliams, 1999). We agree with this,
and think it is a worthwhile habit for all clinicians, junior or senior. We
identify a core problem with all of our patients and develop a formulation, although having done this for a while, we no longer write it out.
Writing the formulation seems especially helpful for those in training.

A close look at the use of psychodynamic formulation began with
Perry et al.'s (1987) elegant review. They presented a format for a concise formulation that we follow here. The four essential parts are (1) a
general summary of the case; (2) a review of "nondynamic factors"; (3)
a description of core psychodynamics using the ego psychology, object
relations, or self psychology model; and (4) a prognostic assessment that
identifies potential areas of resistance. Although Perry et al. (1987) refer
to the importance of including neurobiological factors in the formulation and comment on the relevance of a psychodynamic formulation to
nondynamically focused treatments, they do not provide a systematic
format for including these elements.

The CCRT method developed by Luborsky (1977) provides a very
clear, albeit simpler, formulation. The CCRT can help the clinician focus
and organize clinical material and may usefully serve as component of
the more multifaceted psychodynamic formulation we describe here.

Summers (2002) provided an updated structure and format for the
psychodynamic formulation, building on and extending the concepts set
forth by Perry et al. (1987); that work, along with the CCRT, provides
the basis for this chapter.

HISTORICAL TIME LINE

The first clinical data you will collect are about the patient's current and
past subjective experiences. What has been upsetting and painful and
difficult, and what are the feelings, thoughts, and fantasies associated
with those painful experiences? What are the prominent symptoms and
the repetitive experiences or behaviors?

Your task is to develop a historical time line with a clear picture
of the waxing and waning of symptoms over time, and the experiences
that seem to have precipitated them. Focusing on potential triggers is

extremely important, and one should gently but firmly inquire about this, despite a patient's insistence that the symptoms appeared out of nowhere. Like the character Columbo in the old TV series of that name, a therapist needs to take a modest, understanding, but persistent stance in delving into these questions with the patient. An uncomplicated, direct, curious manner helps to draw patients out. Be skeptical but respectful!

You may gather the developmental history and sweep of experiences over the patient's life by asking more open-ended questions when a patient is talkative and interested in discussing her history. Other patients may require a session or part of a session that is more specifically focused on the early history. Here, the therapist will ask about the family background and each period of the patient's life, starting from the beginning.

The history includes not only symptoms, but also the important experiences of the patient's life. Don't make the common mistake of focusing so much on the patient's symptoms that you neglect the patient's seminal life events and the nature of the patient's strengths. Relevant interpersonal issues and cultural and social context are crucial parts of the picture. For example, a patient who comes to treatment concerned about feeling withdrawn, anxious, and afraid, and whose marriage is breaking up, is understood differently from a patient who has the same feelings, but whose marriage is intact.

The context for understanding a person's problems also includes an assessment of neurobiological vulnerability, which is established through family history or specific psychiatric symptoms. Usually you will rely on the patient's report of symptoms and family history. It will be difficult to determine what is a neurobiological factor, and what is related to psychodynamics. We will discuss this important but thorny issue shortly.

PSYCHODYNAMIC FORMULATION WORKSHEET

We use the Psychodynamic Formulation Worksheet (Figure 7.1) to keep track of the domains of data that are essential to the comprehensive formulation and to remind us to look for information over the longitudinal course of the patient's life. The worksheet makes the task of gathering information more concrete. The boxes need to be filled in over the course of the first four to six sessions. Of course, the unique and complex history of a person requires more than a series of small boxes to express, and sometimes the patient has not discussed important parts of the history. But you should take a first pass at identifying important issues in

	0–5 years old	5 years old–puberty	Adolescence
Seminal life events	Needy mother and aloof father. Two younger siblings.	Teasing, some social alienation.	Rejection by girl and public humiliation. Subsequent rejections by others. Good academic performance but much struggle and procrastination. Leave home for college.
Key subjective experiences, psychiatric symptoms		Social anxiety, low self-esteem, mood fluctuations. Longing for closeness.	Chronic low-grade depression, parasuicidal behavior. Procrastination about academic work. Social anxiety. Suicidal after social disappointments.
Neurobiological factors, syndromal pathology	Shyness, family history of depression and psychosis.	Prepubertal social anxiety.	Depression, social anxiety.
Psychodynamic themes	Attachment problems with mother, some degree of intrusiveness.	Father distant, ambivalent identification. Mother a little enmeshed. Guilt and anger about relationship with mother, also father.	Identity issues, depression. Social alienation and conflicted relationships with friends. Looking for partner, friends, idealizing others, frequently disappointed. Anger and guilt after rejections. Competition.
Treatments and response			Previous psychotherapy with some response. Good response to antidepressant, with decreased mood reactivity and interpersonal sensitivity.

FIGURE 7.1. Psychodynamic Formulation Worksheet for Peter.

each of these building blocks of development. The worksheet illustrated here has notations about Peter's history. We use an additional column for each subsequent decade of life (e.g., 20–30 years old, 30–40 years old).

The top row is for *seminal life events,* including major family changes or disruptions, traumatic or medical events, life-changing developmental events such as starting a new school or leaving home, and occupational or relationship events. This category reflects external reality, the things that happened in the patient's life.

Key subjective experiences refers to the patient's description of frequent mental states or experiences and is connected to psychiatric symptoms such as marked anxiety, depression, or obsessional behavior. It includes both how the patient feels and felt and the symptoms that developed. Examples of entries in this row include more general experiences such as loneliness, fear, contentment, as well as more specific experiences such as worry about physical attractiveness, anxiety about money, or confusion about career. More information is better than less here.

The role of trauma as an external factor in the development of psychopathology is clear, as is its often profound effect on personality development and intrapsychic life. A psychodynamic formulation will need to carefully conceptualize the effects of single traumatic experiences, recurrent trauma, and recurrent micro-trauma on experiences of self and other, self-esteem, and subsequent psychopathology. The traumatic experiences will be noted with seminal life experiences and the associated recurring subjective experiences and symptoms along that row. It is important to maintain a curious and open attitude when inquiring about trauma and not to suggest or encourage memories.

Neurobiological factors refers to those nondynamic aspects of the patient such as proneness to mood disorder, psychosis, anxiety, substance use, eating disorder, and attentional problems, or biologically driven temperamental or personality factors. It is certainly an inference to determine whether there are neurobiological factors in the patient's presentation, but the formulation is an inference and a working document that can and should change with time. We recognize the need to develop hypotheses about the impact of early relationships and conflicts on the patient—we are bold about hypothesizing and modest about concluding—and there is no reason not to take the same attitude when hypothesizing about what is biologically and what is environmentally driven.

Summers (2002) recommended assessment of the following factors:

1. The role of temperament, that innate part of the personality, importantly determines behavior and experience, and surely affects the child's emerging experience of self, and others (Chess & Thomas, 1996; Rutter, 1987). Psychodynamic formulation should attempt to clarify what may derive from intrapsychic conflict and/or developmental difficulties, and what may be temperamental.

2. Better classification and identification of childhood psychopathology has helped to elucidate the potential impact of childhood psychopathology on development and adult psychopathology (Biederman

et al., 1993). This would include identification of learning difficulties and other neurodevelopmental vulnerabilities and their impact on the individual and on personality dynamics (Brown, 2000). Childhood psychiatric diagnosis should be included and its impact discussed.

3. The impact of subsyndromal illness on emotional development has not been well studied (Akiskal, 2001), for example, mild mood syndromes that later become full-fledged illness, or anxiety problems that do not meet severity threshold. The possible subsyndromal symptoms that even young children experience may have a profound impact on the development of self-esteem and may be crucial factors in emotional development (Biederman, Hirshfeld-Becker, & Rosenbaum, 2001). This may be evident retrospectively only when reconstructing an adult patient's development.

4. With the advent of increasingly effective and powerful pharmacological treatments, there are many individuals who have had effective medication treatment over an extended period of time and at earlier critical developmental periods. Surely these interventions, and their effect on patients' experiences, have also shaped their experience of self. These effects must now be considered to be important environmental experiences in their own right that effect subsequent development.

Syndromal pathology refers to the presence of frank psychiatric symptoms that are part of a longitudinal illness. The diagnosis of a syndrome, or the appearance of a neurobiological vulnerability, should be noted when it is apparent in the history. We are aware that collecting information about neurobiological factors may be difficult, and the patient may not be able to provide enough information. In some instances, you may want to include family members in gathering the history. This listing of neurobiological factors is intended as a prompt to ask about these areas; it is not necessary to comment about them in the formulation unless they are relevant.

The row entitled *psychodynamic themes* allows the clinician to note emerging areas of dynamic conflict. These notations are a first take at describing the problems and conflicts as they show themselves. Examples include loss, dependency, competition, guilt, conflict with women or men, authority problems, separation, self-esteem problems, rigidity, anger and impulsivity, or fear of bodily damage. Although these themes do not map directly onto the six core problems—depression, obsessionality, fear of abandonment, low self-esteem, panic anxiety, and trauma—these mini-inferences will help you decide which of the core psychodynamic problems best describes your patient. This row is also the place to make notations of repetitive patterns using the CCRT format.

Previous treatments and the responses to them are noted in the last row of the worksheet, and this includes both psychotherapy and psychopharmacology. Arraying these treatment responses in the worksheet reminds us that treatment takes place over the life cycle. Much can be learned from what worked and did not work before, and transferential patterns are a window into the psychodynamic problems.

WRITING THE FORMULATION

The data you gather and jot down on the formulation worksheet need to be synthesized. You may be able to connect the dots and see the core psychodynamic problem and how it runs through the patient's life, or it may still be obscure.

An optimal formulation would include 750–1,000 words. It should be written simply and clearly, with as little jargon as possible. Specific examples can illustrate the points made. The formulation is not a history, and you should resist the urge to write up all of the information you gather. A good formulation is at a higher level of inference than a history. We describe the four parts of the written formulation, based on Perry et al. (1987) and Summers (2002), and this is summarized in Table 7.1. The example formulation at the beginning of this chapter follows this format.

Overview

Part 1 summarizes the patient's identifying information, events precipitating the illness, and salient predisposing factors. This section sets the scene for the rest of the formulation, so it should summarize critical information such as major historical events, the extent and quality of interpersonal relationships, and a summary of important neurobiological factors. Part 1 concludes with a review of the behavior that will be explained by the formulation. This section gives the reader an overview of the patient and a summary of the core problem, symptoms, vulnerabilities, strengths, and life events that the rest of the formulation will attempt to explain.

Nondynamic Factors

Part 2 details the nondynamic factors relevant to the formulation. This begins with any concurrent syndromal diagnoses, such as major depression or bipolar disorder. This is followed by a summary of neurobiologi-

TABLE 7.1. Elements in Comprehensive Psychodynamic Formulation

Part 1: Summarizing statement

- Patient identification
- Very brief summary of:
  - Precipitating events
  - Most salient predisposing factors in the history
  - Major historical events
  - Extent and quality of interpersonal relationships
  - Important aspects of neurobiology
- Behaviors that the formulation will attempt to explain

Part 2: Description of nondynamic factors

- Current syndromal diagnosis
- Family history of psychiatric illness
- Brief summary of relevant information about:
  - Syndromal psychiatric illness
  - Temperamental factors
  - Childhood psychopathology
  - Subsyndromal illness
  - Psychopharmacology experiences
  - Other factors: medical illness, mental retardation, social deprivation, drugs/physical factors affecting the brain
  - Traumatic experiences

Part 3: Psychodynamic explanation of central conflicts

- Core psychodynamic problem
- Tracing of core problem and associated conflicts through personal history
  - Include childhood example, major life event, recent example
- Explanation of patient's attempts to resolve this problem that have been maladaptive and adaptive
- Formulation of core problems and central conflicts using the psychodynamic models most useful for the problem:
  - Important conscious and unconscious wishes, motives, behavior, defenses
  - Important developmental struggles
- Derive a potential recurrent CCRT
- Key strengths and how they have interacted with problems
- Effect of nondynamic factors in shaping psychodynamic problem via their effects on experience of self, other, and relationships
- Effect of dynamic factors on development and maintenance of syndromal illness

Part 4: Predicting responses to the therapeutic situation

- Prognosis, focusing on patient's experience of treatment
- Probable transference manifestations, expected resistances
- Personality strengths likely to be employed over course of treatment
- Probable reactions to psychopharmacological treatment
- Prognosis for treatment response in phases of treatment

Note. From Summers (2002). Used with permission of the Association for the Advancement of Psychotherapy.

cal vulnerability in the style of a "review of systems": family psychiatric history, temperament, childhood psychopathology from the syndromal perspective, history of subsyndromal or prodromal illness, responsiveness to psychopharmacology, and identifiable traumatic experiences. These factors are described with their essential supporting evidence. Of course, there will be variation in the degree of certainty about these factors, ranging from clearly supported diagnoses with good data to inference and hypothesis. Because the formulation is always a work in progress, which we hope will be modified and refined, inferences are not only permissible, but also necessary to create a comprehensive picture of the patient.

Psychodynamic Synthesis

The psychodynamic synthesis is presented in *Part 3*. This is the hardest section to write, but the most important. It begins with a statement about which of the six psychodynamic problems the patient is struggling with, and the rest of the section will support and illustrate this. The central conflicts associated with this particular psychodynamic problem should be illustrated. Three examples, including a childhood experience, a seminal life event, and an event in recent history should be described and related to the psychodynamic problem and associated conflicts. You must show how each of these three events reflects the patient's core problem and her typical solution to it. The psychoanalytic model that best explains that psychodynamic problem—ego psychology, object relations, or self psychology (see Table 3.1)—will supply the language for describing the problem.

For example, if the patient's main problem is fear of abandonment, the core conflict will likely involve separation and anger; these conflicted feelings will be present in important relationships and emerge at crucial life events. As discussed in Chapter 6 (on fear of abandonment), object relations theory supplies the most useful language. The typical problems with object constancy and split self- and object representations can be illustrated with a childhood experience with a parent, a crucial life event, and something in the recent history. The examples will flesh out the description of the conflict and support it by showing the life data. Viewing this example from the CCRT perspective, the wish is for closeness, the response of other is distancing, and the response of self is anger.

The formulation explains how the patient has attempted to manage these painful conflicts, as well as his or her important defenses, wishes, and identifications. Like a recurring theme, or a "red thread" that runs through the history, a good formulation shows the essential problems, how they have been expressed throughout the patient's life, and how the patient managed them (e.g., defenses). Personality strengths provide resilience and ballast to these problems and their impact, and they should be described here, too.

Because development is driven by many nondynamic factors as well, a modern psychodynamic formulation attempts to integrate dynamic with nondynamic factors in understanding a patient's life. Thus there are two additional tasks you must accomplish in Part 3 of the formulation.

First, you should address the impact of the patient's neurobiology on the form and content of the psychodynamic conflicts. Just as the experiences of self and other are shaped by events, so are they shaped by the individual's neurobiology. For example, the temperamentally active and aggressive child will address the developmental challenges of separation–individuation, the oedipal period, adolescence, and adult life cycle stages differently from the more placid person. The child with a bipolar vulnerability, who develops syndromal illness in the late teenage years, and whose subclinical symptoms were retrospectively present in the preteen years, likely had subtle deficits in affect regulation that made maturation more difficult. The child with symptoms of attention-deficit/ hyperactivity disorder (ADHD) who experienced profound self-esteem injury associated with difficulties in rule-bound behavior may have particular challenges in developing a sense of mastery. Childhood obsessive–compulsive disorder may intensify separation difficulties because of a profound need for reassurance along with a sense of premature autonomy and aloneness. While childhood experiences have particular impact on development, these neurobiological factors undoubtedly affect all of the subsequent development.

Second, you should hypothesize about how the dynamics affected the neurobiology. That is, how have the psychodynamic issues contributed to the development, recurrence, maintenance, or resolution of syndromal illness? Typical examples here would include the triggering of panic attacks and panic disorder by the activation of conflict over aggression in a work setting in a patient with a three-generation history of panic, or the recurrence of major depression precipitated by increased marital tension in a patient with a history of early separation and loss.

The hypotheses about the relationship between dynamics and neurobiology are often more speculative than other elements of the formulation. Some think this is impossible to do. We recognize the difficulty, but feel that developing a formulation is a process of using limited data to develop an overarching explanation, in this area and others. There is an ongoing process of refining, changing, and improving the accuracy of the formulation. If you do not explicitly hypothesize about the neurobiology–dynamic relationship, you (and the patient) will make assumptions about it; then it will be implicit and not discussed and considered. In the end, you are allowed to be wrong!

In summary, Part 3 sets out the core psychodynamic problem, this patient's specific conflicts and defenses, at least three vignettes (childhood, major life event, recent history) that illustrate and support these ideas, and speculations about how the nondynamic factors influenced the patient's dynamics and vice versa.

Response to Therapeutic Situation

Part 4 focuses on predicting the patient's response to the therapeutic situation, drawing on the synthesis of Part 3. This includes how the patient may experience treatment and probable transference manifestations. You may also hypothesize about those strengths upon which the patient will particularly rely during the treatment. Because the defensive style and transference paradigm will inevitably affect a patient's attitude toward medication, the formulation should hypothesize about the anticipated reactions to psychopharmacology, as well as the emerging treatment relationship.

The prognosis should include conjectures about the phases that may evolve in treatment. For example, the treatment of a patient with depression who has been refractory to previous psychopharmacology and psychotherapy may include a prolonged phase of psychopharmacology trials, along with attention to psychological factors that have contributed to treatment refractoriness. During this initial phase, the patient may periodically feel close to and taken care of by the therapist, and this reaction could allow for a better psychopharmacological response. The next phase of treatment might involve more intensive psychotherapeutic work, with a more conflicted transference reaction; the patient may be able to work more effectively in this mode because the depressive symptoms are less severe due to psychopharmacology.

PROBLEMS AND PITFALLS

There is often some vagueness in the initial formulation—it is the picture as you see it after a few sessions. Although there is a lot one cannot understand at this point, a useful formulation commits to a clear way of organizing the data. Then we can focus on the areas of uncertainty and listen carefully to see whether the initial formulation is borne out. It should provide the basis for an engaged discussion with the patient; if not, then you should go back to the drawing board in the spirit of inquiry and collaboration. You should not think of your formulation as a private test of your understanding; rather, it is a work in progress to be discussed, reflected on, and modified.

It is important to commit to one core problem, recognizing that there may be other problems that are relevant, or that may become central later in treatment. The purpose of the formulation is to guide your approach to the patient in therapy. If you cannot distinguish between two or three equally important problems, how will you be able to help the patient begin to understand himself, and how will you decide what to comment on? Most patients cannot work on two or three problems at once, especially early in treatment.

Writing a formulation will expose you (and, ultimately, the patient) to the limitations of current knowledge about development, psychopathology, neurobiology, and how they fit together. In addition, it makes us confront what we do not or cannot know about the specific patient we are treating. It is not possible to know what the patient's childhood was really like, or how to most simply express the essential conflicts. Both patient and therapist have initial ideas, and they will certainly change over time.

In writing Peter's formulation, we speculated about the impact of the patient's social anxiety, and family history of depression and psychosis. We often cannot tell how much temperament or the genetics of personality contributed to the development of an illness, and how much was contributed by a patient's adverse environmental experiences. Although this type of understanding is evolving in our field through the study of populations, in any specific case we rarely know. Yet the formulation calls for an estimate of this. Of course, limited information has never stopped the curious dynamic therapist from hypothesizing about earlier relationships and developmental experiences, so it should not stop us from hypothesizing about the relationship between biology and dynamics. Not only is it important for the therapist to conceptualize this connection, but some patients want to understand their neurobiology as well. Modern narratives of the self include an impression of one's neurobiological fingerprint, and many patients think about their genetic vulnerability, especially if they are struggling with emotional problems.

Peter completed his treatment after 5 years of intensive psychotherapy and medication feeling much more content and stable. He continued to be vulnerable to loss and depression, but managed far better. He understood his acute sensitivity to feeling overwhelmed by women, his urge to connect with strong men, and his tendency to deal with his anger in a guilty and self-defeating manner. He worked through these feelings in the transference relationship with the therapist, and had increasingly healthy positive intimate relationships. He was dating and had several satisfying and close relationships with women. The main themes identified in the initial formulation did turn out to be important and relevant. But his later problem with procrastination and uncertainty about his interests and talents was not so clear early on. It was obscured by his intense depressive symptoms and his attempt to just survive. Subsequently, these problems became a focus in the treatment. Peter was ultimately able to apply and gain admission to a competitive graduate school and launch his career. He finished therapy feeling open and enthusiastic about the future.

We end this chapter on a note of caution in the description of the case. We hypothesize that the patient changed because of the treatment we describe, but we cannot be sure because psychotherapy, like life, is not a controlled experiment. We make choices, we take actions, we learn, and we change. We can never be certain the changes would not have occurred in the absence of therapy.

SUMMARY

The psychodynamic formulation is a concise conceptualization of the patient's problem that begins with the core psychodynamic problem and illustrates the connections between the patient's symptoms, key childhood experiences, seminal life events, and current life issues. A comprehensive formulation combines psychodynamic with nondynamic factors in understanding the patient's life course. The formulation allows the therapist to anticipate the unfolding of the treatment, including the opportunities for change, obstacles and resistances, and emerging themes in the therapeutic relationship.

~

CHAPTER 8

Defining a Focus
and Setting Goals

A person who aims at nothing is sure to hit it.
—ANONYMOUS

The formulation and data gathered in the initial sessions suggest a focus for treatment. The focus will help to jump-start the therapeutic process and build the therapeutic alliance at the same time. With a clearly defined focus, you may be able to shorten the treatment, work more consistently on what the patient offers, and strengthen the relationship. You should be cautious about jumping to conclusions in deriving a formulation, as well as rushing to define a focus. You may not yet have recognized an important aspect of the problem, and, of course, the patient may not yet feel comfortable discussing the whole story. But the advantages of an early focus outweigh the risks, and in our practices, no good day goes without an apology for getting something wrong, followed by a significant change in direction. We define a focus early and change it if needed.

Defining a *focus* means agreeing with the patient on how you will describe the problem, and therefore how you will attack it together. This can be done within the first two to six sessions, after you know the core problems and the formulation is developing. The focus provides the therapist with a way of thinking about what to explore, what to ask about, and how to frame and phrase interventions. It is something that is agreed upon with the patient, and it needs to be collaborative. It is different from a *goal*, which is an endpoint in therapy. The goal is what we hope will happen if patient and therapist successfully focus.

These working definitions of focus and goal are how therapists tend to think about treatment, but not the intuitive way patients do. For the patient, the goal is everything. It is what she wants, what she hopes for, what she hopes to achieve. Usually, the patient expresses ideas and feelings about the goal, and the therapist works backward to define a focus.

For example, a patient who came to therapy complaining that her husband was passive, depressed, and insensitive, and whose wish was for her husband to change and love her more, needed help to come up with a useful focus for her therapy. Needless to say, the therapy was not likely to help change her husband. The therapist focused on why she felt so rejected when her husband was introverted and quiet. Why did she feel so driven to take care of him and so angry about it? What impact did her anger and hurt have on how she treated him, and on their relationship? The focus of the therapy became her needs and conflicts—dependency, caretaking, sacrifice, resentment, fears of abandonment—and what she could do about them. The focus was on things inside her that she could do something about. The goal was to decrease the intrusion of old feelings, needs, and defenses into the current situation, to help her decide whether she should stay in the marriage and have the best relationship she could.

There is a particular feeling a therapist has when the focus of treatment is clear. There is a sense of clarity and purpose about the interaction, and it is like exercising a toned muscle. From the perspective of the therapeutic alliance, a defined focus reflects agreement on goals and tasks and probably helps to promote the bond between therapist and patient. However, defining a focus requires an effort on the part of the therapist, as it does not necessarily emerge on its own.

PATIENT GOALS

Although patients come for help because they want to feel better in some way, their goals for the treatment vary widely. Some want to change something about their internal state—to feel less anxiety, or feel more satisfaction or pleasure. Some want to change an aspect of their functioning—to improve the ability to concentrate, or the capacity to organize themselves in some particular area. They may want to make an important external life change, like marrying or separating, having children, changing careers, or changing relationships with parents or siblings. Some want to deal with life cycle developmental problems, such as adapting to aging or loss or a change in the family. Some want to change somebody else, a goal that needs to be reframed.

Some patients are very ambitious and aspire to marked and dramatic changes. Others have more incremental goals in mind. Some have a more narrow focus, with one thing they want to change, and they are disinclined to work on anything not related to that goal. Whether realistic or not, some want a major personality change.

Sometimes goals are expressed in the patient's "theory" of the problem. Every patient (and every person) has a theory for why they are the way they are. This theory is usually a mix of realistic, accurate perceptions, but it usually also contains rationalizations and attempts to explain things the patient does not understand, and it avoids acknowledging thorny and painful aspects of the problem. Patients' goals usually follow from their theories. Examples of this include: "My anxiety comes from having bad, reprehensible thoughts, and I need to control these thoughts, and then I'll feel better." The patient's implicit goal might be avoidance of stimulating situations and distraction and suppression of thoughts. Or "I've behaved badly, and now I am guilty and deserve criticism and punishment." The goal associated with this theory is to prove oneself to be blameless and good, and not deserving of punishment. Another is: "There is something unlovable about me; I am angry and bad, and this causes others to leave me." The theory is that they are noxious and this is the cause of their loneliness, and the patient's goal is to not feel angry.

UNSTATED GOALS

You must ask the patient about his or her goals, and explore and discuss them. This helps the initial engagement, and it is a key foundation for the development of a therapeutic alliance. But the alert therapist will recognize that every patient comes with important unstated, private goals and unconscious wishes for the treatment. Examples include the wish for protection, the wish to engage in a power struggle and achieve victory, the wish to be admired or idealized, or the wish to be loved. Most patients are unaware of these goals, or have never thought about them seriously. Sometimes dynamic therapy will help clarify their unstated goals as they become more self-aware.

Some patients know very little about psychotherapy, and their initial comments about goals reflect lack of experience and lack of information, rather than important ideas about their conscious and unconscious goals. With more experience in the therapy, they are able to communicate their thoughts more cogently. Some patients are afraid to venture into a discussion of goals out of fear of not achieving them, or because doing so will touch on uncomfortable feelings about the therapist, such as dependency or affection. Sometimes, the very problems they came to therapy for make it hard to communicate clearly about this.

Danielle, a 22-year-old woman, came for treatment after an overdose with over-the-counter medication. In the hospitalization that followed the overdose, she related her lonely and failure-filled history.

Attractive in a waif-like way but extraordinarily shy, the patient had marked social anxiety and a proneness to social avoidance from an early age. She grew up in an upper-middle-class family with seemingly attentive and involved parents. Her older brother struggled with significant learning disabilities and become a great focus of early attention in the family. Her affectionate and socially anxious mother responded to her anxiety with sympathy and a permissive attitude. When Danielle was disinclined to play with children in the neighborhood, the mother accepted this and helped arrange for enjoyable solo activities. When she wanted to stay home from school, this was allowed.

At times, the parents pushed Danielle to become more connected outside the family, but she was adamantly avoidant. She usually felt that she had the upper hand in what evolved into control battles about decisions related to school, summer camp, vacations, and so on. Often she and her parents entirely avoided these conflicts with pleasant but superficial interaction. Ironically, she lost respect for her mother because she could control her so easily.

Danielle had a verbal learning disability and developed increasing perfectionism, obsessionality, and preoccupation with weight and appearance. She became more isolated as the years passed, and had virtually no social contacts outside of school during her high school years. She went to a small college far from home, and felt thrown into closer proximity to others her age than she had experienced ever before. Excited about her prospects yet intensely anxious, she struggled to be "normal," while feeling chronically confused and alienated. Secretly, she hoped to escape the demands of her peer relationships. At the end of her first year, she had the feeling that she had to either have "real relationships" with people or leave school. Unfortunately, she felt overwhelmed by getting close to others students and left.

Following a brief time at home with her parents, Danielle tried again to launch herself. She lived with a group of other young adults conducting an ecological study project in an isolated rural area. Repeating the pattern of wanting but running from social connections, she soon felt she needed to leave, and returned home. However, after this escape from the requirements and demands of peers, she became acutely depressed and made the overdose that resulted in her hospitalization.

Danielle's core psychodynamic problem was fear of abandonment. As she began treatment, her stated goals were to find something that she cared about and an activity or place of some kind that would inspire and motivate her. She felt hopeless and wanted to feel part of something and feel hope about the future. She asked for assessment, advice, direction, and support for doing something and sticking with it. Essentially, she said: "I want a life, and I want advice, support and pushing to make it happen." Eventually, she commented, "You are supposed to give me a life."

Over time, as she talked more about her thoughts, feelings, and fantasies in the therapy, it became clear that she had an intensely held fantasy about the therapy and the therapist. She saw herself as a small, defenseless baby, looking for protection by a large, powerful, and benign mother. She had fantasies about being a baby in the therapist's womb, about being a little bird standing on the therapist's shoulder following him around all day long, and about being a small child standing just behind the therapist "in his shadow."

This example shows a rather dramatic contrast between stated and unstated goals for this patient—she came saying she wanted to find a sense of personal meaning and identity, but longed for an almost symbiotic relationship. Although there is always a difference between a patient's stated and unstated goals, eventually in treatment they must begin to converge. The uncovering process facilitates awareness of the unconscious goals, and after a while Danielle was able to recognize her fantasies about being a baby. She mourned the difference between what she wanted and would always want, and what was more realistic and achievable.

It is not always easy for the therapist to elucidate the unstated goals, and even more difficult to have a patient recognize them. However, when this happens it leads to deeper and more powerful insight, as the patient sees how the unstated goal is usually applicable to other important figures in the patient's life and not just the therapist.

HOW IMPORTANT ARE THE PATIENT'S CONSCIOUS GOALS?

A good coach knows that you must respect a player's level of skill and competence, build confidence, support and encourage improvement, and set a high bar of expectations. Likewise, a good psychotherapist must accept the patient where she is, respecting her stated goals, listening carefully for the unstated ones, and expect as much growth and change as possible.

Patients' stated goals must form the basis for the initial engagement until you are able to collaboratively change them. This is out of respect for their skills, strengths, accomplishments and struggle with their problems, and the recognition that they have done their best with it, and because they know themselves better than the therapist knows them. Also, to do otherwise would be to undermine an essential part of the therapeutic alliance.

If you think the goals should be changed, then it is certainly reasonable to suggest this. For example, you might say, "Would it be more realistic to adapt to the way your father is, and find a good accommodation, rather than try to change the whole tenor of the relationship?" Or, "Maybe the issue is to find a way to start a new relationship rather than rekindle the old one."

Successful therapy involves setting reasonable and achievable goals and accepting that some goals cannot be achieved. Setting unreasonable goals for therapy may stem from a generous appreciation of the patient's potentials, but it will likely result in disappointment, reexperiencing of failure, and frustration.

DEFINING A USEFUL FOCUS

It is not up to the therapist to make the ultimate decision about the goal for treatment, but it is a crucial responsibility to propose a reasonable and appropriate focus. We begin the process of defining a focus by taking inventory of the following five factors: formulation, wide versus narrow focus, ambition and motivation, level of the problem, and the patient's personality characteristics (Table 8.1).

TABLE 8.1. Relevant Factors in Defining a Treatment Focus

- Formulation of the patient's problem
- Wide versus narrow focus
- Motivation
- Level of problem
  - Intrapsychic
  - Relational/systemic
  - Life cycle/developmental
  - Adaptation to neurobiology
- Patient characteristics

Formulation of the Patient's Problem

The treatment must focus on the core psychodynamic problem and the patient's particular conflicts reflecting this problem. You should explain what you think the core problem is in plain English, simply spoken. This makes it easier to understand both cognitively and emotionally.

In the case of Peter, the depression involved guilt, identity problems, low self-esteem, conflict about women, and a pattern of procrastination. The formulation ties these conflicts together, with historical antecedents, and identifies the important nondynamic factors involved. This gist of this formulation is Peter's need to be close, and the upsetting feelings that come up about this in close relationships. The focus of treatment must include this essential conflict.

Our clinical experience leads us to believe that guilt and conflict in intimate relationships are problems psychodynamic psychotherapy is especially helpful for. But we cannot rely on hard data to support this contention because research on treatment efficacy, unfortunately, has focused on diagnoses rather than on the issues that often bring people to treatment.

Wide or Narrow Focus

How wide or narrow to focus the treatment depends on how global or how localized the problem is. Some patients present problems that are relatively circumscribed, although they may be severe, with less intrusion of these problems into other areas of their lives. Others relate a picture of more pervasive difficulty, where most or all important areas are involved.

One wants to be parsimonious in defining goals for psychotherapy, treating only what needs to be treated. This makes sense from an efficiency perspective, but it is also important because dysfunction in one area may cause fallout and difficulty in others, and if the primary area of difficulty is ameliorated, there may be improvement in other areas without specific therapeutic attention. For example, a person with difficulties in intimate relationships may have relatively less conflict and minimal symptoms in occupational function, but the misery and preoccupation that results from conflict in their personal life may spill over and affect work and work relationships. Attention and improvement in personal relationships would result in improvements at work even without specific therapeutic attention.

Some patients tend to stay focused on one area, talking only about their family life, or only about their somatic symptoms. The clinical judgment you must make is whether this is a manifestation of anxiety and resistance to looking more deeply, or whether it is simply a more focal problem. There are patients who intuitively connect disparate areas of thinking, feeling, and functioning; for them everything is related to everything else. Is this wide ranging and probing, or inefficient, meandering, and nonproductive? It is frustrating to trainees that there is no clear way of making this determination. But the guiding principle for evaluating the success of the focus you have defined is whether the patient's self-awareness is developing further and getting clearer. Knowing when progress is being made is sometimes only apparent later, and this validates the clinical judgments.

Motivation

This hard-to-define quality is essential in thinking about how ambitious the therapist should be. Some patients seem to be truly willing to go the distance in struggling, thinking, and collaborating to try to get better. Some are certainly suffering, but they have less perseverance and focus in enduring the rigors and difficulties of psychotherapy. Although some therapists reduce the idea of patient's motivation to something about the patient's pathology (e.g., less motivated because of rigidity of defenses) most experienced practitioners would consider there to be a motivational factor that is independent of the patient's problems. This factor may be the same quality that allows people to delay gratification, to focus and persevere in work and sports, and overcome physical problems.

Which Level to Focus On?

Each patient's problem can be studied and understood at many levels of analysis—individual, relational, developmental, and neurobiological. Defining a focus means choosing one level to work on primarily. Things get too complicated for patients if you try to do too many things at once. There are four possible levels to focus on:

1. *Intrapsychic.* This is the traditional psychodynamic individual psychotherapy model in which the patient's problems are understood to be based on conflict within her own mind, with subsequent compromise formations and behaviors. The problem is seen as a consequence of dysfunctional adaptation to conflict, and the goal of therapy is to understand the constituent parts to the conflict in order to arrive at a better adaptation to it. The therapist recommends that the patient try to understand the intrapsychic conflict in order to bring about a change in experience, perception, and behavior. Focusing on the CCRT (see Chapter 3) as the core of the intrapsychic conflict is one way to formulate the problem in a manner readily understandable and palatable to the patient and easily achievable by therapists in training.

2. *Relational/systemic.* Here the focus is on the relational level of the patient's problem. The focus is still on the patient's own psyche, but it is on how an important relationship affects him or her. What determines the patient's responses, and how does his behavior then affect the relationship? Essentially, the therapist proposes to help the patient improve his adaptation to a relationship or system, and thereby improve his subjective state and his behavior. Here, too, focusing on the CCRT could be helpful.

3. *Life cycle/developmental.* The emphasis in this type of problem is on the usual developmental stages through which children and adults progress, the anticipated transitions and crises, and the ubiquitous life cycle events such as loss of a parent, illness, children growing up, and relationship maturation and change. Here the patient's problem is seen as resulting from normal life cycle events and difficulties in adapting to these events. What makes this a psychodynamic perspective is the conviction that intrapsychic conflict and compromise can be obstacles to the effective management and resolution of these life cycle challenges. The impetus for psychotherapy is to allow the patient to deal most effectively with these normative developmental issues.

4. *Adaptation to neurobiology.* This fourth level of explanation, and of focusing the therapy, is based on adaptation to neurobiological

constraints. These constraints may include temperamental vulnerabilities such as shyness and social sensitivity, or proneness toward temper and impulsiveness. It may also include adaptations to genetic vulnerability to psychiatric illness such as mood disorders or anxiety disorders. This focus helps the patient understand the brain-based causal aspect of her experiences, the meanings she attributes to her way of responding, and attempts to find an improved adaptive response. For example, a patient may recognize her temperamental equanimity, low reactivity, and affective reserve, or emotionality and tendency to feel intensely.

These four different levels of understanding—intrapsychic, relational/systemic, life cycle/developmental, and adaptation to neurobiology—are distinct from one another. Each level of explanation has strengths and weaknesses, and of course, one may be closer to the patient's own way of thinking about the problem.

The intrapsychic provides a clear focus for treatment and clear rationale for individual work, but it may be more anxiety provoking, more likely to induce resistance, and make the patient feel "pathologized." The relational/system level of explanation is likely to resonate well with the patient's complaints, but limits the focus of the treatment to that relationship or system. The life cycle/developmental level usefully supports and validates the ubiquitous problems of adolescent and adult development and helps the patient to see herself in a larger context. However, by "normalizing" the problem, it can lessen the potential for exploration and understanding of the individual conflictual background for the patient's problem. Therefore, it may somewhat reduce the motivation for therapy. Finally, the adaptation perspective is essential to help a patient with significant neurobiological vulnerability to illness, yet the extent of the neurobiological and psychodynamic contributions is not always clear. This focus runs the risk of inadequately working on the dynamic issues or trying to modify biology, which may be rather difficult.

Patient Characteristics

Evaluating patient characteristics that predict good response to psychodynamic psychotherapy (and psychotherapy in general) has been the subject of exhaustive research. We do not discuss this in great detail here, but summarize the findings. The following characteristics seem to be associated with the ability to respond to psychodynamic treatment: psychological mindedness, curiosity, introspection, ability to utilize metaphor and symbols, verbal ability, intelligence, and ease of or capacity for closeness in relationships (Gabbard, 2000; Ursano, Sonnenberg, & Lazar, 1998; Beutel, Stern, & Silbersweig, 2003). However, we do not want to leave the impression that dynamic psychotherapy is only a treatment for the worried well. The patient characteristics discussed are associated with but not required for good outcome. For example, Milrod, Leon, Barber et al. (2007) reported that the presence of Cluster C personality disorder (as opposed to no personality disorder) predicted a better response to psychodynamic treatment of panic.

In addition to the patient characteristics that traditionally predict psychotherapy responsiveness are the resources the patient has available to him in contemplating treatment. These include time for the treatment, emotional energy to give to the process, financial resources, and support by others for the process.

BRINGING THE FACTORS TOGETHER

The therapist attempts to synthesize all of the factors just discussed into a focus that combines understanding of the patient expressed in the formulation, the patient's motivation and resources, an awareness of the breadth or narrowness of the focus that would be useful, the patient characteristics, and the level of the problem. The focus should offer the most parsimonious way of working with the patient's problems. The patient's conscious goals, impressions about the unconscious goals, and a sense of the initial interaction between therapist and patient must also be synthesized into the focus.

Of course, we are describing a process that is, of necessity, highly individualized. By taking an inventory of all these factors, the novice therapist will learn how to take charge of this essential part of beginning the treatment. Rather than wait passively for the patient to define a focus, you can take a more active approach. We will illustrate this synthetic process with two examples describing the patient and problems, the inventory of factors, and the proposed focus. One will be an example of a successfully defined focus, and one not so successful.

> Carrie was a 53-year-old woman who came for evaluation because of depression and concern about her college-age daughter's emotionality. She was worried that her daughter had a personality disorder and it was her fault. Carrie was a tall, attractive woman with a brunette ponytail and an easy smile. She seemed a little embar-

rassed about seeing a therapist, and was polite, eager to please, and deferential.

Carrie's daughter was in therapy and seemed to depend on her mother for advice and help with surprisingly basic life decisions, all the while successfully managing a demanding academic load. She was resentful of her mother and critical of her. Carrie felt burdened by looking after her daughter and guilty that somehow her daughter's problems must have to do with her mothering. She was quite insistent on this last point; after all, she argued, what other explanation could there be for her daughter's problems? There were two younger children, both of whom seemed to be quite well adjusted.

Carrie was the younger of two children born to the second marriage of a dashing but unfaithful lawyer and his beautiful but critical and insecure wife. Carrie's mother disliked her older brother, the product of the father's first marriage, and was overly attached to her older sister, an academically precocious and socially inept scholar. Her father died a year before Carrie came to treatment, and this was a great loss. Growing up, the father was engaging, lively, affectionate, and nonjudgmental, while Carrie felt her mother was insecure and angry. Later as an adult, she saw her mother as competitive and bitter.

Rather quickly, the flow of topics began to shift toward vignettes about the mother. Practically every phone call, visit, or interaction felt irritating and rejecting. Her mother never said the right thing; she seemed to need to get the last word in, or she left longish pauses on the phone to indicate her disapproval. She talked endlessly about herself, her health, and her loneliness. But Carrie felt compelled to listen and be helpful.

By the third session, the therapist had begun to organize the formulation around the core problem of depression, noting the prominent self-criticism, guilt, and powerful ambivalence toward her mother and her daughter. It had also become clear that although the daughter certainly had her difficulties, and perhaps there was some earlier disruption in the mother–daughter bond that had contributed to this, Carrie had certainly tried very hard and done quite a good job as a mother. The therapist's impression was that this worry about her daughter was symptomatic of the core problem, rather than a serious realistic concern.

Further exploration of Carrie's current life revealed that she had a loving relationship with her husband, who was fun-loving and high-spirited but irresponsible. He did not seem to pull his weight in managing the kids, taking care of the finances, and working around the house. Carrie laughingly commented that it was really like having four children.

More childhood history came out, too. She felt that she was an afterthought in the family. Her sister was the apple of her mother's eye because of her academic prowess, and the brother was sweet to her but older and involved in other things. Her mother expected her to be available and responsive to her demands for attention, and was critical of anything that was emotionally "messy" or complicated. Early on Carrie developed a strong group of friends and felt that she lived much of her life with them. She tried her best to gain her mother's love and interest, but usually felt the best she could do was avoid too much criticism.

By this time, the formulation was even clearer. Carrie's depression had to do with an early attachment problem with her mother, leading to anger, self-criticism, and guilt, and she dealt with this by taking care of others—her mother, her husband, her children, and especially her troubled daughter.

Carrie's therapeutic interest was in her daughter and her mother, and the problems there. She had issues with her husband, but mostly she felt pleased about their relationship. Her other two children were a source of great joy. She enjoyed and was very successful in her career. Her ambition was to feel better about herself and especially find a way to manage these two troublesome relationships. She had a relatively narrow focus on what she wanted to change, and a more global change in her functioning was not her goal. She was strongly motivated and made it clear that if she felt she was getting somewhere, she was very committed to the appointments and to working hard.

Carrie's difficulties were best conceptualized at the intrapsychic level. One could have worked with her problem at the relational/systemic level, but the issues were not confined to one relationship or even one generation, and seemed to be part of what Carrie brought with her to each relationship. In fact, she had chosen a career that combined public service and pleasing clients. Although the life cycle level of the problem was relevant—her children were growing up and leaving home, and her mother was ailing—approaching her problems from this angle did not seem like it would help her get a handle on the powerful internal dynamic that seemed to be affecting her quality of life.

This patient had the classic characteristics of someone who will do well in therapy. She was verbal, bright, able to think in a flexible way, and naturally introspective. She also had the resources, time, and support from her husband to do the work. It is an interesting, and perhaps unfortunate, observation that when it comes to psychotherapy, those with the most psychological health often get the greatest benefit from treatment. This idea that "the rich get richer" should not be understood to mean that those with fewer psychological resources will not benefit from treatment, but rather, that the treatment of those who bring less resources to treatment may require an approach that is especially well organized, focused, and effective.

> In the fourth session, the therapist described his impression of the core problem—depression, self-criticism, guilt—and the sense that these feelings were organized around her feelings about her mother. He proposed that the focus of treatment be working out and understanding her ambivalence about her mother to allow her to find a better way to get the most she could in the relationship, and prepare for her ultimate death. This would give a clear and finite scope to the therapy, and the benefits of work would surely spill over into her other relationships. Carrie was tearful and upset in hearing this. It made her sad to realize how central the problem with her mother had always been, but she felt some relief at having it clearly spelled out. She was also relieved as it helped her see that her main struggle was with her mother, and that her guilt about her daughter was just a reflection of that—maybe she had had some problems as a mother, and if so, it was because of her own upbringing, not because she was so bad.

The focus was agreed on collaboratively. Having the focus allowed the therapist to encourage the patient to explore her feelings in a more vigorous active manner. The patient felt like she knew what she was working on and why. The treatment continued for slightly less than a year on a weekly basis. At the time of termination, Carrie was able to view her mother dispassionately, with more empathy and also more ability to assert and protect herself. She had pushed her husband to take on more responsibilities around the household, and had been able to let her daughter take greater distance and live independently after graduating from college.

But defining a focus does not always work out so well! When psychotherapeutic treatments are not very successful, there is a tendency to note the patient characteristics that prevented this, the intransigence of the problem, or the possibility that more time was needed to be able to make progress. But it is also possible that the treatment was not successful because there was not an appropriate focus. The next vignette illustrates this and involves some speculation about what might have been more helpful.

> Margaret was a lawyer in her late 30s who was referred for treatment because of depression and anxiety. She had previously been in an extended psychotherapy, which had not been terribly successful.
>
> Successful in her chosen career, she had unfortunately developed rheumatoid arthritis in her late 20s, and this had progressed recently, causing some physical limitations, especially in her exercise regimen. She had a long history of dating and conflicted relationships with men, including multiple experiences of feeling that men turned out to be dishonest, unreliable, and self-centered. She seemed to feel that she needed to be in a relationship.
>
> After being encouraged to "shop around" and meet with several therapists, Margaret chose the one she liked most. The early sessions involved much painful emotional detail about the multiple prior relationships with men, including the most recent experience of betrayal and hurt.
>
> The crucial aspect of Margaret's earlier history was a feeling that her parents were loving and supportive, but that her mother was unrealistically and indiscriminately positive about everything she did. She felt that her mother was afraid and upset when anything bad happened to her, and that she was supposed to live out her mother's "unborn wishes." She loved the unlimited support, but felt suffocated by it.

The therapist proceeded with an inventory of factors in defining a focus. The core psychodynamic problem and formulation suggested problems with self-esteem. The conflicts revolved around dependency and independence, as well as the need to please others. Her chronic illness must have exacerbated this. Margaret's problems seemed confined to personal relationships, and she had many of the characteristics predictive of a good psychotherapeutic response. Since she had had so much difficulty with men, the level of the problem that seemed most immediate was relational/systemic. The focus of the treatment would be a better understanding of the issues involved in intimate relationships. The goal was to have a successful relationship with a man. Margaret hoped the therapy would improve her ability to choose a potential mate, decrease behaviors that might contribute to conflict and strife, and help her to communicate and resolve problems that might come up.

The suggested focus resulted in an initial bounce in the patient's mood, and more motivation to consider her issues. There was also a medication change at the same time, so it was unclear which accounted for her feeling better. There followed an extended discussion of the painful feelings involved in her disappointments with men. It became clear that Margaret had a tendency to choose men who could be selfish, and then test and almost provoke them to express their limitations. As she described her painful experiences of hurt, rejection, and abandonment associated with this, she became more angry and frustrated with the therapist. Attempts were made to understand her anger and interpret it as a transferential reaction, that is, noting that she felt the same kind of encouragement and support that her mother provided, which led to hopeful optimism and then disappointed rejection. The patient experienced these interpretations as accurate but even more reason to feel depressed and rejected. Support and continued attempts to help the patient see her frustration with the treatment in this context, along with medication changes, were to no avail.

Margaret told the therapist that the focus of working on intimate relationships made sense, and the goal of helping her get into a good relationship was certainly what she wanted. But she felt this implied there was something the matter with her, and this was very upsetting and undermining to her. It reminded her of her parents just wanting her to be happy, and their wish for her to find a solution to her unhappiness rather than be herself. She expressed tearful appreciation for the help she had received early on in the treatment, but made it clear that she felt that just talking about men made her feel bad. Why did therapists always think that all a woman needs is a relationship with a man? She announced she was going to end the therapy.

When she ran into the therapist in a public setting approximately three years later, she volunteered that she was feeling much better, had met and recently married a man whom she felt relatively content with, and despite some progression in her physical illness, things were going pretty well.

Could more have been done? Were the limitations inherent in the technique of psychodynamic psychotherapy, the patient's history and the nature of her problems, aspects of her character, or the contribution of her neurobiology? What did the therapist fail to see? Did her progressive illness affect the way she saw treatment? Was she really as happy as she said she was later on? Had the treatment helped? There are no clear answers to these questions, but the patient had a specific criticism at the time the treatment ended that had to do with the focus of treatment and the goal that had been mutually agreed upon. This needs to be taken seriously, and one wonders whether defining the goal as a relational one, finding a good mate, was most helpful. Did it promote a replication in the discussion, and in the treatment relationship, of her mother's need for her to be normal, happy, and healthy? She was very sensitive to criticism.

Should the focus have been more on the development of her capacity for independence, self-awareness, and self-acceptance? That is, perhaps the therapist should have defined a focus related to the development of independence and self-sufficiency, based more on the life cycle/developmental metaphor, rather than on improved capacity to manage an intimate relationship. Undoubtedly, she could have complained that this would be unhelpful in her quest to find an intimate relationship, but it might have had been a more enduring legacy.

CONTRACTING FOR TREATMENT

Defining a focus and establishing goals fall under Bordin's (1979) concept of task and goal (discussed in Chapter 4). We see the identification of specific goals and recognition of specific tasks for patient and therapist as essential elements of the therapeutic alliance. Indeed, defining a focus constitutes a kind of therapeutic contract. The patient proposes what he or she would like to try to accomplish, and the therapist indicates what might be a good focus. Then they discuss this. Treatment can proceed if there is a measure of agreement. This agreement between therapist and patient becomes an essential building block in the alliance.

From a practical perspective, we recommend that you summarize the core problem and suggest a focus for the treatment by the third or fourth session. By then you are likely to know the core problem, although the formulation may not yet be clear. This succinct presentation should be made with clarity, vigor, and confidence, but with openness and curiosity about the patient's reactions and ideas about how to proceed.

INEVITABLE TENSION

Just because a contract is struck, it does not mean that both parties will abide by it. For the patient, there is the inevitable tendency to employ characteristic defenses, play out old interpersonal scenarios, and not do as promised. For conscious and unconscious reasons, the patient may not work on the agreed-upon focus, or may propose and hold to a view of it that is not conducive to deeper understanding. She may throw up her hands in helpless frustration that progress has not been made. An alternative focus may be proposed.

This difficulty in getting to work on the problem is captured in the term *resistance,* which we discussed earlier in Chapter 4. If the patient could easily and comfortably think about her problem, it would have happened before coming to treatment. The pragmatic psychotherapist will listen to and reflect on the patient's feedback about the work, the focus, and the goal, and will constructively reassess the focus and goal that have been proposed. Is the difficulty in moving forward just the inevitable resistance, or is it a reflection of a goal set too high or not optimally defined? Is the focus too broad, or too narrow? Is the formulation accurate? Could it be reworked? Is the problem defined as intrapsychic, when a life cycle focus would be more effective, for example? The therapeutic contract is not set in stone, and it needs reevaluation and affirmation or modification.

The therapist may also stray from the defined focus. Lack of attention, interference from personal issues, enactments with the patient, or practical matters may cause the therapist to lose the focus. A little loss of focus results in flexibility and sometimes creativity, but too much can result in sloppiness, disorganization, or boundary crossing.

TRANSPARENCY

Our approach involves directness and transparency about the therapeutic alliance–building process and defining the focus and goals of psychotherapy. These issues are best discussed directly with the patient, but only in as much detail as the therapist can be honest about. We cannot anticipate how much change will occur, because we cannot possibly know. Patients know the uncertainties too, and they generally appreciate trustworthy openness about the therapist's realistic ideas about the focus and goal. A balance between optimism and realistic recognition of how hard it is to change is difficult to maintain, especially in the highly charged emotional field of the psychotherapeutic relationship. But that is exactly what patients need.

SUMMARY

The patient's expressed goals for therapy initiates a discussion between therapist and patient about the focus of the treatment. Using awareness of the psychodynamic formulation, the patient's goals, both stated and unstated, and the patient's degree of ambition and capacity to effectively use treatment, the therapist proposes a focus of treatment that becomes the subject of discussion and compromise in the therapeutic relationship. The resulting treatment plan may define the problem as intrapsychic, relational, related to life cycle challenges, or adaptation to neurobiology.

PART III

MIDDLE PHASE

CHAPTER 9

The Narrative

Building a Personal Story

The narrative was too constricted; it was like
a fetus strangling on its own umbilical cord.
—JOHN GREGORY DUNNE

The Freudian model of sifting through layers of history for deeply hidden archeological prizes that are priceless and demonstrably true has given way to an awareness that there are multiple truths about oneself, discovered at different points in the life cycle, with different therapists, using different models of psychotherapy. The concept of narrative offers a new way of studying the content and structure of psychotherapy stories, transforming the process from a scientific pursuit of verifiable personal history to a more subjective enterprise.

Narrative has traditionally been studied in the context of literature, the telling of stories, and the reading of texts. Application of these ideas to patients as texts, and psychotherapy as a shared reading of these texts, forms the essence of the study of narratives in psychotherapy. Indeed, developing new narratives that are more therapeutic is seen by some to be the essence of psychotherapy, and some psychotherapeutic approaches focus exclusively on the writing and rewriting of a personal or shared narrative (Josselson, 2004; Singer, 2004).

Roy Schafer (1981), Donald Spence (1982), and others departed from the objectivist tradition of psychoanalysis in their emphasis on the co-created understanding that comes out of the psychoanalytic process. These authors emphasize the presence of multiple narratives and the difference between objective and narrative truth. This emphasis presaged the development of interpersonal psychoanalysis and the recent increased interest in the experiences that emerge from the therapeutic dyad. Lieblich, McAdams, and Josselson (2004) review the literature on narratives in psychotherapy in their edited collection. They conclude that the work in this field emphasizes the value of multiple explanatory frameworks beyond the psychological, the variety of types of narratives used in psychotherapy, and the special application of narration in psychotherapy to address issues of power, abuse, and gender.

From our perspective, a narrative is a life story that includes and summarizes crucial biographical information in a coherent way. It can be more comprehensive and global, including early childhood, all important relationships, major life events, important transitions and epiphanies, individual biological factors, and major adult experiences and why they were perceived as they were. But narratives are not always so epic in scope; they may also be more focal, like a short story that illuminates an aspect of the patient's character and provides a brief sketch of the history and context. Usually, the more intensive and enduring the psychotherapy, the more comprehensive the newly developed narrative will be.

Patients begin therapy with self-constructed narratives and, with the help of the therapist, form new and (one hopes) more useful, complex, and self-aware narratives. Even behavioral therapists suggest that one of the goals of CBT for patients with posttraumatic stress disorder is the construction of a more complete, detailed, and smooth narrative (Foa & Rothbaum, 1998).

We believe that new narratives are therapeutic when they are accurate enough to contain new understandings about the past and present (consistent with the core problem and formulation) and are organized in such a way as to lessen excessive blame and guilt. There are certain formal qualities of narratives that are helpful, so patient narratives have much in common. They are typically stories about self and others and include tensions and conflicts that arise and are then resolved. For example, the Core Conflictual Relationship Theme (CCRT), discussed in Chapter 3, is a systematic method for deriving central relationship narratives about wishes, responses from others, and responses of self.

In addition to describing others about whom we care deeply, narratives are propelled by internal logic. They are about how we manage disorder, conflict, and chaos in order to achieve greater mastery, freedom, and security in our lives. There is always an arc of tension and resolution that defines a helpful narrative. Although the constraints on the structure and content of psychotherapy narratives are not as strict as those of a good Hollywood movie, there do seem to be certain features that make for a good narrative. Without rich and interesting characters, complexity, and salient events, there is no tension and no resolution; thus there is no good story, and a good story helps make a narrative therapeutic.

Paul, a Catholic priest, sought treatment after the outbreak of the Church sexual abuse scandals awakened his own personal childhood experiences of sexual abuse. He knew these experiences were important, but he was unsure of how and why. Paul also struggled with spasms of intense and overwhelming guilt, feelings of inferiority despite his achievements, and a powerful need to be liked and respected by others.

Paul felt ashamed of his experience of abuse and could not look at photographs of himself, particularly recent ones, because he felt he was ugly. His initial narrative, the story that summarized and made sense of the troubled part of his life, was that he had always felt insecure, and this had led him to seek out the abuse because he was so needy. He felt he had been wrong in letting a priest touch him inappropriately, and even worse when he let another man do the same thing shortly thereafter. He was deeply convinced that he had been evil, and continued to feel in adulthood that there was something bad about him. His experiences made him doubt his sexuality; the thought that he might be homosexual frightened him. This was the narrative he had of his life when he started treatment.

As Paul began to talk in therapy, he started to see other, stronger connections between his early experiences and how he felt now. He felt guilty, blamed himself, felt ashamed, and was convinced his mother held him responsible for the abuse he had undergone. He thought about how he felt as a priest now, how the abuse affected his life by making him quiet, incapable of accepting compliments, and unable to interact socially with others because he felt loathsome and inferior. He was embarrassed to be a priest and felt horror that someone could manipulate and seduce a boy.

Paul began to empathize with his former insecure and lonely self. He was the youngest boy in a large family where the mother was the dominant influence and the father worked long hours to support the family. As the youngest child (he was 9 at the time), he felt loved, despite the fact that his mother was not particularly affectionate. But after the abuse everything changed. He felt different from his older brothers, who were athletic, socially popular and more at ease with themselves. He felt ashamed, lonely, and depressed, but did not know why.

As therapy unfolded, a new narrative began to emerge. As a boy he was religious, served Mass daily as an altar boy, and looked up to the clergy in his parish. This made him vulnerable to the abusing priest who took advantage of his piety. Yes, Paul succumbed to affection from the priest, but his goal had not been sexual, although it was intriguing to him that someone was giving him attention, money, and other gifts and at the same time was ingratiating himself with his mother. He did not know how to handle the uncomfortable feelings and experiences that came with the sexual contact. He secretly blamed himself and felt deeply ashamed. As he reflected further on what happened, he saw that the priest, the authority figure, was the person who had transgressed boundaries, who had been wrong. Why would the priest have done this?

Whereas the old narrative had emphasized the patient's evil intent, lifelong suffering, and attempt to never again lose control over his bad impulses, the new narrative was more complex and empathic in the picture it painted of Paul's childhood. He was lonely, struggling in competition with his siblings, longing for attention and affection, and looking for a mentor or teacher, as do so many early adolescents. He had the misfortune to find this attention in a priest who used it to his advantage, soliciting sex. He felt scared, ashamed, confused, and trapped in this—not wanting to lose the man's special interest in him, but feeling uncomfortable and degraded by continuing. His shame contributed to his withdrawal and distance from his family.

Paul felt increasingly comfortable talking about what had happened, and shared more details. Ultimately he and the priest were caught; he was deeply ashamed when his family learned about his secret experiences. The priest was sent away. The second abusive sexual relationship, very brief, made him feel even more guilty, as he felt he could not explain it by coercion and manipulation. In the old narrative, this second experience cemented his sense of being bad and worthy of humiliation and punishment. In the new narrative, he saw this as his a repetition of an overwhelming and frightening situation; he was unable to manage the feelings about the first time, not able to live with himself for what had happened, and he simply repeated what he could not manage emotionally.

The patient's new narrative about his early history also allowed him to revise his view of his current life. He connected his present shame about his appearance and devotion to being liked by others to his childhood self-loathing. He saw his continuing insecurity and guilt about his successes as a result of this. With a more forgiving and understanding perspective on why he did what he did as a child, he saw these self-critical symptoms as a reflection of old feelings that were not realistic in the current context. He was able to see that he did not have anything to be ashamed of, that he was likeable and lovable without having to work so hard for it, and that his successes were deserved.

The essence of psychodynamic psychotherapy is that the past is prologue, and early experiences shape later ones. A psychodynamic narrative is a story about early relationships, and a coexisting story about the current experiences of adult life. That is, a narrative is always a double story—what happened in the past and how it affects what is happening now, which leads to a clearer picture of the present. The tension between these two stories forms the arc of the therapy, commanding attention and helping the patient move forward in a healthy way.

The pretherapy life narrative usually has not worked well enough to help the patient live a well-adapted life. Because of the limitations, inaccurate views of self and others, and misperceptions implied in the narrative, the patient is prone to make poor choices. He may feel confused and uncertain about himself, or work extremely hard to contain intense emotions, leading to loss of flexibility, freedom, and satisfaction. During therapy, a new narrative is constructed, which is neither rosier and more optimistic than the patient's genuine experience, nor too bleak, providing little incentive or purpose to go on. As this new narrative takes shape, the patient begins to believe it. In this chapter we describe the essential elements in useful psychotherapy narratives, and the useful techniques for helping patients develop new narratives.

THE NARRATIVE AND INTERPRETATION

Interpretation is the traditional psychodynamic and psychoanalytic intervention for conveying more profound understanding to the patient, emphasizing deeper truths. Interpretations reflect the therapist's contribution to the new narrative. They should be focused on the core problem and formulation and help the patient see himself in new ways. But the concept of interpretation is therapist-centric, while narrative is the patient's language for thinking about himself and telling his story. Thus we see the writing of narratives as a more parsimonious and useful concept for talking about new understanding because it stays close to the patient's experience, avoids distancing jargon, and uses our natural, inborn proclivity for telling stories.

NEW NARRATIVES AND SUCCESS

A patient's motivation to come to therapy is a result of natural curiosity and the wish to be rid of painful symptoms; but these reasons wear out pretty quickly. The real spur for doing narrative work is succeeding in feeling different or better. Self-understanding gives a feeling of coherence to uncomfortable situations, which decreases anxiety and helps a patient feel more in control. Does the new narrative do this? Does it decrease confusion, correct misperceptions, and open the door to new behavioral solutions? This is crucial, because if it does, the patient learns how psychodynamic psychotherapy can help and develops further motivation. If not, there seems to be no point to the therapy, and patients will request focal symptomatic treatment, whether that comes from psychotherapy or psychopharmacology.

WRITING A NEW LIFE NARRATIVE

Building a narrative is an iterative process. The new narrative will arise from the old, but the old version must first be confronted. The therapist's job, using the formulation that suggests deeper motivations, more pervasive themes, and attempted solutions to conflicts, is to challenge this initial narrative and provide a stimulus for change. If you help the patient see the implicit narrative he brings to therapy and point out ways that this explanation is limited, or limiting, there is an increased motivation to understand more and to change the narrative.

As it develops, the new narrative will include a more comprehensive and articulated view of the patient's developmental experiences and major conflicts, the way he experienced those developmental problems, and a more adaptive and multifaceted view of his contemporary experiences. Essentially, the patient will come to say, "This is what happened, this is how I experienced it, this is how it shaped my current experiences, and this is what is really happening now."

> Jeff sought treatment after the breakup of his marriage, wildly anxious, agitated, hyper, and angry. He was often 15 minutes early to his early-morning appointments, having been awake for hours, ruminating and desperate for company. He wanted to unload his upsetting feelings and to be soothed and reassured. His initial narrative was that he had loved his difficult and quirky wife, but felt frustrated by her disorganization and selfishness. She left because

she found him so rigid and controlling. He felt that he had worked so hard, done so much for her, providing the financial support for the household and the necessary organizational energy to make the household function. He saw her as unendingly demanding and egocentric, and felt that not only was he the last bastion of standards and reasonableness in their chaotic home, but he had catered to her beyond what anyone could expect. And now she had left him!

The moral outrage was powerful. A deep belief in his helpfulness and reasonableness, his ability to save and rescue, and of the untrustworthiness of others (especially women) were the dominant features of his narrative. The essential plotline was, "I worked hard, gave a lot, and was screwed."

After taking the history and talking with the patient during the initial sessions, the therapist came to the following formulation: Jeff had felt loved, indulged, and supported, but controlled and subservient in his intense relationship with his mother. This shaped his experience of all relationships, especially those with women. He had longed for his mother, but needed to get away from her. He needed to control women to protect himself, and he expressed his anger through criticism. He needed to find women he could dominate and take care of, lest he feel their needs to be overwhelming, causing him to feel subservient and small. This was evident in his marriage, his relationship with his daughters, and his friendships.

The therapist's dilemma was to support him in his grief, confusion, and rage, but at the same time to begin to challenge the initial life narrative—his hard work, her selfishness, his struggle with needy and difficult women. Each of the cornerstones of his story—his selflessness, his wife's difficult nature, his mother's personality—had to be questioned. This is not to say that these perceptions might not be entirely reasonable and accurate. The question is how these perceptions fit together, and what other views might round out the story and help him see things in a more useful and flexible way.

ESSENTIAL NARRATIVE ELEMENTS

Every life is different, but there are certain elements that are frequently present in all helpful psychodynamic psychotherapy narratives (Table 9.1). We describe those elements first and then discuss how to challenge the old narrative to get there.

TABLE 9.1. Essential Components to Narrative

- Explanation for one's life course (e.g., why life happened this way)
- Most important life events and experiences
- Multidimensional picture of important relationships
- CCRT—description of wishes, responses of other, and responses of self
- What can change (mutability)
- Hope and compassion
- Cultural context
- Narrative voice

Explanation for One's Life Course

"*Why it happened*" is always central to the patient's story; it is the glue that connects all of the elements. The central causal explanation is a reassuring kernel of sense that rests at the heart of a narrative and gives it its therapeutic value. It makes a coherent account of a complex life that feels accurate and sensible enough to help the patient organize him or herself and function better. We have identified five types of explanations used in narratives; usually they are combined in some fashion. We do not elevate these explanations to the level of scientific causality; in therapy the goal is to come up with a useful narrative, not an objective truth.

These explanations fit our universal need to tell a story about ourselves to ourselves and answer the question of why life took the direction it did. They reflect positive views of the self, as opposed to negative ones, and we suspect this is part of what makes them therapeutic. We derived these types of explanations by looking at patients' narratives at the end of psychotherapy and looking at what their central causal explanations were. We asked what drove the arc of the story.

1. "*Past experiences* are repeated." Templates are laid down by early experiences, and we tend to repeat the past, ideally making it better, but often repeating our misperceptions and mistakes. The notion that past experiences are repeated is inextricably part of every psychodynamic narrative, and most patients find this intuitive. The narrative explanation takes the form: "I had X, Y, and Z critical experiences in the past and since then I have been repeating those experiences and trying to change them."

2. "*External events* affected my life." Here the focus is on events producing understandable results and effects. The patient's experience

is: "I am this way because of what happened to me. I see things this way because of what happened." This is probably the most frequently employed narrative device, especially early in psychotherapy, and implies the impact of difficult events and a patient's attempt to manage them. It makes clear that the patient's self is relatively untainted by negativity and blame. This narrative explanation can be employed in a defensive manner or as an evasion of responsibility, but we know that useful narratives help patients see themselves as basically good but struggling. Maintaining flexibility and an open mind about when we are responsible versus when an external situation has greater weight is a complex existential task, and this causal explanation stakes out a claim of less personal responsibility.

3. "I am this way now because it was the *best survival strategy* I could come up with." The central explanation in the narrative is the persistence of an old coping mechanism that is now dysfunctional. This explanation is an attempt to create a synthesis between externalization of responsibility and self-blame. It says: children do the best they can with the cognitive and emotional capacities they have available, and they often come up with strategies for dealing with upsetting feelings and insoluble conflicts that work in a limited way, and then these strategies get repeated forever. Jeff's narrative was based on this explanation.

> Jeff did a fine job of managing his childhood and adolescent separation from his family, despite his conflicted and enmeshed relationship with his mother. He wanted to be close to her but was overwhelmed by her, and he dealt with this through a kind of controlling independence—he superficially complied with her wishes, kept his private feelings secret, and chose to go off to camp in the summer.
>
> This survival strategy worked well enough when he was a child, but when brought to his marriage, it led to problems. He was seemingly responsive to his wife's needs, indeed almost too much. But he resented it all the while, and expressed this indirectly through thinly disguised contempt or passive–aggressive behavior. His wife often felt he was angry and controlling, and his children reacted negatively to this tendency, especially when they became adolescents.

Jeff came to see this old pattern and its repetition, and it became the central theme in his narrative, which opened the door to new possibilities in the present, for example, he could assert himself in his new relationship with his girlfriend and not worry about being rejected, and he could respond to his children's needs only when he thought they were appropriate.

4. "We are all *fallible*." People know and can accept this in general, but not always about themselves. Sometimes this idea helps to build a coherent narrative. The patient sees what happened in his life, and the potential causal factors, sees that he might have made better decisions or enforced more impulse control. But people are fallible, and sometimes they just don't do the best thing. The sense of this narrative explanation is that attempts and failures are the essential dynamic of life, and acceptance of this explains and justifies why a life went the direction it did. This is a healthy kind of self-blame, recognizing that we all make mistakes.

5. "*Personal choice and freedom*" is a narrative explanation that is just the opposite of those we have discussed. Here the patient is not the passive actor, the recipient of the effects of the past, or of limited coping skills, important relationships, and accidents. Rather, the patient is the protagonist, having marshaled his resources, creatively surmounted his situation (perhaps with help), evolved a new way of managing things, and had new experiences. In this narrative, there are moments of personal freedom and transcendence of circumstance whose explanation cannot be further reduced.

Important Life Events and Experiences

If the explanation for why things worked out is arc of the life story, then the patient's seminal life events, what they meant, and how they were experienced, are its contents. Who were the characters, what were the crucial moments, and when were the points in time when the individual's course in life changed drastically? Which were the important relationships, including those with parents and other early caregivers, what happened in those relationships, who was constant and available, who was disappointing, who died, and who left? Later relationships, loves gained and lost, family, friends, comrades, and coworkers are the substance of the story. Traumatic events and positive experiences are included. If a narrative is the story of who we are, and we are essentially social, then it is a story of our relationships, how they developed, changed, and were internalized.

A Multidimensional View of Parents

In contrast to the unidimensional view of parents described by many patients early in therapy, a multidimensional, articulated picture of the most important early relationships, usually with the parents, is essential for a mature (posttherapy) narrative. The parents can be viewed from a distance. They have strengths and weaknesses, motivations, and needs; they are givers and takers, nurturing and needy, independent and dependent, transcending their own circumstances and limited by them. This is hard-won territory in building the new narrative. It comes from the detailed, safe, and thorough exploration of childhood memories and the patient's own experiences as a parent, lover, or friend.

For example, Jeff came to see how extraordinary his mother was only later in his treatment. He recognized her limitations, her need for him to be a narcissistic extension of herself, helping her to get the attention and admiration she craved. He saw, too, her capacity to manipulate and control him when he did not give her the response she wanted. But through therapy, after he had done so much work on his relationship with his children, he came to see her energy, enthusiasm, affection, and remarkable ability to create wonderful experiences for her family. She was a wonderful conversationalist, hostess, and entertainer. By late in the treatment, Jeff saw his mother's strengths and weaknesses; she gave him a lot but figured prominently in his struggles.

Core Conflictual Relationship Theme

The life narrative must capture the essential conflicts using whatever language is comfortable for the patient. The CCRT provides another way of organizing a narrative. The patient's wishes, responses of others to these wishes, and responses of self are the essence of a relational conflict, and the story is constructed around these central repeated elements. In our example, Jeff wished for love and support from his mother, and he perceived her response as demanding, controlling, and potentially punishing. His response of self was to become compliant and resentful. As a result of this core conflict, and especially because his responses of self, Jeff developed secondary wishes (Wiseman & Barber, 2008) to escape elsewhere, or control the relationship so he did not feel in danger. These secondary wishes led to further problems.

What Can Change

A therapeutic narrative is hopeful but realistic about change. Of course, one cannot know with certainty what will change. Perhaps one of the most difficult parts of treatment for Jeff was accepting the reality that he would likely not be able to change some of his visceral feelings and perceptions about women; he could see their origins, notice their repetition, and develop his ability to distinguish between those perceptions based on the past and those based on more contemporary considerations. He had to accept that he would feel controlled at times, resentful and distant; he would need to find the woman most suitable for him in the present, with whom he could most comfortably tolerate these feelings when they came up. He realized that this template was part of him, immutable, but able to be lessened in degree; he could not obliterate the uncomfortable feelings, but they could be much less intense, and he could find a satisfying relationship.

Hope and Compassion

A sense of hope about the future is essential to a therapeutic narrative. But how does this happen in a genuine way? Usually it is tied to hope about relationships, or about the possibility of new relationships. So often, early in therapy, a patient's one-dimensional understanding of a spouse, partner, parent, or boss is suffused with painful feelings—hurt, anger, betrayal, or disappointment. The intensity of these feelings is usually proportionate to the fixity with which they view the other person.

Hope can come from the recognition that these painful relationships can be experienced differently. New understanding of others allows patients to realize that the situation is more complicated than initially recognized. In the face of a more complex picture of the other person, it is possible to feel more empathy and more affection. Sometimes hope comes from realizing that the relationship is beyond salvation, and divorce or estrangement is the best option. This too allows for new possibilities for better and more loving relationships.

In either situation, a narrative that has more hope and more compassion is more likely to bring out positive responses in others than one suffused with bitterness and anger. Hope is a self-fulfilling prophecy and more likely to bring about that which is hoped for.

Cultural Context

Cultural values and struggles are important causal elements in the narrative, but they are also the medium for expressing more universal issues. Many patients find that embracing important cultural concerns and references in their narratives lend verity to their stories. For example, Jeff's upper-middle-class Jewish background was part of the story of attachment to his mother and part of his struggle with his daughters. His relationship with his mother especially was consistent with the Jewish cultural theme of close mother–son relationships. This cultural subtext probably contributed to their interpersonal dynamic, and it also served as a kind of shorthand that could be used to refer to the more complicated psychological truth in their situation, the enmeshment of mother and son. Important events in a group's history, issues of power, subjugation, discrimination, and alienation are irrevocably part of an individual patient's story and are an essential narrative element.

Narrative Voice

Using traditional literary concepts to analyze therapeutic narratives is the converse of humanities scholars using psychoanalytic principles to analyze works of art. In analyzing patient narratives, Alon and Omer (2004) describe "psychodemonic," "tragic," and "comic" narratives. We describe these below and suggest that most successful psychotherapy narratives are tragic narratives.

The psychodemonic narrative portrays the patient as fundamentally bad, evil, and negative, and describes the effects of these qualities on his life. The "bad seed" explanation could refer to the patient's genes, soul, or something more inchoate than that. The rest of the narrative, the relationships with others, life experiences, the why, all derive from this explanation. Mutability is limited, and hope and compassion are at a minimum.

This is in contrast to the "tragic" narrative, which emphasizes fatal flaws, accidents, limitations and mistakes, and the elaborate circling out of control that these small past deviations can cause. In the "tragic" narrative, current suffering is seen as the result of prior events. Pain and suffering are the patient's lot in life and have an understandable cause. The fundamental innocence implied in the tragic narrative allows for a rich and complex story of change and transcendence and, thus, hope. Most psychotherapy narratives take the tragic format, with many variations. Jeff's story certainly does, with the central theme of his early difficulty with his mother, the painful later effects, his limitation in being able to experience her otherwise, and her inflexibility toward him.

Comic narratives rely on accidental events, misunderstandings, and fundamentally good motivations that are misunderstood, with the triumph of love in the end. It is interesting to consider whether psychotherapy narratives ever follow this format. Our impression is that this type of narrative, as reasonable, accurate, and helpful as it might be for many people, is not uncommon in life, but less frequent in longer-term psychotherapy. Most therapeutic narratives involve loss and suffering, but often more successful treatments that have brought significant change cause patients to look back and see a change in fortune from bad to good with a triumph at the end.

Late in treatment Jeff felt he had found a narrative understanding of his life that helped him. With his increased understanding of his relationship with his mother, he was able to assert himself more with her, letting him feel less controlled and therefore less angry. He could more fully appreciate her many positive attributes. But it was in a new relationship with a woman and in his relationships with his children that he really saw the therapeutic impact of the new narrative. With his earlier narrative, his relationship with his teenage children was an accident waiting to happen. As they were stretching their wings developmentally in adolescence, alternating in their closeness and distance with him, he was deeply upset.

Jeff worried that he would be left alone when they grew up, knowing that he was dependent on them. He was especially angry with the older one, the daughter, who was temperamentally headstrong, assertive, and impulsive. They were locked into control battles over and over again. A reasonable sleep schedule, cleaning up the kitchen, helping out around the house, attention to schoolwork; almost anything could become a subject of controversy. She would not give in, and the more they argued, the more he felt he had to win. He tended to perceive the problem as: if I give in, I will lose her because she will do whatever she wants; if I win, she will stay at home, be well-behaved, and remain close to me. As the narrative understanding of his life got clearer, he saw that this was a repetition of his experience with his mother, in which he was controlling to protect against rejection.

Each time he successfully resisted repeating the old pattern he was thrilled, and knew this was healthy for him and for his daughters. He might fall into it again, but he became more able to climb out of it, more able to do so quickly, and even to forestall conflict. In a parallel fashion, his new relationship with his girlfriend was healthier than any one before. He could tolerate differences of opinion and honest communication with less of the old emotions, and found a degree of closeness he had not had before.

TECHNIQUES FOR CREATING A NEW NARRATIVE

Challenging Perceptions

There can be no new narrative, and no relief, until the old version loses its power. There are always alternative perspectives, explanations, and dimensions of understanding that can add to or change the old narrative. For example, was Jeff actually as good, hard-working, and upstanding as his initial narrative presented? Or was he also critical and competitive, with a holier-than-thou attitude? Was his moral outrage based on a healthy adult sense of imbalance of commitment and love, or something else? Was it really true that he had given endlessly to his wife and not received much in return? Was his intrusive mother truly so self-centered in their interactions, or did he not tell her what about her behavior bothered him?

Working from the Surface

Before Jeff could begin to question his own narrative, he needed reassurance about his pain and fear. Empathy and support in therapy allow a patient to feel the security and freedom needed to verbalize unsettling thoughts and reflect on them.

This security, along with the instillation of hope, is an essential prelude to changing in the old narrative and creating the new narrative. For the therapist working with Jeff, there was a cyclical quality to the process of psychotherapy. The cycle would begin by elucidating old perceptions and questioning them, then providing support, and then exploring more, then support, and so forth. But with each cycle, Jeff moved deeper into his feelings and experiences. Beginning with more surface concerns and explanations, he could start to acknowledge more complex feelings and less reasonable and realistic explanations. For example, early on, Jeff felt so convinced of his giving qualities and reasonableness that he was not able to see that every bit of help he gave his family came with an indirect expression of his anger and a need to detach.

After a patient has talked about an important experience in the past or present, the therapist's goal is to bring out the patient's initial narrative understanding of the event. Typical questions that allow patients to unpack their implicit narratives are:

- "How were you feeling in that situation?"
- "What were you most afraid of in that situation?"
- "What did you think was going to happen?"
- "Why do you think that happened to you?"
- "What do you think caused the other person to react to you that way? Why do you think the other person did that?"
- "What do you think it is about you that made the other person react or behave that way?"
- "What did the situation remind you of?"

- "If your fears had come true, what would you have felt, and how would you have reacted?"
- "How did you feel about feeling that way?"
- "What is your idea about why these kinds of things keep happening to you?"

When you ask these questions, patients often do not really know the answers, but they usually have some ideas or suggestions. Working from the surface implies asking questions about matters that are close to the patient's awareness, not the deeper thoughts, feelings, motivations, or conflicts you as a therapist hypothesize about. Working from the surface means starting from what the patient already knows or thinks, pushing and exploring, suggesting alternatives, listening carefully, and wondering aloud for what else might be there.

For example, Jeff only began to question his initial narrative after he began to see how his feelings and explanation for his feelings were inaccurate and inappropriate. Repeated probing about this helped him to get in touch with his anger and hurt and begin to see his repetitive attempts to get distance from or control others as his adaptation to these feelings. This laid the groundwork for the new narrative.

Some patients find it helpful to work on their narrative utilizing a more concrete format. Journal entries, brief autobiographies, poetry, artwork, and diagrams can all be useful. Some patients prefer text and actual written narrative and will come to appointments with new versions of their narrative, allowing for collaborative discussion and review.

How Much Emphasis Should Be Given to the Past?

Psychodynamic psychotherapy deals extensively with the past. Malan's triangle (Malan, 1979) suggests that the patient's central conflicts can be expressed in past relationships, realistic present relationships, and in the relationship with the therapist, that is, transference. Likewise, a comprehensive narrative includes all of these elements. The story begins in childhood, traces the important life events, twists, and turns along the way to include important relationships, and ends up in the present. The transference expresses the same conflicts and can be included in the narrative.

Some patients are filled with memories and easily reflect on past events, while some are fully planted in the present and less inclined to look back. Some like talking about the therapeutic here and now and their feelings and thoughts about the therapist. It is best, if possible, to flesh out all three areas of Malan's triangle with patients, because they reinforce one another, and understanding in one area builds understanding in the others.

Some patients ask whether talking about the past is essential in psychodynamic psychotherapy. We think that it is possible to do useful psychotherapy focusing primarily on the present or the transference and spending less time on the past, but it is probably harder and may be less effective for the patient. The greatest potential for change comes from a broader exploration and a more comprehensive narrative. For briefer treatment it is often more useful to have a present-centered focus, as the single domain of data will allow for greater clarity and consolidation of the narrative. In more extended treatment, with broader objectives, there will likely be work in all three areas. Because narratives fundamentally involve a timeline, they are most powerful and convincing when they start in the past and come up to the present.

THE NARRATIVE AND THE THERAPIST

As we have advocated elsewhere, transparency in the therapist's role helps strengthen the therapeutic alliance and educate the patient. The therapist should explain the value of elucidating the implicit narrative that the patient has been using and the potential benefit of developing a new life story. Although this will likely affect a patient on a more cognitive and intellectual level, it will resonate emotionally as well and serve as a reference for understanding the therapist's behavior and attitude.

So many of the typical questions and concerns that patients have about therapy can be answered using the framework of the life narrative: "Why do we have to talk about the past? Is this therapy going to end up blaming my parents; isn't that just complaining? What difference does it make if I understand the past when my problems are in the present? How can I ever know what really happened? I feel this way about my family, but my sister (or brother) sees it so differently, how can I know which is right? Therapy seems so subjective, how do I know if what we are talking about is true?" You can respond to each of these questions with an explanation of narrative development as the central task of psychotherapy, and the ideas behind narratives we have tried to convey in this chapter. We tell our patients that our collaborative work on a new, clearer, and more complex narrative of their lives is the main task of therapy. The new understanding will need to feel right to them and incorporate awareness of things that have been hard and painful to think about. The narrative is their story of what and how things happened and may not be accurate for others, even other members of the family. The standard of truth is whether, with deep and sustained consideration and input from the therapist, the narrative seems true to them. A new narrative should also open up new possibilities for living a better life.

Because therapy is essentially a learning process, with a focus on changing the way one sees and experiences the self and others, repetition and review are very important. Many patients will express the feeling that something important happened in a previous session, but not remember what it was. Although this may reflect the power of repression and the avoidance of anxiety, it may also remind us of the difficulty of learning new things about oneself. People forget what they have not yet fully learned. It can often be anxiety-reducing, stabilizing, and soothing for a therapist to repeat the narrative that has been constructed so far. This is especially useful at moments of upset and crisis. Summarizing the narrative has a different and equally powerful effect in moments of quiet, when gains are consolidated.

SUMMARY

The elaboration of a comprehensive narrative, built up through questions and hypotheses that start from the surface of the patient's awareness and move deeper, helps to increase the patient's self-awareness. The narrative, which is a collaborative effort, is verbalized frequently over the course of treatment as it becomes more complicated. This new self-understanding is the essential prerequisite for therapeutic change.

CHAPTER 10

Change

People grow through experience if they
meet life honestly and courageously.
This is how character is built.
—ELEANOR ROOSEVELT

Change is inevitable, except from
vending machines.
—ANONYMOUS

The ultimate purpose of psychotherapy is to help a person change.
This is where the tire meets the road for patients. How do we know
whether our work with a patient is leading to healthy change? We are all
shy about evaluation of our performance, and while stockbrokers and
Olympic athletes get immediate and ruthless feedback about their work,
teachers and artists and therapists do not.

There are quantitative yardsticks for assessing psychotherapy outcome and process, but many factors enter into the real psychotherapy
situation that make it humbling to plan for, observe, and assess change.
Patients are often unclear about what and how much they want to
change. The therapist's and patient's conceptualizations about what has
changed, their observations on change as the therapy is ongoing, and
how they each see it weeks, months, and years later are all fairly fluid
and hard to pin down. Therapists make judgments (sometimes biased)
about what *can* change, what *should* change, and ultimately what *has*
changed. Objective behavioral outcome assessments are certainly the
cleanest measure, but they may not be aligned with patients' goals or
aspects of the patient's subjective experience.

215

Although the psychodynamic psychotherapy literature has been rich in its discussion and explication of how patients experience change, it has been less explicit in describing how therapy and the therapists facilitate these changes. Perhaps this is why so many of our patients say, "I am understanding myself better, but how is this going to help me change?" As a field, we often have not had a concise, common-sense answer for them!

Traditionally, the field has viewed insight as the silver bullet that, in and of itself, facilitates change. The transformative power of insight is part of what originally defined psychoanalysis and psychodynamic psychotherapy. But we have not been precise in describing how the therapist facilitates change, other than by facilitating insight. Years of practical experience with doing dynamic psychotherapy and the positive impact of cognitive and behavioral therapies on thinking about change have led us to expand and reconceptualize change in psychodynamic treatment. This chapter proposes a model of change and elaborates the strategies used in PPP to facilitate change.

Michelle was a petite, vivacious woman who swept into my office with a big, warm smile. She was successful as a salesperson for a national cosmetics firm, and she told me she had a son in middle school who was increasingly restive, and she was worried about him. But the main she reason she came for treatment was that she was terrified that her marriage was breaking up. She was angry at how negative and empty her relationship with her husband had become. The painful drama of their difficulty communicating tumbled out, and it was hard for me to respond much initially.

Michelle described her husband Jack as a quiet, creative man, who had become subsumed into his family's business, and left behind many of his own ambitions. She had spent 3 years struggling with a hard-to-diagnose medical illness, and now was finally feeling healthy. She was ready to pick up her life, only to find that her husband seemed ready to leave it. Jack refused couple therapy and had just begun to see a therapist of his own. When Michelle met with Jack's therapist, she learned that he was working on finding himself and was unsure about whether to stay in the marriage.

Michelle was the older of two daughters, her father's favorite. She loved her father deeply, and when she heard his voice at the other end of the phone, her spirits rose. But their history was complicated. He had bullied, cajoled, and demanded excellent school performance and good behavior, and in turn had made her his confidant and taught her everything about how the business world worked.

He, too, was a top-performing salesperson. Michelle's mother was quiet, affectionate, and loyal.

Michelle believed she could not tolerate the rejection from Jack; she was convinced she could not be alone, and she felt like a "big fat loser." It was hard to take this in as she sat in my office, elegant, outgoing, and engaging. She seemed to have so much going for her. But she felt it was just luck that had allowed her to snare her husband. She felt she worked for a second-rate company, and she lived in a second-rate city.

The deterioration of her marriage made her feel like a failure. It also made her angry, and she was a fighter. She created scene after scene at home. She berated Jack, criticized him, and demanded time, attention, and gifts. Needless to say, the more she demanded, the more passive, stiff, and unresponsive he became.

Michelle's core problem seemed to be low self-esteem, and the dynamic formulation revolved around the exciting but painful relationship with her father. She felt both criticized by him and valued by him; this intense entanglement had left her overly vulnerable to how she was treated by Jack. She looked to him to complete her and make her feel loved, and she felt devastated and angry when he failed to do so. Although this had always been a tension in their relationship, the stress of her illness and symptoms and associated exhaustion had left him depleted and angry. The focus of the treatment was on her experience of the relationship and what she could do to feel better and contribute more productively to the marriage. Her self-esteem in other areas was lower than what it could be, but this was the area causing the greatest distress.

WHAT CHANGES IN THE PATIENT?

Effective psychotherapy changes patients' subjective experience as well as their objective functioning. Mood, affect, cognition, life satisfaction, and capacity for pleasure can all be positively affected. Theoretically, change in one or more of these areas can "trickle down" to other areas. Is the patient functioning better at home, work, in relationships, cognitively, in the ability to organize and focus? Does the patient bring flexibility and creativity to problem solving? Does she feel greater satisfaction and capacity for attachment and closeness? Has there been improvement in the capacity to observe, understand, and consider alternatives—has there been an internalization of the "psychotherapy function"? Do significant others notice changes that the patient might not be aware of?

Much of the contemporary debate about the efficacy of psychodynamic psychotherapy and its comparison to more symptom-based treatments hinges on the issue of whether the treatment should only remove symptoms. Reducing symptoms is clearly important and certainly makes an individual feel better, but should the treatment also actively facilitate improved mental health and functioning? Should we simply take out the lesion and let the patient heal, or should we provide training and rehabilitation as well?

Michelle's symptoms—loneliness, anxiety, anger, and impulsive outbursts—were a problem for her and the marriage, but she also exhibited limitations in her healthy emotional functioning. She had difficulty being alone and finding her own sources of satisfaction and fulfillment. She looked to her husband and son, as she had earlier looked to her father, for validation and approval, and she did not develop a sense of confidence, or even interest, in herself. Even if she patched up the marriage, she was going to need more emotional strength as she got older, lost her parents, watched her son leave home, and lived through other key transitions. Can (and should) psychotherapy seek to help her build that emotional strength, even after her presenting symptoms have diminished?

We list below some of the traditional (and not-so-traditional) "targets of change" in psychodynamic treatment (see also Sharpless & Barber, 2009).

- Less emotional upset and more ability to handle stressful and painful situations and not be derailed by them.
- Decrease in symptoms.
- Positive self-esteem, with a sense that one's life fits with one's expectations. Feeling one has made the best of one's opportunities, with the feeling of mastery (and acceptance) that comes with this.
- More stable and sustaining relationships, with the connection, sharing, support, stimulation, and validation that comes with these relationships.
- Improved ability to function in the world, in vocational and leisure activities, in ability to meet basic needs.
- Better capacity to creatively adapt to new situations that arise. Ability to deal with life cycle demands and find good solutions.
- Greater ability to use contemporary and realistic thinking to

make decisions and find pleasure, meaning, and value in life. Greater creativity.

- More positive experiences and positive affect, and less negative experience and affect, with improvement in the skills necessary to promote positive experiences.

Most of the entries on this list are probably familiar and noncontroversial. The last item deserves some additional explanation. A patient once said that his goal was to "get [his] smile back," referring to the then popular movie, *City Slickers,* about three middle-aged men who went out west to have fun and solve their midlife crises. At the time, this seemed like an understandable therapeutic goal. But it was vague and disconnected from the obvious family problems that brought him to treatment. It seemed wishful and not very practical. Nevertheless, this patient put his finger on something that is important for almost everyone. The theory underlying positive psychology, with its focus on the enhancement of experience and positive emotion, is that positive experiences are both an end unto themselves and they also help to buffer against negative experiences. Studies suggest that the capacity to create and sustain positive experiences can be developed and improved and yields highly desirable results (Seligman et al., 2005). This is relevant to the case of Michelle. Of course, she will need to figure out why she gets so hurt and so angry at Jack, and do something about that. But unless she also figures out how to have some pleasurable and positive experiences with him, their marriage is going to be a lot of hard work, and not very satisfying.

MECHANISMS OF CHANGE

The extensive literature on mechanisms of change in psychodynamic psychotherapy shows an evolution from the early model of a cathartic cure based on accurate and rapid interpretation of the patient's unconscious to an appreciation of the importance of the therapeutic intimacy that develops between patient and attuned psychotherapist, and then most recently, to the importance of new tools and skills that promote healthy adaptation. How do we make sense of this literature: is it new insight, a new and better parental figure, or new skills that promote change?

Early psychoanalysts, including Freud, believed that increased self-understanding and awareness of conflicts was responsible for change. Insight was both the goal and the mechanism of change. The emphasis in classical analysis on understanding the seemingly incomprehensible (e.g., dreams, hysterical symptoms) or picayune (slips of the tongue, jokes, etc.) demonstrates the premium placed on insight into one's self. How this insight brought about change was not so clearly described.

Strachey (1934) articulated the classical mechanism of therapeutic change in psychoanalysis. For him, accurate interpretations made by the analyst constitute a superego mitigating force, allowing the patient to see herself in a less critical light, leading to greater intrapsychic flexibility and decreased conflict. Based essentially on an ego psychology model, Strachey regarded the patient's identification with the analyst's understanding as leading to a less self-critical, punitive, and anxious experience of self. Understood from the patient's perspective, "I am okay because I understand myself through appreciating my analyst's well-tempered understanding of me." With Michelle, this means she will be less self-critical and less prone to seeing herself as a "loser" as she takes in the therapist's interpretations about her relationship with her father and her ambivalence and dependence on him. She will be more aware of her feelings and conflicts, understand herself better and judge herself less.

Alexander and French (1946) radically departed from earlier psychoanalysts. They believed that a "corrective emotional experience" helps the patient to change. That is, the patient is able to reexperience old conflicts in a new way and can have a new kind of experience with the therapist that does not follow the historical pattern. This concept generated tremendous controversy in analytic circles, but proved to be an important influence on subsequent thinking.

Winnicott (1965) and others of the object relations school (see Chapter 3) emphasize the therapeutic relationship as the lever for change. The connection with the therapist, modeled on the mother–child bond, serves as a safe container for the patient's noxious, disturbing, and unacceptable feelings and impulses. Through a process of projection and reintrojection, the therapist detoxifies these painful and disturbing feelings, like a mother bird who predigests food for her young. The experience of containing painful feelings, and borrowing the therapist's strength to do so, allows for increased tolerance on the part of the patient for these feelings and a greater ability to live in the present. "I am OK because my analyst has been able to tolerate and contain me, and I am now able to tolerate and contain myself." In the therapy, Michelle could express her need and her fury at Jack, and the therapist could help her contain this anger. Usually she felt awful about being so angry and felt that she could hardly control it. But the experience of talking about anger, and accepting and understanding it, will help her manage her emotions more comfortably.

Loewald (1960; see also Cooper, 1989) speaks to the importance of the therapeutic relationship in facilitating change, but makes a different point. He describes the development of a new kind of connection, where the closeness with the analyst allows for new and creative solutions to conflicts. The real availability of the analyst and the unconscious attunement with the patient result in a new relational field that facilitates the patient's openness to her unconscious. This renewed connection with the unconscious restores her to the normal developmental path, which had been previously blocked by the neurotic illness. Simply put, "I am OK because I can now be open to myself and to my analyst, and this experience allows me to accept myself and be open to others and other new experiences." Loewald would say that Michelle will get better if she feels that her relationship with her therapist allows her to feel strong, valued, creative, and special. She will be able to take in this new relationship and be changed because of it. These concepts are similar to the selfobject relationship the patient develops in Kohut's self psychology model (Kohut, 1984).

The relational perspective, articulated by Greenberg and Mitchell (1983), Renik (1993), and others, builds on the work of these earlier object relations theorists. The relational school sees the therapeutic enterprise fundamentally as a two-person unit, breaking down the old distinction between an ill patient and a healthy therapist. Rather, the relational psychoanalyst recognizes that the therapist inevitably engages unconsciously with the patient, enacting scenarios from the patient's past, and also from the therapist's own past. These factors from the therapist's subjectivity cannot simply be ignored, or even subtracted out through analytic awareness. They are seen as an integral part of the relationship, and therefore of the therapeutic relationship. Healthy change comes out of understanding this inevitable entanglement, and this understanding is importantly aided by the therapist's participant-observation in the experience. Relative transparency about the therapist's role in the relationship is part of the therapeutic technique here. The relational perspective emphasizes how Michelle's relationship with the therapist reflected not just her transference responses (worry about being judging, hoping for approval), but also the therapist's own personal background, and how these two subjective experiences come together to create something new that can be experienced and understood.

Gabbard and Westen (2003) synthesize much of this literature, proposing that we move beyond single-mechanism theories of therapeutic action to an awareness of multiple types of therapeutic action in psychoanalysis. They also remind us of the importance of distinguishing between the aims of treatment and the techniques used to facilitate those changes. We agree with this position as it applies to dynamic psychotherapy, as we regard each of these mechanisms as important.

In all of the psychodynamic models discussed above, treatment aims to change internal experience, and this is thought to result in new thoughts, emotions, and behavior. But most nondynamic psychotherapies take the opposite approach. For example, cognitive therapists believe that the modification of thoughts leads to changes in behavior and emotion. Similarly, behavioral therapists posit that internal changes are a result of trying out new behaviors, rather than the other way around. Thus CBT, which subsumes both of these strategies, focuses on dysfunctional patterns of thought and behavior and helps the patient try out new cognitive and behavioral responses to old situations. The feelings associated with these behaviors are observed and subsequently used as sources of data in the therapy.

Skill development is seen as a central mechanism of change in CBT. For example, Barber and DeRubeis (1989) emphasized that developing awareness of one's cognitive processes and coping skills is responsible for the prophylactic effect of cognitive therapy for depression. Other adaptive skills are relevant (Badgio, Halperin, & Barber, 1999), including the ability to develop close personal and work relationships. Flexible problem solving, maintenance of health, and management of time and resources are also skills. Patients may not have developed skills, such as assertiveness, adequately because of ongoing symptoms or because of developmental deficits in learning (see also Wachtel, 1997). Trying a new problem-solving approach that turns out to be successful is a powerful reinforcer and helps to generate valuable information that allows a patient to go back and reexamine unrealistic thoughts and perceptions.

SYNTHESIZING MODELS

Michelle came for weekly therapy appointments for about a year and a half. Early on, she was sad, fearful, and angry as she tried to steel herself for the impending breakup of her marriage. She and Jack were not communicating, he was distant and angry, and sex was infrequent. She learned that Jack had rented an apartment and had not told her.

As she talked about this over the weeks, Michelle realized she was terrified of feeling alone; she felt she could not manage and contain this fear. Her daughter was scheduled to go to camp for almost 2 months, and she was distraught about how quiet and empty the house would be.

Through the painful work of talking about her relationship with Jack, Michelle started to be able to distinguish between her childhood feeling of sadness and aloneness when her father was disappointed with her, and the reality of her marriage. Her father had been loud and demonstrative in his affection. She craved activity, noise, and conversation because they made her feel engaged and loved. She realized that her terribly lonely, rejected feeling in the marriage was stirred up by her husband's distance, but really it was an old feeling from childhood and had a different basis from what was going on currently in her life. Following these discussions, it occurred to her that if the marriage were to end, she would survive and would find a way to be independent and take care of herself. In other words, she was better able to catch herself when she reacted to the present like it was the past.

With an increasing awareness of her sensitivity to rejection, Michelle started to look at the situation from Jack's perspective. He was exhausted and drained by her several years of being ill; she had been demanding and needy for much of the time. He had done everything around the house and tried to tend to her. He was fed up. Now that she felt so well, she was ready to move on, but he was not. He was angry about what he had been through and was now doubly angry because she was demanding intimacy and time together. For reasons of his own, her anger was especially intolerable, and this precipitated his crisis about continuing in the marriage.

Her ability to see the situation from Jack's perspective helped Michelle soften her feelings about him. For the first time, she began to realize that she needed to be patient and let him be. She could not expect him to be like the good side of her father, always ready to jump in with support and help. Neither was he always like the bad side of her father, critical and judgmental. Instead, he was the same man she had been attracted to and married almost two decades before, but who was now going through a harrowing reappraisal of himself and his life.

It took a fair amount of convincing for Michelle to work on giving her husband space, supporting him, and not asking for more than was reasonable. She often reverted to her wish to be treated like a beloved, remarkable daughter. But now, she needed to support Jack and wait to see if his love became clear to him. If she demanded it, it would necessarily come with resentment and all of his subtle rejecting behaviors.

Ultimately, Michelle learned how to stay in the present with Jack and keep on a more even emotional keel. Jack began to feel better, too. Michelle's therapy schedule drifted down to monthly meetings, and she began to feel that she and Jack were off to a new and different start. She felt more independent and separate, and he was acting more like the quiet, loving, and attentive man she remembered.

All three of the above-mentioned mechanisms—new insight and emotional awareness, new relationship experiences, and new skills and behavior—were operative in Michelle's treatment, as they generally are in pragmatically oriented psychodynamic psychotherapy. Michelle clearly gained important new insights into herself and her past; she saw that her overwhelming fear of separation was based on old experiences (e.g., Castonguay & Hill, 2007). She had a new relational experience—with the male therapist she felt even and steady support, without indulgence or criticism. She also developed new relationship skills involving patience, empathy, and restraint in her needs (Badgio et al., 1999). Thus the three above-mentioned mechanisms were operative in Michelle's treatment, as they generally are in pragmatically oriented psychodynamic psychotherapy (see also summary in Table 10.1). Some might suggest that our model departs from psychodynamic psychotherapy because of its emphasis on teaching new skills and thus represents an integrated, or eclectic, psychotherapy. If by integrated or eclectic therapy, one refers to the use of a mélange of techniques employed in an intuitive and unplanned fashion rather than the systematic application of various techniques, then

TABLE 10.1. Psychotherapy Mechanisms of Change

	Mechanisms of change		
	New insight and emotional awareness	New relationship experiences	New behaviors, skills
Strachey (ego psychology)	++	+	
Alexander and French, Winnicott (object relations)	+	++	
Loewald (similar to self psychology)	+	++	
Relational	+	++	+
Cognitive-behavioral therapy	+		++
Pragmatic psychodynamic psychotherapy	++	++	++

Note: + and ++ denote degree of emphasis.

our approach is not eclectic. In contrast, we are describing the multiple mechanisms of change that are, we believe, operative in psychodynamic psychotherapy, and we will enumerate specific techniques that exploit these mechanisms to facilitate change.

FACILITATING CHANGE:
A SEQUENCE OF THERAPEUTIC TECHNIQUES

Three mechanisms of change give rise to three broad groups of PPP techniques for facilitating change: (1) emotional exploration, where the therapist helps the patient explore feelings and thoughts, identifying repetitive scenarios that underlie the current problems and allowing for an increased emotional awareness of feelings; (2) finding more accurate perceptions, where the patient is encouraged to compare and contrast old traumatic experiences with alternative views of similar current situations; and (3) trying new behavioral responses, where the therapist supports the development and testing of new behavioral responses.

These three groups of techniques do not have a 1:1 relationship to the three mechanisms of change. For example, increased insight and emotional awareness as a mechanism of change can be achieved through the technique of emotional exploration, but also from finding more accurate perceptions because that will inevitably deepen understanding of old feelings. New behaviors generate new feelings and perceptions that also become part of the patient's new insight and emotional awareness. New skills help to bring about change, and this is seen not only when new behaviors are developed and tested, but also when the patient develops increased skill at self-observation and increasing self-understanding, or when there is greater facility at testing and refining perceptions. In successful treatments, these mechanisms of change are exploited by a variety of techniques, and each technique has the potential to invoke several mechanisms of change.

Emotional Exploration

New understanding and emotional awareness often arise from the exploration of the self that pushes the bounds of what the patient knows or is comfortable with. Exploration implies there is an unknown that can become known, and the therapist is both a goad and a guide in this process. Michelle had to learn that she had powerful old feelings about her father—love, need for admiration, insecurity, anger at rejection— that were on the edges of her awareness. But their power was felt in her experience of her marriage, specifically her reactions to and perceptions of Jack.

The patient will benefit from experiencing old feelings with intensity and immediacy and experiencing the thoughts that go with them. If psychotherapy is a specialized form of learning, then it is emotional learning and the patient is engaged with deep feelings along with new insights. Our job is to find the old painful emotions the patient is struggling with, help the patient give voice to them, experience them again, and develop an understanding of their original context and meaning. The patient will feel some relief and distance from painful emotions when these techniques are successfully employed.

TECHNIQUES FOR EXPLORING EMOTION

The specific techniques for exploring emotions include:

• *Open-ended interviewing*: Open-ended questions—exploration of current, past, and transferential feelings, fantasies, memories, thoughts, and perceptions—allow the patient to experience these feelings as fully as possible. This is the classic psychodynamic approach, aimed at helping the patient get in touch with affects previously unexpressed, or amplifying affects that are suppressed, disavowed, denied, or ignored. A classical psychoanalyst might do this and not provide reassurance, specific support, or concrete answers.

• *Guided exploration* of known areas of conflict. As the areas of upset and the painful feelings become more known, regular returns to these parts of the patient's experience allow for more and more full experience of disturbing affects.

• *Micro-level approaches* in the interview for encouraging the patient to maintain awareness of painful feelings include (1) direct encouragement, education, and support; (2) empathic validation; and (3) silence and space to experience and reexperience.

• *Addressing anxiety.* Approaches to dealing with patient anxiety and disinclination to talk about painful matters include: patience and support, attempts to understand and validate the nature of the patient's discomfort, and interpretations about the patient's discomfort in the session and how this may be similar to feelings about other relationships.

• *Clarification.* Collecting instances of a repetitive scenario adds weight and depth to a patient's awareness of his or her experience, causing greater recognition of the power of earlier experiences.

• *Interpretation.* Providing a full explanation of the upsetting feelings—identifying and describing the repetitive traumatic scenario that underlies the patient's problem—increases the patient's understanding, but it may increase the patient's anxiety and upset first. Interpretations bring out new aspects of feeling, and this causes anxiety; but soon enough accurate and helpful interpretations decrease anxiety, because the explanations are true and understandable and tolerable. A number of empirical studies have found interpretations to be beneficial interventions (e.g., Orlinsky, Ronnestad, & Willutzki, 2004).

Painful affects are often kept at bay through the utilization of defense mechanisms (see Chapters 5 and 6). The analysis of defenses is a core component of psychodynamic therapies, and psychotherapy has been found to improve defensive functioning (Hersoug, Sexton, & Høglend, 2002; Hersoug, Bøgwald, & Høglend, 2005). Furthermore, improved defensive functioning has been associated with symptom relief (e.g., Coleman, 2005). Interestingly, though, there is some evidence that improvement in defenses may actually *follow* symptom change (e.g., Akkerman, Lewin, & Carr, 1999) instead of preceding it.

It is a big responsibility to dig deep and encourage patients to express what they feel. For the therapist it is an exciting sign of progress and intimacy, but also somewhat intimidating. New therapists may seek this experience but be afraid of it. There may be moments when a patient begins to experience intense emotion, and you will remember that old saying, "Be careful of what you wish for, because you just may get it." Newer therapists must learn to tolerate the anxiety they experience when patients feel and express intense emotions.

Some have suggested that repeated exposure to painful old emotions helps to diminish their intensity, and emotional exploration allows for "desensitization" (McCullough et al., 2002). Thus, this first technique involves focusing on and intensifying the experience of painful affects, with the expectation that this will bring about a subsequent decrease in anxiety and upset as the patient becomes more habituated. This "desensitization–habituation" process may take place over minutes within sessions, over an entire session, and over the weeks, months, and perhaps years of the psychotherapy.

Success in eliciting emotion and supporting the patient's experience of hitherto unexpressed or intolerable feelings gets the psychotherapeutic process started, but is often confused with the entire approach. Stopping here leaves the patient on the operating room table, so to speak. Patients often ask (and rightly so!), "What is the point of getting me to think about painful things, and how does that help me get better?"

In fact, it helps in the development of the therapeutic alliance, and in educating the patient, for this question to come up. The answer is that these painful feelings have been the cause of difficulty. Before a better solution to them can be found, one possibility is for the patient to understand them, tolerate them better, and find new ways of looking at them. That will pave the way to finding new behaviors to respond to the same old affects and perceptions.

Over time, experienced clinicians develop a sense of how much can and should be accomplished in a session. Every session should move toward a clearer picture and a more direct confrontation with painful emotion. Otto Kernberg said to us in a case conference when we were trainees: "I am impatient in every session, and very patient over time," referring to his attitude about progress in uncovering painful emotion in patients.

For example, the first third of Michelle's treatment involved frequent use of techniques to elicit her emotion about Jack's threatened separation, and the old feelings of loss and aloneness related to her father. She was able to let herself feel the traumatic sense of being cut off by her father, and the clearer that became, the less scary the marital issues were. No matter how much she wanted to keep the marriage intact, she began to realize that if it did not survive, she would have to pick up the pieces. However bad that would be, it would be different from the old experience with her father.

TECHNIQUES TO FACILITATE SOOTHING AND SELF-AWARENESS

Feeling previously warded-off emotions, recalling disavowed thoughts, and remembering troubling earlier memories are all results of good uncovering and exploratory psychotherapy. They increase anxiety, but remarkably, they also help make patients more comfortable. Anxiety decreases because painful affects typically have a finite life span, and they diminish in intensity.

The intensity of upsetting feelings is decreased when one discusses them aloud with another person. It is one of the mysteries of therapy (at least for us) that there is something curative and uplifting about feeling and sharing painful emotions in therapy. What else can we do to help a patient tolerate intensely felt emotion other than encourage her to express it?

• *Painful affects must be validated as normal human reactions.* Beginning therapists confuse this attitude with just being nice and warm, but it is different. The therapist must understand enough about the painful emotions and their context for them to make sense. Almost anything the patient feels is understandable and can be seen as the best possible response in the moment, given the circumstances. The therapist's intervention can take the form of verbalized empathy and understanding, or it can be the nonverbal silent communication that together expresses understanding. For Michelle, this meant simply affirming that her fear of rejection by her father was understandable, given how much she idealized and loved him. Because this feeling evolved when she was a child, she really did depend on him.

• *Connect the individual painful experience with a larger context of meaning.* For example, getting in touch with a deep sense of loss can make a patient feel worse and more hopeless. If this is understood as part of a ubiquitous human experience, or the kind of tragic circumstance others have suffered, or part of a personal trial, there is a larger meaning to the individual experience. The purpose here is not to convince the patient of something simply through encouragement or optimism, but rather to try to find a context for larger meaning that makes sense to the patient. For example, the therapist pointed out to Michelle that the intense bond she had with her father contributed to some of her best qualities, but also came with a lot of extra baggage.

• *Understand and empathize with the painful feeling in its historical context.* The therapist should encourage the patient to understand her pain as the remembered upset that has remained, ready to be reexperienced when the traumatic scenario from the past is restimulated. Patients find solace in the recognition that their intense feelings are part of their past, not part of their present life experience. This is reassuring because it acknowledges that the feelings may be strong, and they may be immediate, but they are finite and limited because they do not represent a current reality. Michelle actually started to feel the fear of aloneness as less overwhelming and as more of an old feeling than something connected to Jack. Indeed, many patients believe that self-understanding is a main curative factor in psychotherapy (Lilliengren & Werbart, 2005).

• *The intensity of upsetting feelings is decreased when their realistic basis is explored.* Helping the patient consider alternative perceptions, which we discuss in more detail below, reminds the patient that she has, metaphorically speaking, a foot in the past with the intense and upsetting experiences, and a foot in the present, seeing the same situation in another way. Generating new and possibly more adult and realistic perceptions of current situations helps the patient to see how much is present and how much historical baggage she is bringing to the situation. Therapists of many backgrounds help patients consider alternative interpretations to negative perceptions, but Beck and subsequent cognitive therapists have put this intervention at the center of their work (Beck et al., 1979).

• *Reminding the patient of the feeling of tolerance and containment experienced in the therapist's office* provides buffering and support. Identification with the therapeutic situation, and with the therapist, allows for increased tolerance of painful affects. So often, a patient in an effective psychotherapy will have a difficult time and will contain the emotion through the reassurance that she will talk about it at the next psychotherapy appointment. Even after therapy ends, some patients find it helpful to continue to have an internal dialogue with their therapist (Geller & Farber, 1993). Experiences such as these are not necessarily signs of an unhealthy dependence, but rather indicate a technique for managing, soothing, and containing painful affect.

TECHNIQUES TO DEAL WITH OVERWHELMING EMOTION

These techniques just discussed help to stir up old emotion and process it, allowing for habituation to painful inner experiences and increased understanding. They allow patients to tolerate themselves and their own feelings better. The repetitive experience of eliciting emotion and then putting it in context, sharing it in the therapeutic relationship, and leaving the office only to return again, represents the essence of emotional exploration, leading to increased insight and emotional awareness in the patient.

For some patients the techniques just described, which are designed to help the patient gain distance from painful emotions, may not be sufficient. Patients with overwhelming emotion reexperience but do not detach and get relief. Decreased session frequency, more cautious elicitation of painful affects and memories, and more focused exploration are all useful, but these techniques are not enough. Instead, these patients can take advantage of specific behavioral approaches that are more immediately soothing and supportive, such as breathing and relaxation techniques, meditation, guided imagery, journal writing, and other cognitive-behavioral strategies involved in dialectical behavior therapy (Linehan, 1993). These very helpful techniques are outside the scope of this book. Not everyone who is suffering is best treated with psychodynamic psychotherapy, and those who find it disorganizing to explore their emotions are probably more appropriately treated with skill-building and psychopharmacology, approaches that do not stir up painful feelings to the same degree.

Finding More Accurate Perceptions

Once Michelle could identify the old feelings and put them in their original context, she was less anxious and the old feelings were less intense. The second strategy for facilitating change is to help the patient adapt better to what she feels. We encourage the patient to develop new perceptions based on a here-and-now, more objective, multidimensional way of seeing things. The therapist asks and encourages speculation about the motivation and experiences of others in the patient's life and helps to consider a variety of ways of understanding difficult situations. These discussions often have a kind of "detective work" feel to them, with collaborative back-and-forth about possibilities and weighing and accepting or rejecting perceptions, responses, and realities.

Traditional psychodynamic psychotherapy is often unwavering in its focus on the patient and tends to eschew speculation about the motives and experiences of others, seeing this as often unknowable and distracting. In contrast, we regard this type of discussion as highly valuable. We think that talking about others in the patient's life improves the ability to perceive and understand interpersonal experiences. It was essential to Michelle's recovery that she became able to understand her husband better and see his behavior from a new perspective. The recognition that he was drained and hurt, which led to his detachment (rather than being basically cold, critical, and unloving), allowed her tolerate this period in their relationship much better.

We do not know, and our patients do not know, exactly what the objective reality is, in comparison with their repetitive scenario-based perceptions. Michelle's therapist met with the couple on two occasions, and this helped the therapist understand Jack better. As therapists, we do not set ourselves up as the arbiters of reality, because that is ultimately a capacity we want our patients to develop and improve. We obviously do not just want to replace one rigid way of viewing the world with another. However, we are often able to think of and suggest alternative ways of perceiving the situations our patients tell us about—what we think might "really be happening." Our role is to suggest alternatives, model flexibility (Borkovec & Sharpless, 2004), and help patients improve their own abilities to generate and evaluate these alternative ways of experiencing their lives.

Thus this second strategy for facilitating change helps develop the patient's skill at simultaneously perceiving the world in two ways, based on old scenarios and current realities. The old scenarios have a particular feel to them, and patients learn to recognize these feelings and put them in their place: in the past. New perceptions are based on current adult realities, and are often recognized by the fact that they feel different from the same old experiences. In the beginning, patients notice the difference between their old perceptions and new realities considerably later than the moment when the feelings are triggered. Further along in treatment, they come to recognize the disparity soon after the triggering experiences. Ultimately it becomes a more instantaneous process. This skill, like the ability to ride a bike or catch a ball, is something that can be developed with repetitive practice, and it requires discipline and focus. Initially it requires much conscious attention and a sense of hard work. With time, it becomes a part of the patient, a capacity that is present even when the patient is not aware of it. Michelle became adept at distinguishing between her old feelings of rejection and the perception of Jack as rejecting, and her current feeling of being a little bored and a perception of Jack as involved in his own life in a healthy way.

Trying New Behavioral Responses

The third technique for facilitating change is encouraging the patient to try out new behaviors. With a greater ability to tolerate painful feelings, and new and more contemporary perceptions of the repetitive trouble situations, the patient can try new behavioral responses. These new responses will often call upon social skills and capacities that may be evident in the areas of the patient's life less pervaded by conflict. Patients will often be able to come up with new strategies themselves, but we are not afraid to suggest new behaviors for patients to consider. Traditional psychodynamic psychotherapy tended to let patients struggle with their difficulties and encourage new behaviors when patients tried them. In contrast, we encourage collaboratively hatching new plans and guiding and encouraging patients to try them out.

Of course, there is a concern about stimulating a power struggle, infantilizing the patient, and reproducing earlier traumatic situations by "telling a patient what to do." New behaviors are considered, not forced, and attention is paid to the potential for deforming the treatment relationship in a way that will undermine the therapeutic alliance. Nonetheless, we believe the potential therapeutic impact of working actively to develop a new behavioral repertoire outweighs the risk of the therapist enacting old patterns.

Trying new behavior involves three steps: developing new behavioral responses, testing new behaviors, and learning from new behaviors.

DEVELOPING NEW BEHAVIORAL RESPONSES

With an increasingly clear picture of old scenarios and their repetition, it is much easier for the patient to break out of the old behaviors and try something new. Decades of behavioral research demonstrate that learning is easier in new environments. Indeed, therapy can constitute a novel environment, in a sense, and can serve as a means of stimulating new responses to old stimuli. Sometimes patients come up with new behavioral ideas themselves, sometimes they result from the therapist's suggestions, and often it is a collaborative process. The therapist actively counseled Michelle about the need to de-escalate her demands on Jack when she was hurt and anxious. She developed more patience and learned to ask for less and wait to see what came her way more naturally. She let him be, and worked hard to tone down her usual effusive emotional style when she knew it would push Jack away.

Using the opportunity created by a strong therapeutic alliance, the therapist can gently suggest the need for new behaviors, pointing out that feeling differently only takes a person so far. What are some possible ways of handling the same old situations differently? Ideas can be considered and evaluated for comfort, effectiveness, and appropriateness.

EVALUATING NEW BEHAVIORS

When the patient tries something new, then therapeutic attention is focused on how it felt, what was different, how the patient perceived things differently, and how the others in the scenario acted differently. This is empowering for the patient and often a moment of significant therapeutic change. It is the cart before the horse, in the sense that the patient has tried a new behavior that feels strange and foreign, and not natural to the situation. The patient can consider what was different from the usual response. Was there less distress, a different result from the interaction? Often trying one new behavior opens up the possibility of other approaches. An interpersonal situation that had seemed immutable and fixed starts to be a problem that can be solved—the patient is emboldened to bring attention to bear and improve it. Indeed, trying new behaviors often enhances patients' motivation in treatment.

LEARNING FROM NEW BEHAVIORS

A positive cycle develops when new behaviors succeed. They support and extend the patient's sense of self as capable of change, effective, and able to manage painful emotions. They validate the more adult and realistic aspects of the patient's perceptions and further reinforce the childhood origins of repeated upsetting experiences. A successful new behavior further supports the patient's capacity to effectively distinguish between the old scenarios and the current reality. New and more realistic ideas about others in the past and the present develop under these circumstances. All of these trends give rise to increased flexibility in thought and feeling and a readiness to embrace the world in a more positive light. Michelle felt better about herself when she felt she was behaving in a less needy way. She also felt she got more genuine attention from Jack.

A special circumstance of this type of learning occurs when a demoralized patient experiences a breakthrough in subjective experience. Sometimes this happens by design; a planned new behavior produces a surprising and positive result. Sometimes accidents occur. Either way, the new positive affect has the effect of shaking the patient, causing a kind of motivational tipping point and creating a new openness to change. Martin Seligman (2002) has referred to this "break in the clouds" as an important element in the treatment of depression.

Different techniques may work better for different patients. We do not know in advance who most needs increased insight and emotional awareness, who needs help with alternative perceptions and adaptations, and who needs work on new behavior. We are not taking a postmodern relativistic position that such information is unknowable, but rather that we simply do not know enough at this point in the development of our field to individually tailor the treatment in advance. Research has rarely focused on these techniques for facilitating change or on matching techniques to specific patients' problems. We hope that new data will illuminate this area.

We suspect that great therapists employ all of these strategies, figure out quickly which one is working best when, and tailor the treatment to the patient's strengths. Skilled psychotherapists make intuitive judgments and frequent changes in technique that tilt their work in one direction or the other—more awareness and insight versus more finding new perceptions versus more adjustment of behavior. They make these decisions based on observations about what helps in the therapy on a moment-to-moment and session-to-session basis. Following from this hypothesis, the PPP approach to psychotherapeutic change is to clearly identify the three strategies available to promote change and flexibly try them out while carefully observing the patient's response.

SUMMARY

The inexorable sequence of psychotherapy starts with creating an atmosphere of trust, where patients can uncover and explore painful feelings and understand their origins and context. This results in greater openness in considering new perceptions and trying new behaviors. Our discussion tries to clarify the confusion in the psychodynamic literature between mechanisms of change and techniques for facilitating it. These techniques make the inchoate "working through" process more clear and specific.

CHAPTER 11

Moments in Psychotherapy

We do not remember days,
we remember moments.
—CESARE PAVESE

Psychotherapy is a series of moments of attachment and engagement. It is a new kind of relationship for the patient (and the therapist). There are moments of particular intensity that stand out and account for much of the impact the treatment has on the patient. The empirical literature speaks of the therapeutic alliance as the most robust predictor of outcome (Martin et al., 2000), and the bond component of the alliance in particular is built up through moments of contact. In this chapter we describe some of the characteristic moments that occur and suggest how to facilitate them. Although every patient–therapist pair is different, there are some characteristic moments that occur when therapy is going well.

CLOSENESS

There are moments of *closeness and understanding*. The patient is open, expressing himself, feeling engaged in the here and now, and the therapist is responding fully. There is a quality of immediacy. It feels good for both participants, and they feel that something important is going on. This closeness usually occurs because a patient is talking about himself,

236

in specifics, about something emotional and particular (not global and observational), and the therapist feels she understands what the patient is feeling (Luborsky, 1984). It is about particulars, not generalities. Something mutual develops in the verbal interaction.

> Owen, a mistrustful young man who felt constantly inferior, manipulated by women, and one-upped by men, had been in therapy for 2 years. He was tall and thin, with short, reddish hair and an intense gaze. He worked as a lab technician and wanted to be a research scientist. He began to recognize that his feelings of competition and manipulation were projections of his own insecurity and anger. As vignette after vignette was discussed, he began to catch himself and genuinely understand that his reactions to others were driven by his old feelings about his father, mother, older brother, and stepmother.
>
> One day, after Owen described a workplace intrigue, I commented that his coworkers certainly had their personal motives, but he was interpreting their behavior according to the old template. I agreed that the older man in the office did treat him like he was at the bottom of the pecking order, and there was a woman who seemed secretive and scheming. But he was doing a good job, I said, and it seemed that in reality he was safe from his coworkers. I said I thought the problem was his own feelings about his work, his tendency to see things according to his relationships with his parents (and stepmother). I said I thought he was able to see this now, and in seeing this, now he really had to face his dreams and aspirations and uncertainty about fulfilling them, instead of complaining about others.
>
> There was a long silence, during which Owen looked at me, and time seemed slowed down. I thought maybe I had overreached, said too much, or made him feel criticized. Maybe he was hurt and had detached, or maybe he was just very moved. Finally, he said softly, "I'm scared because I don't know if I will be ever able to do what I really want." This time, I left a long pause. I did not know what to say, and then realized that I did not have to say anything. It was his moment, his facing his own fears, and I was there with him. I felt like I knew what he was feeling, and that I'd seen inside his mind more clearly than ever before. I felt an intense sense of closeness and bonding. The room seemed to disappear, and for a moment, it was just the two of us contemplating what was before him.

Moments of intense closeness such as this are exciting and potentially anxiety provoking for both the patient and the therapist. One hopes they allow the patient to feel known, accepted, affirmed, and perhaps loved. The therapist, too, may experience something redeeming and transformative about these moments, making her feel special and unique, yet humbled by the commonality of people's struggles. These moments of increased rapport indicate that therapy is on the right track (Malan, 1979).

Whatever specific content is being discussed, there is a powerful positive emotional valence to these moments. The positive feeling of closeness and understanding usually improves the mood and level of attention of both parties. Fredrickson's (2001) experimental studies suggest that positive mood is accompanied by an increased capacity to consider alternative strategies for problem solving, and this undoubtedly also contributes to the therapeutic effectiveness of these experiences.

Moments of closeness and understanding may seem ineffable and hard to reduce scientifically, but as Louis Pasteur said, "Chance favors the prepared mind." Ongoing attention to the patient's feelings, awareness of one's own, a consistent effort at understanding the patient's repetitive patterns, and enough flexibility and spontaneity will allow the therapist to make the most of these moments when they occur, and perhaps make them more likely.

LOSS

One therapist described being with a patient who is experiencing loss as follows:

> "Much of the time in sessions (but certainly not always) I feel calm and emotion-filled but not overwhelmed or confused. There is a sense of being a vessel that fills and empties—I listen, empathize, imagine, feeling but not reacting too much. If I am sad, I will be sad with the patient; if I feel loss, I think about things I feel like I have lost. If irritated, I usually realize it is my limitation, though stirred up by something the patient is doing. Above all, I try to stay close, connected, feeling, engaged, but aware that what the patient is feeling is not me."

When a patient is *contemplating feelings of sadness, loss, or limitation,* the therapist has a poignant, sad feeling, too, prompting her to reflect on her own losses, separations, traumas, and the passage of time. These moments usually have a fresh feeling for the patient—until now, the sadness has been avoided, but the patient lets it in, realizing that it hurts but that it is not so bad. Most patients are frightened of feeling sadness and loss. Feelings of loss are no more and no less than that—they are feelings about something that has already happened.

A young man suddenly lost a father-like figure who was a steady source of support during his childhood and early adulthood; this was just a year after losing a favorite aunt. This patient's mother died when he was a young child, and he was alienated from his father. When he told me about the sudden death, I teared up, experiencing these losses with him. In this case, I did not say anything, I simply sat there with him for a few minutes quietly.

Patients will usually see a gradual diminution in the intensity of sadness and loss. The feelings will become more of a familiar companion for the patient, present but not disruptive, less of a terrifying and overwhelming experience. The therapist will often feel a sense of satisfaction and comfort in observing this trend in a patient, and it is usually a sign that the therapy is moving forward.

But sometimes the sadness is so intense, and so deep, that it does not get better after talking about it. This is often the case in patients with attachment problems, self-esteem problems, or those who are so mired in depression that there is no way out yet. The biggest challenge for the therapist here is tolerating the shared feeling of sadness. We are all vulnerable to feeling overwhelmed by loss, we all feel it, and it might be the hardest emotion to keep in perspective. There may be plenty of moments when some of us who are merely mortal therapists will have difficulty tolerating this, and we defensively avoid the feelings of loss.

Most patients do not want to be convinced out of their sadness too quickly—others have usually tried to encourage them before. Some degree of empathic mirroring and encouragement is necessary for them to get somewhere. Intense sadness gets either better or worse with therapeutic attention. If it is not getting better, likely it will get worse; affect-amplifying, empathic attention to feelings of sadness and loss may be stressing the patient's ability to cope, and the therapist must find another path. The strategies for change described in Chapter 10 include a range of alternative approaches for this. The therapist must make a strategic decision in moments of loss about how much to empathize and share the feeling, and how much to help the patient manage and mitigate it. These are not mutually exclusive, but it can be confusing to do both at the same time.

JOY

On the other side of the continuum are *experiences of positive emotion*— laughing together, sharing joy at a fortunate event in the patient's life, feeling intense admiration or respect for the patient, even a form of love. Sometimes these moments come in the context of closeness and intimacy, but they may occur simply because of the positive emotional tone of what is being discussed or because something positive has occurred between patient and therapist. One patient discussed some wonderful career successes and moments of breakthough positive feelings about his wife and family. His pride, joy, and love were palpable in the session and caused a similar response in the therapist. Another patient had a remarkable daughter, and news of her latest successes was always a shot in the arm.

Joy is open, inclusive, emotional, and arises from union, connection, serenity, and acceptance (Vaillant, 2008). Joy reflects adaptation and acceptance, and should increase with therapy.

> Ann was in her mid-50s, and her mother had several bouts of depression during Ann's childhood. Over the course of therapy, Ann realized that she loved her mother and felt very close to her, yet she had tremendous buried anger toward her because of her unavailability during long stretches of her childhood. She was anxious about any angry or critical feelings in herself, fearing that such feelings were unacceptable and dangerous to others. She worked terribly hard to maintain an upbeat attitude toward her mother, and indeed toward everyone, and pushed herself to care for her now-aging mother despite her negative feelings. In fact, she was a model daughter. But she wondered whether she really loved her mother, or was just doing her duty.
>
> Ann was a warm and kind woman who maintained a careful distance in the therapy. After several sessions in which I confronted her directly about her ambivalence toward her mother and her fear of acknowledging any anger lest she feel like she would explode with rage, she unexpectedly saw her mother at a distance in the local supermarket. Ann's mother was at the far end of an aisle, and Ann watched her unobserved for a moment. As though seeing her anew, Ann felt a powerful surge of love and affection, seeing this elderly gray-haired woman carefully choosing groceries. Gone were the burden and obligation. Instead she felt, and knew instantly, that she really did love her mother. She was deeply contented, indeed joyful, to realize with certainty how much she loved her mother, and how fortunate she was to have her. As she described this experience, her love emanated from her, and I was filled with a similar feeling. I simply commented that she seemed to love her mother very much.

Positive emotion can come from the patient or the therapist. It is almost always infectious and shared. We know that patients can have strong positive feelings toward therapists, that is, positive transference based on positive relationships from the past, or based on ambivalent relationships that are too painful to experience in their entirety. Positive transference is transient and unstable. Joy in the therapeutic relationship is irreducible, based in the here and now, and usually increases over time.

The culture of psychoanalysis, and its trickle-down into the culture and technique of psychodynamic psychotherapy, does not place great stock on the value of expressing positive emotion in treatment. It is seen as risky because the patient may misunderstand, the therapist may take license in expressing private countertransference feelings, and boundaries may be crossed. When it comes to positive emotion, the traditional view seems to be that less is more.

We question this view and wonder whether it cuts off the therapeutic lifeblood of positive affect. Positive experiences are often what patients remember, what they like, and what cause them to refer others for psychotherapy. We suggest that moments of positive emotion help to grease the wheels of change. This may be particularly powerful with a therapist who generally restricts expression of positive emotion, but perhaps it is just as effective when the therapist is frequently warm and positive. Certainly there are limits to appropriateness, and the mutual experience of positive feelings should respect the boundaries of the relationship, a professional one determined and limited by the goals of the patient feeling better. The warmth and affection of a good therapist is more like the love of a grandparent than the emotional intensity of a parent or partner.

The positive emotional experiences that occur in psychotherapy are just not written about much or talked about in professional venues. In fact, they are probably an essential staple of good psychotherapy (whether psychodynamic, cognitive, or behavioral). They are part of the art, not the written procedure.

DIFFICULT DECISIONS

The psychotherapy relationship is generally a collaborative one (e.g., Bordin, 1979), and optimally each partner does his or her part. The patient talks about feelings and thoughts, stepping back and reflecting, trying to consider alternatives and new behaviors; the therapist listens, focuses, and empathizes. But there are particular moments when there is a sense that the patient is at a fork in the road, with an important decision to make, or struggling with whether and how to approach a situation in a new way. The patient wonders whether to sleep with someone for the first time, to quit a job and pursue something new, or to take a stand against an old familial pattern. The therapist may or may not have an opinion, but has a feeling of great responsibility. What she says might really matter.

There is a particular poignancy to this moment. The feeling that something very important is at stake, and a choice to be made, is powerful and even awe inspiring for the therapist. It is a moment of potential change. Like other emotional moments, this one is so resonant because both participants feel the significance of time passing, directions chosen and forgone, and hope for the future tempered by sober respect for the unknown.

In the end, it is always the patient who makes the decision, yet what the therapist does is never entirely neutral or dispassionate, nor should it be. The more your patient is choosing among reasonable alternatives, the more hands-off and facilitating of her independent decision-making process you can be. The more the choice the patient is leaning toward is unhealthy or unreasonable and the patient's perceptions and reasoning is distorted, the more important it will be to exercise your responsibility by offering guidance and advice.

THE ABSURDITY OF LIFE

Life is not fair, and sometimes patients are served such a big helping of bad fortune that it triggers a powerful feeling of meaninglessness and recognition of the absurdity of life. This is usually a therapeutic moment, too, because to experience absurdity means to feel that there is no dark and personal reason for unfortunate events (the kind of perception that is usually the basis for a psychological problem).

The therapist's stance is to enthusiastically recognize and appreciate the patient's experience of absurdity; this is not usually difficult because it is so palpable. This moment does not require anything complicated from the therapist; it has a built-in therapeutic quality to it. The patient is feeling a release from the sadness and pain of whatever has happened, liberated by recognizing the absurdity of it.

A more superficial version of this occurs when you and the patient smile together about something absurd in the therapy situation, such as an elevator in the building that takes a long time to come, bad traffic, running out of Kleenex, or dealing with insurance companies.

ABOUT THE THERAPY

There is a wonderful moment that comes when you and the patient see a new life narrative together. Sometimes the narrative follows the therapist's interpretation of an event and its connection to the patient's larger developmental arc, and sometimes it follows from the patient's own synthesis. The feeling of seeing the same thing together and the sense of satisfaction that results from seeing clearly a deep, pervasive pattern, come together in a moment of collaborative closeness. This is not the deep emotional resonance of empathic communication; it has a different feel. It feels more like the satisfaction coworkers feel about a difficult job well done.

Sometimes patients are frustrated with therapy because it is slow, uncomfortable, expensive, and the results are uncertain. They may have transferential reactions that make the therapist seem rejecting, cold, or unhelpful. This leads the therapist to feel anxious, defensive, or frustrated in return. The therapist can respond with increased conviction, feeling that this frustration is the patient's problem, certainly not the therapist's. This retreat to arrogance is, sadly, a common reaction. Learning not to engage in this automatic response is one of the most important interpersonal skills novice clinicians must develop. Alternatively, therapists can become anxious and uncertain and try to appease the patient by placating and minimizing the conflict.

Paying close attention to what the patient is feeling, empathizing, and connecting affectively is the reparative response to a frustrated patient. It will help the patient calm down and identify the source of the discontent and consider what to do about it. Appropriate apologies from the therapist about errors, slights, and misunderstandings help to decrease the hot emotion of feeling misunderstood. When a patient feels hurt, then a hurt has occurred. The challenge for the therapist is to feel this and express it genuinely, not as a manipulation. That is, when a patient feels slighted and hurt, it is important to understand how and why this came about. But in the moment, the slight simply feels true. The therapist must intervene to help the patient feel better first to help her gather a larger sense of perspective. Respect for the patient's emotional reactivity, which we all have, will allow the therapist to express this with sincerity.

How should the therapist respond when it becomes clear that the patient is getting better? Improvement in the patient may be apparent in a new level of contentment, a new ability to perceive a relationship or situation realistically, or a typically troublesome situation handled in a new way. Admiration, respect, and positive feedback are the appropriate responses. The patient will usually notice the changes, but it will help for the therapist to point them out. Not only does this validate the change and increase the motivation for more change, but the positive emotion leads to further problem-solving flexibility.

EMOTION ABOUT YOU

Telling another person how you feel about them is usually restricted to close, personal relationships. But our patients have feelings about us, and it is important to help them share these feelings. Therapy is an unusual opportunity for honesty and directness; you and your patients will talk about things that are present in ordinary conversation but unacknowledged. It is a privilege and a skill for a patient to be able to express her feelings about the therapist in therapy.

It can feel awkward for new therapists to inquire about patients' feelings about them. It seems presumptuous, like indulging in narcissism or fishing for compliments. But simple inquiries about how the patient is feeling can be followed by encouragement that discussing such things is not weird or inappropriate. A patient's expression of emotion about you is a moment that is different from closeness, loss, or the other moments we have discussed. It is less mutual than some of these other moments. You are likely to be either reacting and absorbing the patient's affect, or feeling detached and conceptualizing what is going on.

Patients' feelings about you are related to the here-and-now relationship, the therapeutic alliance, and to revived old feelings (i.e., the transference). It is gratifying when the patient expresses trust, respect, and confidence in the therapy and in her relationship with you. But there may also be criticism, either direct or implied. Observations about your personal characteristics are as likely to be positive as negative. You will need to listen carefully and accept what is said, with the assumption that it is true because it is how the patient feels.

Sometimes patients consciously withhold their feelings because they are embarrassed or frightened. Often, they unconsciously withhold because they fear rejection, dependency, vulnerability, or competition. When the patient's reaction to you is based on something painful she is feeling but not able to name, articulating the feelings often helps. It may be therapeutic to reflect back to a patient that she seems to feel rejected by you, or irritated with you, or misunderstood; your awareness of those feelings helps the patient to feel understood. This can help diminish the patient's fear about expressing herself.

When a patient is talking about you, you need to step back, simultaneously feeling and observing. The best way to respond to a moment of emotion about you is to feel your response, know what it is, and not act on it right away. You will have your own personal emotional reaction—pride, pleasure, hurt, anxiety, sadness, anger. But feelings you have about the patient that are not based on admiration, respect, and empathy are best held in awareness and felt, rather than expressed or acted on. Of course, it is impossible, both theoretically and practically, to not act at all; we are human and have feelings, and these are inevitably communicated. But it is our solemn responsibility to hold our reactions in check, to reflect and not to act out. It is our responsibility to make the patient comfortable exploring himself, while we find ways of tolerating it.

MISTAKES

As therapists, we inevitably make mistakes, such as forgetting important information, mixing up the appointment schedule, and making insensitive comments. Mistakes can often be subtle, too, such as attending to one issue over another that might be important, or being distracted and not paying full attention for part of a session. Although these errors are inevitable, they often cause therapists much guilt and self-questioning. Therapy can look easy—you just sit and talk with someone—but it requires consistent focus that is hard to maintain. We therapists have moods, subjective responses, waxing and waning attention, personal interests and sensitivities. It is valuable to examine a mistake to see whether there is any new information that it brings to your attention. Mistakes may reflect countertransference. For example, did you mix up the appointment because you had an urge to avoid the patient, and if so, why would you feel that way? Did the patient communicate disinterest in the therapy or dislike of you? Did you forget to charge a patient, hoping it would induce them to like you more?

A mistake and its discovery causes both therapist and patient to stop and pay attention. In fact, part of why attention to mistakes is so valuable is because immediately afterward you are both paying close attention to each other (Casement, 2002). A mistake and its repair is a therapeutic moment when the mistake is rare. When mistakes are frequent, they are not therapeutic and there is a problem with the therapist.

It is almost always the best course to acknowledge a mistake. In the discourse of everyday life, when one makes a mistake, one apologizes.

This signifies recognition of the impact the mistake has had on the other person and acknowledges responsibility. Apology usually helps to set the therapeutic relationship right, but it does not mean you cannot also ask the patient how she felt about the mistake and about your apology. But if therapy is fundamentally about helping a patient develop a new, better, and more accurate narrative, truth-telling and acknowledgement of responsibility are essential qualities. If the therapist cannot do this, the patient will be less emboldened to try. Of course, apologies should not be made for the therapist's sake, to decrease guilt or avoid thinking about what drove the error. You should think about what would comfort you if you were a patient, and what would repair the breach of confidence and safety. It is usually helpful to ask the patient how she felt about your apology.

> A teenager with repeated self-defeating behaviors was so stuck in a cycle of depression, resentment, and rejection that I became frustrated; I lost my composure and got angry. Feeling guilty, I discussed my outburst with several supervisors, teachers, and colleagues. I knew it had been a mistake, and my degree of frustration indicated that I had lost my focus on empathy and let my personal feeling of ineffectiveness come to the fore.
>
> I was ready to apologize at the next session when the patient showed up 15 minutes late. She looked depressed and disheveled. She had difficulty saying much. I expressed my regret and remorse at being short-tempered in the previous session, and the patient cheered up remarkably quickly. Later in the session, she said that my anger made her feel like I cared for her. No one else took her feelings that seriously. This was a turning point in the therapy and subsequently she began to understand more about why she was so self-defeating, and began to make changes in her behavior.

Of course, we do not advocate that therapists yell at patients or make other therapeutic mistakes. Rather, we should be open to seeing that a mistake may have important implications for an individual patient when it is part of a consistent, understanding, and accepting treatment. It is our job to do our best to make the mistake into something positive and useful.

The old worry about apologizing is that it might preclude a deeper discussion of motives and reasons and make it harder to understand the patient's conflicts. But expressing something positive, like apology, support, and validation of harm, does not preclude the exploration of something negative, such as the patient's hurt or anger.

SELF-DISCLOSURES, BEING PERSONAL

A favorite supervisor once said that a therapist should show a patient the same courtesy, respect, and interest you would show to someone you are seated next to at a dinner party. Above all else, be normal! This advice extends to handling personal questions and self-disclosure. Of course, the therapy is for the patient and about the patient, but you cannot expect a patient to become comfortable talking openly and honestly if you do not show some signs of getting engaged.

Another way to say this is that any interaction is like a song, with words and music. The words are literal part of the interaction, but the music is that part which is emotional, attached, and rhythmic; without the music, the song is just a bunch of words. The therapist must experience and express feelings to make the therapy more than a bunch of words. The therapist should say as much as is necessary, but as little as possible to avoid distraction. One therapist said:

> "When patients ask where I am going on vacation, I tell them. When they ask who is coming along, I will usually answer that, too. Leave-taking is part of life, and this topic is more likely to be shut down if I don't provide the information than if I answer it. If a patient goes on to ask what I will be doing, what the place is like, and so on, then I will ask how they are feeling about the vacation, what they are wondering about me and my life. Telling the specifics about my vacation is not likely to help the therapy much, and it might make for distraction; also I've already answered some questions, so I have maintained a genuine engagement with the patient. When questions are pursued to this degree, it is usually based on the transference and fantasies about the therapist, and that is probably where the attention should then be focused."

Comments about here-and-now aspects of life, what neighborhood the therapist lives in, whether she's seen a recent movie, whether she has children, where education or training took place, are all part of "being normal." Furthermore, by answering some of these questions, the therapist can justifiably inquire about the meaning of the patient's curiosity.

Expressing sad, affectionate, joyful, and concerned feelings about the patient is appropriate when genuine. Positive emotions are almost always appropriate to express, while negative ones are rarely constructive. Irritation and resentment are usually problems of the therapist, not the patient. The therapist needs to work these uncomfortable feelings out, and it is rarely useful to express them. Sometimes it is possible to constructively express negative feelings about a patient's behavior, asking whether others may have reacted this way—for example, "I felt like you pushed me away after you broke down and cried; I wonder if others have felt this."

The traditional approach has been to be very careful about self-disclosure. Too much personal information can be a burden on the patient and can distract from what the patient is there to work on. It can also make it harder to see the transference.

If your negative feelings are powerful and interfering, then consultation with a colleague is invariably the best course. Usually, discussion and understanding will be enough to tame these negative emotions so that you will be able to use them constructively. If not, then the patient should probably be referred to someone who will like her more; at that point, it's just not a good match.

SUMMARY

The experiences of emotion and connection we have discussed here do not do justice to the many types of experiences you can have. They are some of the most common and powerful ones. These moments in psychotherapy help to increase the bond between the patient and therapist. Because they are new experiences for the patient, they also reflect new relational experiences, one of the three mechanisms of change in psychotherapy.

CHAPTER 12

Therapist Strengths, or Managing Your Countertransference

> People seem not to see that their opinion of the world
> is also a confession of their character.
> —RALPH WALDO EMERSON

In the last few chapters we focused on the building blocks of therapy—formulation, goal setting, facilitating change, and therapeutic moments. But to be effective, a therapist must be able to move beyond these building blocks. It is the instantaneous reactions you have that will transform a conversation with the patient into therapy. The therapist's personality strengths and how they are applied will make for a "therapeutic" demeanor and will help to bring about therapeutic moments.

Marjorie was a 63-year-old widow suffering from depression and anxiety. She called initially for medication advice and then began to call for reassurance approximately three times a day. She complained when phone calls were not returned promptly (i.e., within an hour or two). She repeatedly described her fear, aloneness, and terrible nausea, often like she was telling me about it for the first time. Sometimes she was irritable. She seemed to have a great deal of difficulty feeling self-sufficient. She had a weekly appointment, where we focused on her difficulty functioning while addressing her sadness and loss. She wanted multiple appointments over the week, feeling that this was the only thing that would help her. She also needed to know that I was there, and would be able very quickly to answer her calls. Often, she brought up the possibility of seeing a different therapist.

I could certainly see Marjorie's ongoing depression and anxiety, and her pattern of repetitively seeking encouragement. I understood that she was resentful about being denied constant comforting reassurance. I felt compassionate and concerned, and I returned her calls and responded to her worries, hoping this would reassure her and decrease her anxiety about starting treatment. I had the feeling that the calls would slow down as she felt that I was responsive. I met with her twice a week for a few weeks.

But the calls kept coming, sometimes three or four times per day. I was more and more annoyed by the number of calls and the complaints she made. Hers was a dependent transference, and at times even a hostile dependent transference (she was both dependent on and angry at me). After a while, it evoked an irritable and rejecting countertransference feeling in me.

Several times I tried to tactfully bring up the possibility that this pattern was similar to what happened in other relationships (her grown children from whom she was estranged). She was very insulted and almost quit treatment. I was sure it was not going to be helpful to discuss my negative feelings about the interaction with Marjorie, and I realized that any continuing attempt to provide this insight to her was really just an outlet for my irritation.

Instead, I expressed support and reassurance and reminded her that the symptoms would probably get better, as they had in the past. I gave firm guidelines about how she should take her medication and answered most but not all of her calls. She seemed to feel better when I was warm and reassuring, and appreciated greatly the sense that I was trying to take care of her, despite the fact that she frequently felt upset that no one was helping her.

I reassured her that I thought she would feel better and suggested that the terrible loneliness and the physical symptoms of nausea were how she felt when she was dislocated, lonely, and worried about the future. I told her I would help her to feel better and find better ways of dealing with the loneliness and misery, and I tried to do so in a direct, calm, unpatronizing tone. I kept one foot in the relationship, feeling worried about her intense loneliness and anxiety, and one foot outside, regarding her as a patient who was going through something she would look back on in 6 months with a different perspective. I expressed optimism and hope about the future and said that she still had so many things to look forward to and enjoy. All the while, I encouraged her activity, social life, and healthy time alone.

Marjorie took these comments in and continued to express her feelings of loneliness; she continued to call, but less frequently. She picked up her social activities a little and started playing golf again. She insisted she felt as badly and complained that I was not really helping her enough. But she also expressed her appreciation for the therapy, and said, "Thank God I've at least got this to come to each week."

In this vignette, the therapist's personal qualities—his steadiness, knowledge, warmth, genuineness, optimal distance, and optimism— were used to stabilize, support, and "contain" the patient. The strengths were present in the therapist's tone of voice, body language, and informal comments. These qualities helped to provide Marjorie with a considerate responses to her distress, unlike the frequent responses of others in her life. The therapist was able to resist becoming part of a destructive and rejecting enactment, and Marjorie had a new and more positive experience. Although this example involved a primarily supportive phase of therapy, these strengths are just as useful in more directly exploratory work.

EFFECTIVE THERAPISTS

Given how important the personal qualities of the therapist seem to be, it is striking how little is known about what makes for an effective psychotherapist. We summarize some of the findings from a thorough review on this topic by Beutler et al. (2003). Therapist gender, gender match, and race seem to have little impact on patient outcome despite a widespread belief that this is important. The type and amount of professional training a therapist has received, and his or her skill in facilitating therapeutic processes, have not shown meaningful effects on therapy outcomes (Beutler et al., 2003). There is even conflicting evidence for the positive impact of therapist experience on outcome (Blatt, Sanislow, Zuroff, & Pilkonis, 1996; Propst, Paris, & Rosberger, 1994; Hupert et al., 2001).

There is, however, increasing evidence for the relation between competent delivery of a treatment and good outcome (Barber, Crits-Christoph, & Luborsky, 1996; Barber, Sharpless, Klosterman, & McCarthy, 2007). A few studies report significant effects on treatment outcome of adherence to a treatment manual (Bein et al., 2000; Feeley, DeRubeis, & Gelfand, 1999; Kendall & Chu, 2000). But others have found a curvilinear relation between adherence and outcome (Barber et al., 2006); that is, there is better outcome with a medium degree of treatment manual adherence than a low or high degree of adherence.

Therapist self-disclosure showed statistically significant but clinically weak positive effects on outcome (Barrett & Berman, 2001; Piper, Joyce, Azim, & McCallum, 1998; Piper, McCallum, Joyce, Azim, & Ogrodniczuk, 1999). Although therapist emotional well-being was found to be significantly related to patient outcome in some studies (e.g., McGuff, Gitlin, & Enderlin, 1996; McCarthy & Frieze, 1999; Williams & Chambless, 1990), the research reviewed by Beutler et al. (2003) did not suggest a causal relation between the two. Therapist racial attitudes have been investigated through research on therapist cultural sensitivity training or the use of a culturally sensitive treatment to patient outcome. These studies found consistently high effect sizes (Evans, Acosta, Yamamoto, & Skilbeck, 1984; Thompson, Worthington, & Atkinson, 1994; Wade & Bernstein, 1991), as reviewed by (Beutler et al., 2003).

As we discussed in Chapter 4, studies indicate small effect sizes for the relationship between quality of the therapeutic relationship and outcome (Martin et al., 2000). Although a causal link remains to be confirmed (see Barber et al., 2000; Barber, 2009), the therapeutic relationship quality is still considered a strong predictor of outcome.

Summarizing what is known about psychotherapist qualities, Beutler et al. (2003) concluded that there has been a precipitous decline in attention to therapist variables, and many promising earlier findings have not been pursued. This seemingly important question has been difficult to capture and study in empirical research. It may be that the research designs have been insufficiently powerful to yield conclusions, or perhaps the right questions have not yet been asked. Perhaps it is hard to get therapists to agree to be studied.

This brief review shows how little we know about the qualities of the therapist that make therapy more effective. Our focus on therapist strengths provides a way of addressing the needs of early-career therapists to not simply learn a technique, but to learn a way of being. We begin by looking at how a therapist pays attention in therapy sessions and move on to therapist personality strengths and specific approaches for using these strengths to manage the difficult emotions you will experience as you work with patients.

PAYING ATTENTION

When the telephone rings during a psychotherapy session, we should let the voice mail pick it up. To do otherwise would pull the therapist's attention away from the patient, and this might be upsetting. But what else do we know about where the therapist should direct his attention in effective psychotherapy?

Freud spoke of the "evenly suspended attention" (1912b) of the psychoanalyst, characterizing a kind of relaxed and flexible shifting of attention to what the patient says and does, and the internal feelings, thoughts, and fantasies of the analyst. The Freudian analyst is caricatured as a distant and unengaged presence, but this concept of listening to the patient and to oneself is actually quite strenuous and requires a lot of engagement.

The patient's emotional state is the most important thing to pay attention to. Emotions may be expressed verbally or nonverbally. There is usually one dominant emotion experienced at any point in time, and the therapist should focus on this—whether it is sadness, loss, anger, longing, anxiety, or pleasure. The therapist should be aware of it, observing it and watching for shifts and changes. Usually the patient is aware of the feeling the therapist senses, but not always.

Like the faith healers who held their hands over the sick person's body, "feeling" for the illness, we metaphorically try to sense the emotional hot spot in the patient's experience. Learning to do this is learning to simplify one's perceptions; there is an overwhelming amount of detail to observe about a person, and there are momentary shifts in topic, attitude, and body language. Sensing the dominant affect is like squinting while looking, so that only the broad outlines are clear. Patients get lost in their own complexity, and it is up to us to help them simplify and focus. Close attention to emotions is important, because at a moment of readiness, the therapist will want to help the patient name the feeling and connect it with what he is thinking about.

Simultaneous with the empathic attention to emotions, the experienced therapist listens to what the patient says, keeping track of the story, the characters, and the facts. These data fit into patterns, and the therapist thinks logically, rationally, and sequentially about the clinical information, organizing it in different ways. This occupies a certain amount of the therapist's attention, generating hypotheses about the formulation, trying to fit the pieces together, and modifying and trying other ideas. The therapist's attention to patterns also includes considering various interventions and imagining the patient's response to them.

Thus there is an oscillation in attention between feelings and thoughts, between the patient's emotional experience, and the words, facts, and ideas the patient is talking about, and how they are conceptualized. (Our minds enable us to keep track of multiple incoming feeds of information, so this dual attention is not a new or alien ability. It just takes practice to develop.) There are periods when the patient is speaking and the therapist is thinking hard about exactly what is being said and how it fits with the history. At other times one is looking "through" the words as they are spoken, focusing instead on the dominant feeling the patient is experiencing.

The intensity of attention that occurs for both patient and therapist fluctuates. There are times when the patient is deeply attending to himself and looking at himself in a new way, seeing new aspects of himself and new meanings to thoughts and behaviors. There is a particular look of activation, a slight widening of the eyes, loss of focus, and a quality of distraction we can see in the patient who is paying especially close attention to his thoughts and feelings.

Often, the therapist zeros in on the patient's experience at a moment like this, trying to imagine exactly what the patient is feeling. This type of rapt attention, with a loss of a sense of time because of immersion in the moment, has been referred to as "flow" in the general psychology literature (Csikszentmihalyi, 1991). The state of flow involves such attention and engagement that nothing else exists for the moment. Such moments occur episodically in therapy, and when they occur, they are usually valued highly by patients as well as therapists.

The opposite of flow is wandering attention on the part of the therapist. Just as we are looking for disparities in the patient's communication, we are also looking for evidence of our own unconscious at work in how we listen. Thus the wandering attention may be due to an enactment in the relationship with the therapist, or to some problem in effective communication between the two. An example of an enactment would be a patient who is very reserved and careful, and who reveals so little of himself that it is uninteresting and hard to pay attention. Another would be a patient who overpowers the therapist with the intensity of his affect or the violence of his language. Sometimes the content of what a patient says is overwhelming; for example, hearing about abuse or acute psychological pain is often so upsetting that it is hard for a therapist to listen. Alternatively, perhaps the patient's communication style is not congenial to the therapist's because of cultural, temperamental, or language differences.

These problems with wandering attention can only be addressed by confronting and working out the issues themselves. The self-protective patient needs support, encouragement, and help expressing himself; the aggressive patient needs tactful confrontation to understand why he needs to be so aggressive and help him find a way of developing a collaborative relationship.

Of course, the difficulty in focusing attention may truly be the therapist's, and not the result of something about the patient. Too little sleep, hunger, preoccupation with personal problems, illness, depression, and imminent vacation are all common reasons for this. The therapist must try to address and manage these concerns. The abused patient must be heard, and the therapist needs to reflect on his personal emotional responses to the upsetting material to make sure he is able to be empathic.

THERAPIST'S INNER EXPERIENCE

One patient impishly inquired as the therapist was keeping notes during a session, "What are you writing down now, your shopping list for dinner?" She was being funny, but she expressed her worry (and, perhaps, her annoyance) about not being listened to. She was also acknowledging an obvious fact: Therapists have their own feelings and thoughts, they are human, and it is only natural that they will spend some of their time daydreaming and thinking about themselves. Most of us fantasize about a day in the sun when listening to a patient glowingly recall a beach vacation.

The psychoanalytic tradition has creatively mined the remarkable fact that the therapist's feelings and thoughts reveal much not only about himself, but also about the patient he is listening to. The therapist who feels comfortable and satisfied during his 8:00 patient appointment, anxious and insecure at 9:00, irritated and impatient at 10:00, and daydreaming of love at 11:00, may just be having a busy day, but more likely these feelings reflect something of the interaction with each of the patients. The therapist brings some consistent vulnerabilities, interests, and strengths to all interactions, and is the same person in each hour, but like a set of tuning forks that vibrate sympathetically with sounds in the environment, different feelings and thoughts in the therapist will be stimulated by different patients. The challenge is to use these feelings effectively; you do not want to suppress them, but you cannot be immersed in them.

The best and worst part of being a therapist is the constant emotional experience. You feel open and reactive, stretched in many directions by powerful feelings about the patient, about the therapy, or about yourself; or closed and struggling, wondering why you are closed, why you seem to want to be. These "in your face" emotional experiences are an essential part of therapy and usually enable therapists to sense early on whether this is their calling.

Maintaining perspective on your emotions while letting yourself go to feel whatever you feel is the challenge. If you try to control your emotions you will be exhausted, irritable, and unempathetic. Ultimately, it will not work anyway. If you let yourself go and forget to observe and reflect on your feelings, you will lose the focus on the patient, and your responses might be spontaneous but not professional and helpful. Honest self-scrutiny is what we ask of our patients, and we try to do the same ourselves. It is endlessly challenging, and appreciating the difficulty of self-observation will help you to keep your empathy for patients' struggles in doing this.

It usually takes a few years of learning therapy and observing yourself before you recognize and clarify your individual and unique responses to patients: particular enjoyment when patients are affectionate, fear of upsetting an already upset person, or a tendency to criticize and chastise. Certainly these feelings arise because of something the patient feels toward you. But you have some tender areas and some old templates that are always ready to be stimulated by particular patients. This is fine, and to be expected, although most early-career therapists feel guilty and inexpert because of it. You will get better at doing therapy by knowing and accepting who you are, not by trying to change yourself to someone who does not feel and react this way.

The feelings stirred up in the therapist by the patient in the following example illustrate the shifting nature of these emotional reactions and the therapist's continuing challenge to stay aware of them.

> David was a 42-year-old professor with dark, wavy hair, whose countenance darkened into worry and doubt or brightened into a broad smile depending on what he spoke about. He came for consultation because of depression and anger at his wife.
>
> David felt hurt, rejected, and resentful of his wife's behavior. She was brusque and cold at times, and not as tactful and gentle as he wanted and needed. Her casual comments cut him to the quick and left him angry and puzzled. He wondered why didn't she understand his need for kindness and special attention? Why didn't she recognize his hard work to support her and the family? A thoughtful, kind, intelligent and reasonable man with a good sense of humor, David was easy to identify with. It was easy to feel his hurt, and I asked myself the same question—why was she so insensitive to him?
>
> But as the therapy progressed, it was striking how hard it was for David to give up his feelings of resentment. He saw this, too. When there was an argument and an attempt to make up, it took

days for him to "bury the hatchet." David's wife came in for a joint meeting, and she pointed this out quite clearly. He brought deep feelings of disappointment and hurt to the marriage and often perceived her behavior as more critical and dismissive than how she actually felt. Maybe he was not so easy to live with, I began to think. I found myself identifying with her—he treated her like she was so difficult and troublesome. It's hard to feel that you are never doing the right thing to make your partner happy.

I felt David's wife was affectionate and loving, but her way of communicating was different from what David wanted. He wanted someone who went out of her way to be warm and to avoid hurting him. She loved him, but this was not her way. It turned out that he was particularly sensitive to criticism, having grown up with tremendous sibling rivalry and a lot of negative emotion expressed in the family. His experience of his wife was shaped by this early upbringing, and he was prone to read her as distant and unloving and often felt criticized. He could be prickly at times, and this did not make her feel open and affectionate toward him.

My initial feeling of irritation and criticism toward the wife was based on identifying with David and his hurt and anger. Only with some distance from these feelings—which were based on identifying with him, not on a full, accurate view of their interaction— did it become clear that he could be distancing and difficult to live with. Then the identification switched to her. Just because he was kind and interested and easygoing with me did not mean he was this way at home. David felt wronged, ready to see anything she said as hurtful, and he was openly derisive at times. His attitude was part of why she kept her distance.

Over time, my feelings switched back and forth, and soon enough settled into a kind of overarching identification with both and with their affection for each other, their needs, and their disappointments. Experiences from my personal life, present and past— rejection, resentment, affection, intimacy, forgiveness and making up, peaceful satisfaction, compromise and accommodation—were stirred up by these experiences and formed a basis for the empathy and various identifications.

Later in the therapy, David began to more fully understand his needs and his wife's affectionate attempts to fulfill them. He was less angry, more loving himself, and more aware of the need to enjoy himself as much as possible. He was less worried about how much affection he would get in the future. I felt respect and admiration for David as well as his wife, optimistic about their future together, and a sense of both the satisfactions and compromises of close relationships.

A feeling is just that—it is a feeling, and it feels palpably true. Feelings often seem reasonable and accurate in the moment. There is an urge to simply react to them, thinking that they reflect "reality." Recognition of what part of the situation was the patient's, what part his wife's, and what part was the therapist's own life experience helped the therapist determine how to respond to the patient and what to do in the therapy.

STRENGTHS

Each therapist comes to the work with personality strengths that will help in their therapeutic work. By developing your own personal strengths, you can increase your ability to help your patients develop theirs.

Hope, love, kindness, social intelligence, flexibility, and curiosity are probably chief among the strengths you will call upon. Hope is essential because of the therapeutic value of optimism; we never know what therapy (and life) will bring, and a positive outlook makes a positive outcome more likely because you can stay open to new possibilities. Love and kindness are the active ingredients that allow a patient to feel safe, appreciated, and held. Social intelligence allows for the effective processing of complex psychological data; this helps to understand what is going on with the patient and in the therapeutic relationship, observing from multiple points of view. Because we never know all of the important data, and life throws curveballs at our patients and us, flexibility in conceptualization, perception, and behavior is important; otherwise we will be stuck in quickly outdated perceptions of our patients. Curiosity helps increase understanding and facilitates building a new narrative with the patient; because we spend so many hours hearing about others' lives, we had better be curious if we are to remain engaged.

In their taxonomy, Peterson and Seligman (2004) describe other personality virtues and strengths that are probably helpful as well: creativity, open-mindedness, and perspective, persistence, integrity, humility, and humor. Without discussing each one in detail, it is clear that each of these will contribute to the flexible, emotional, open, reflective relationship that we seek with patients.

We do not know much yet about how to specifically increase therapist personality strengths, or even how much this is possible. Developing personality strengths is a major area of research in positive psychology, and it appears that aging, maturation, and challenging circumstances are usually important ingredients. Personal psychotherapy may increase character strengths as well as point out potential transference–countertransference problem areas. There is some evidence that psychotherapy, especially dynamic therapy, increases reflective functioning of borderline personality disorder patients (see Levy et al., 2006). Thus perhaps therapy may be helpful at increasing reflective functioning of trainees. Surprisingly, there are few data yet on this simple question. Education, social support, and some degree of personal travail may also help to promote personality strengths. Positive psychology interventions such as gratitude exercises and positive experience journals may also help.

Therapists are sometimes drawn to helping others because of their own difficulties. Loneliness, fatigue, frustration, and depression sap therapists of their capacities, and social engagement, rest, satisfaction, and enjoyment increase them. It is important to take good care of yourself to be able to help others. The very work of doing therapy challenges character strengths and provokes self-reflection, and for many this results in further strength development. If every career and every life path causes a development of some personality strengths more than others, we suggest that those strengths listed above that help make therapists effective—hope, love, kindness, social intelligence, flexibility, and curiosity—are probably also increased as a result of our long hours of attention, concern, and facilitating optimism. Many of us hope that doing psychotherapy is a virtuous cycle of trying hard to manifest these qualities in ourselves that help others, all the while helping ourselves learn and develop further.

USING STRENGTHS TO MANAGE YOUR EMOTIONS

Moving beyond the scant available data, we have tried to describe some of the strengths that we see as important for therapists. But most important is how those strengths may be used to help you manage your emotions and react in healthy and helpful ways with your patients. The particular character strengths you have will likely be the basis for your best strategies for managing the emotional intensity of being a therapist.

Of course, the traditional mainstay technique for dealing with powerful emotions about patients is to *understand* (Table 12.1) the situation. Making oneself think about the patient's situation from a variety of angles, trying to imagine how it would feel to be the patient's husband or wife, child, parent, friend, or lover helps to put the therapeutic relationship in a clear context. Using knowledge about the patient's history and typical psychodynamics and awareness of one's own personal concerns

TABLE 12.1. Therapists' Techniques for Managing Emotion

- Understanding
- Optimal distance
- Positive emotions
- Empathy
- Personal painful feelings

and vulnerabilities (learned through previous therapy and life experience) helps to fully understand the patient. It also helps the therapist contain the feelings experienced in the session. This technique helped the therapist in the vignette above place and conceptualize his confusing and disparate emotional responses to David's story.

Staying clearly focused on the therapist's role—listening, understanding, supporting, collaborating, and educating—helps to keep an *optimal distance* from the patient's experience. Being close enough to feel what is happening, but far enough to know that it is someone else's life and issues, helps to manage the emotional turmoil of being close to a patient going through a hard time. Optimal distance prevented the therapist from empathizing too much with David to the exclusion of his wife, and then when he was identifying more with the wife, from taking too critical a perspective on David.

You will usually feel admiration and respect for your patients because you know what they are struggling with and how they have borne up and dealt with crises and challenges. Typically, these feelings are felt and expressed infrequently, and it seems like the business of the therapy is to deal with problems and upset. A focus on these *positive emotions* not only supports the patient, but also reminds the therapist of the patient's strengths. This helps the therapist manage the intensity of the negative emotions he might be experiencing. In the example above, recognizing David's daily struggle with his problems, his frustration and loneliness, admiring his stoicism, sense of humor, affectionate parenting, and wise and thoughtful scholarly work helped the therapist weather the patient's frequent feelings of irritation and hopelessness.

Conversely, attention to the patient's pain, even a determined focus on it, helps to deal with negative feelings toward a patient. Someone who is critical, demanding, or very needy of the therapist can trigger resentment or various defensive maneuvers for dealing with resentment—detachment, passive–aggressive behavior, or reaction formation. Conscious attention to the patient's pain and an explicit focus on *empathy* can cut through some of these understandable therapist responses. Make yourself imagine what it feels like to be the patient, how difficult it may be to go through just one day feeling that way. This will increase your ability to reflect on the meaning of the patient's behavior and delay the automatic responses we have to upsetting or annoying interpersonal behavior.

Finally, the therapist's own personal sources of sadness, distress, or anxiety for the therapist may be stirred up by a patient's difficulty. The therapist can *use these personal feelings* as a source of strength and wisdom. The humility, feeling of immediacy, and genuineness that come from experiencing painful feelings in therapy—in the privacy of the therapist's mind—can bring gravity and focus to the ongoing discussion. It is striking that what the therapist is feeling, even if unspoken, will affect the relationship with the patient. The facial expressions, body language, and speech give away the therapist's depth of emotion, and this will often instantly calm a patient down, helping him tolerate his feelings, and therefore helping the therapist tolerate his.

SUMMARY

The therapist's personality strengths help to transform dialogue with the patient into therapy. These strengths are reflected in the therapist's way of paying attention to the patient and how he uses his inner experience. Specific strengths are helpful for managing intense emotion in the therapeutic encounter: understanding, optimal distance, positive emotion, empathy, and personal painful feelings.

PART IV

COMBINING TREATMENTS

CHAPTER 13

Psychopharmacology and Psychotherapy

All roads lead to Rome, but our antagonists think we should choose different paths.
— JEAN DE LA FONTAINE, "Le Juge Arbitre"—*Fable XII*

Words are, of course, the most powerful drug used by mankind.
— RUDYARD KIPLING

Sometimes dynamic psychotherapy does not take root until the patient gets pharmacological relief from disabling symptoms, making it tolerable for him to discuss painful issues. The power of psychodynamic psychotherapy lies in its ability to isolate and focus on internal conflict, using the therapeutic setting to throw into relief feelings and patterns obscured in everyday life. But if the symptoms are too severe, constructive self-reflection may not be possible. Clinical wisdom and some limited data suggest that many people will require more than one type of treatment to be at their best.

There has been a sea change in perspective on combined psychotherapy and psychopharmacology, questioning old notions like the concern that medication treatment will decrease symptoms and thus decrease motivation for therapy. The practice of combined treatment is remarkably common, even in the treatment of psychoanalytic trainees (Roose & Stern, 1995). Wright and Hollifield (2006) suggest that the efficacy of combined psychotherapy and pharmacotherapy may be more than additive and result in therapeutic interaction that is greater than the sum of the two individual treatments.

A psychodynamic understanding of the patient and the treatment relationship can enhance combined treatment in a variety of ways. There can be better communication between doctor and patient, and this leads to more genuine conversation about anxieties and concerns about the medication. The dynamically aware prescriber may be able to elicit a better history because of the depth of understanding; the prescriber can grasp the meaning of the symptoms to the patient and get a clear picture of the actual symptoms as opposed to what the patient is trying to communicate through a description of the symptoms. For example, awareness of one patient's tendency to be stoic and underreport or another patient's history of having to make dramatic gestures in order to be heard will allow the clinician to more accurately assess the severity of whatever symptom or side effect the patient is talking about. Clinicians will be able to explain the value of the medication, the target symptoms, and the rationale for taking it in the context of the patient's worries and fears. Psychodynamic clinicians can discuss the psychological significance of the medication along with its medical and biological significance.

There is a vast literature on the placebo effect (Harrington, 1997; Mayberg et al., 2002), which is another way of conceptualizing the impact of the doctor–patient relationship and the patient's psychological history on the nature of the drug response. More favorable medication response occurs in positive relationships than in negative ones. The dynamically oriented clinician is in a position to understand and affect the placebo response, improving the potential for medication response.

INTEGRATION OF MIND AND BRAIN

Patients tend to lump their problems into those that are personal, psychological, or arising from their environment, and those that reflect a "chemical imbalance." As therapists, we rather quickly fall into this perspective as well. But as a field, we are searching for a unifying and integrative model of mind and brain to support the integration of a variety of treatments and suggest new areas of investigation.

From a conceptual perspective, some unifying theories have been proposed, such as Damasio's (2000) model of consciousness, but there is not a dominant model embraced by the field. Kendler's (2005) review of mind–body philosophy nicely elucidates the philosophical frameworks used to grapple with the problem of integrating mind and brain. He concludes that most clinicians use the philosophical framework of explanatory dualism to cope with this problem on a day-to-day basis. Explanatory dualism holds that mind and brain are best understood by using simultaneous psychological and biological explanations. Neither explanation is supraordinate, neither is secondary; mind and brain are not the same thing, but rather different ways of explaining and understanding the same thing. We tell patients something like:

> "How you feel has to do with both your feelings and the things that have been happening to you, and it also has to do with your brain and how it processes what is happening. Psychotherapy can make you experience things differently and see the world differently, and medication can help to reset circuits so that you will not have such extreme reactions. They can work separately or together, depending on what is going on with you."

These perspectives on mind and brain come together in research on the neurobiology of psychotherapy. Researchers are studying the relationship between mind and brain by looking for the neurobiological correlates of psychotherapeutic interventions (Beutel et al., 2003; Etkin et al., 2005; Mundo, 2006). We know that some conditions, for example, depression and panic, are treatable with either medication or psychotherapy (for depression see Salminen et al., 2008; for panic see Barlow et al., 2000). If treatments as different as psychotherapy and medication both produce therapeutic results, are they similar interventions understood differently, or different interventions? Goldapple et al. (2004) suggested that verbal psychotherapies for depression may involve a "top-down" treatment mechanism, targeting the cortex and cortical modulation of subcortical structures as its mechanism, while pharmacological treatment might modify limbic structures leading to less cortical interference, a "bottom-up" effect. There may be other situations in which therapy and medication work using the same mechanism.

As pragmatists and explanatory dualists, our perspective is that psychotherapy and psychopharmacology are different interventions based on parallel and equally important perspectives on the mind and brain. The important and pragmatic questions ask which patients should get which treatments, and how they should be delivered. The comments that follow reflect our clinical experience and observations; as little information as there is about the efficacy of combined treatments, there is even less about just how they should be combined—that is, specifically *how* the interaction between psychotherapy and medication can be exploited to bring about the greatest possible benefit.

We start with a discussion about combining treatments when a psychiatrist is both therapist and prescriber. Then we discuss the more common situation in which the treatment is split between a therapist and a psychopharmacologist and provide a framework for facilitating an effective collaboration.

INDICATIONS FOR COMBINED TREATMENT

Research studies of the treatment of depression have shown some synergistic effects of psychotherapy and pharmacotherapy (Keller et al., 2000), especially for severely depressed patients (Thase et al., 1997). Maina, Ross, and Bogetto (2009) found that adding psychodynamic psychotherapy to medication decreased the relapse rate in depression. However, the number of studies showing these synergistic effects is relatively small. The situation is a bit more complex for anxiety disorders, where some studies have shown that combined medication and CBT are no more effective than CBT alone for obsessive–compulsive disorder and generalized anxiety disorder (Foa, Franklin, & Moser 2002). It is interesting to note that other studies of combined treatment for anxiety (especially social phobia and panic disorders) raise the possibility that psychopharmacology may interfere with the effectiveness of behavioral approaches (e.g., Basoglu, Marks, Kilic, Brewin, & Swinson, 1994). Most impressive was the finding from the multisite collaborative panic disorder study (Barlow et al., 2000) that showed that the addition of medication interfered with long-term maintenance of gains arising from CBT. Thus there is some evidence to suggest that medication combined with CBT is not the treatment of choice for panic disorder, or perhaps for social phobia. It not clear whether these findings generalize to psychodynamic psychotherapy.

MEDICATION AND THE PERSON

Sandra was a 36-year-old married professional woman who came to treatment because of low energy and depression. She described a stable but distant relationship with her husband, and complained of exhaustion in looking after their 2-year-old daughter. Sandra was thin and fragile-appearing, and she gave a careful and halting history. There were several episodes of being beaten by her father in early adolescence and an experience of being raped while she was in college. She felt extraordinarily "jangled" and needed a lot of time alone to regain a feeling of safety and wholeness. Her feeling of safety and integrity was easily eroded by the demands, expectations, and interpersonal stimulation that she felt in virtually every area of her life—her daughter, her husband, and her coworkers.

Sandra described an intense attachment to her mother, whom she thought was committed and well-intentioned. Her mother was often critical and needy, and Sandra felt pressure to please her mother, but was resentful of her demands. Her father was an affectionate but volatile man who drank too much. On several occasions, just after Sandra went through puberty, her father lost his temper at her for minor misbehavior and beat her. Sandra could recall vividly the circumstances of each beating, including the smell of alcohol on her father's breath. She complained to her mother after the second beating, and her mother seemed to respond with understanding and promised to make it stop. But it occurred again, and Sandra was shocked that her mother had been so ineffective or uncaring. Her deep disappointment drifted into guilt and self-criticism, and she had occasional moments of cold fury toward her mother, when she would pull back and punish her by rejecting her.

The rape in college occurred when she went to a frat party that got out of control. Sandra drank too much and was cornered by a student. She felt it was her fault for having had so much to drink, and she felt ashamed and told only one friend.

Sandra had subsequent boyfriends, but felt best when she was independent. Four years before Sandra came to the initial evaluation, she met and eventually married her husband, a somewhat detached and mildly depressed but kind man. During their engagement, she realized that she was depressed and she sought treatment with a psychopharmacologist. She tried several antidepressants, but experienced uncomfortable and unacceptable side effects with minimal benefits, and she decided to give up on medicine.

This time when she came for evaluation, she felt anergic, depressed, and was worried about her daughter and her ability to be a good mother. She knew that she was depressed and wanted therapy, but she wondered whether she needed medication, even though she was anxious and skeptical about it. She was worried about side effects and afraid the medication would be too powerful.

After a series of trials and dosage adjustments, Sandra ultimately found benefit from a very small dose of a benzodiazepine antianxiety medication and a nonsedating antidepressant. During the initial medication trials, Sandra had exquisite sensitivity to a variety of side effects, including sedation, anxiety, appetite suppression, nausea, and a sense of derealization. She was able to work quite collaboratively with the psychiatrist–therapist, giving feed-back about the benefits and side effects of the medication. During this time, the psychotherapy was mostly supportive, as she was too upset and felt too fragile to do any exploratory work. She was fre-quently concerned that the medication would hurt her or it was too powerful and would damage her in some way. Ultimately, the medication doses for both the antidepressant and the antianxiety medication were stabilized to balance benefit and side effect. San-dra had a clear response that helped her to feel less depressed, more energetic, and more resilient.

Sandra felt less depressed within the time course expected for anti-depressant response, and she was less anxious with the low dose of anti-anxiety medication. Reducing her acute symptoms allowed a shift in her psychotherapy from support and education to exploration and nar-rative development organized around the core psychodynamic problem of trauma.

Helping a patient construct a new narrative, reexperience old feel-ings, rework perceptions and try new behaviors is action enough in the therapeutic relationship. But prescribing medication, a tangible object that the patient places inside the body, and which diffuses throughout all of the tissues with specific unseen effects at neurons and synapses in the brain, is likely to evoke transference and countertransference that are much harder to recognize because of the complexity of the situation. How did medications make Sandra feel—both positive and negative feel-ings—and how did that affect her subsequent treatment? Was Sandra's sensitivity to medication related to her biology or to her interpersonal sensitivity and expectation of being hurt? Just as patients have transfer-ence to the therapist, they bring transference to the medication.

Medications can change a person's self-experience. Where psycho-therapeutic change tends to be incremental and continuous with previ-ous ways patients have felt about themselves, pharmacological response is sometimes discontinuous and more foreign. The patient feels changed and different, and feeling different can help her to begin to think dif-ferently about herself. A patient who has been chronically irritable and becomes less so with medication starts to question the old assumption of being difficult and unlovable. A traumatized person who has felt fright-ened and anxious, and becomes less reactive and more confident, may see herself as stronger and more in control.

New and more complex ideas about the self also begin to emerge, taking into account the newly evident sense that how one feels depends on one's brain and its biological workings, as well as one's mind, self, and history. In an intuitive and visceral way, patients start to factor their understanding of their biological vulnerabilities into their views of themselves—their neurobiological fingerprint. Sandra realized that if medication could be so helpful in decreasing anxiety, then perhaps her feeling so vulnerable was just a little bit less her fault and a little bit more just the way she was wired.

MEDICATION AND TREATMENT GOALS

Sandra complained of low energy, depression, fatigue, career dissatisfaction, and worries about her parenting. Which of these symptoms was likely to respond to psychotherapy and which to medication? It is tempting to simply define physical symptoms like fatigue, or sleep disturbance when it is present, as targets for medication, while attitudes, function, and relationship problems are the domain of psychotherapy. But often the correlate of a better relationship is sleeping better, and one certainly has more energy when one is satisfied with one's work. Likewise, improvement in fatigue makes one more fun to be with, and this will increase the enjoyment of close relationships.

It is important to provide patients with a framework for understanding why you are offering combined treatment and what results might occur from the treatments, even though they can be difficult to predict. Generally, we do regard the psychotherapy as targeting the life narrative, changing and reworking it to make experience and perception different, which then leads to behavioral change. It is incremental, top-down in the sense of higher thought affecting visceral experience, and focuses on contrasting new and old modes of experience. Medication, bottom-up, affects experience too, but is more discrete and specific in its impact and changes subjective experience without the split-screen quality of feeling old reactions and new reactions at the same time.

Thus we explain to patients that therapy will help them think about and change how they experience themselves and others. We hope they will come to see themselves in a new light, leading to new ways of experiencing and new behavior. They will substitute the old and dysfunctional for the new and more adaptive. Psychopharmacology will decrease symptoms that are abnormal effects of vulnerable biology. We point out to them that having fewer symptoms will help them draw on their strengths and deal with stresses more adaptively. We note that combined treatment can offer two pathways to improvement. Medicine will help the syndrome, whether it is a mood disorder, anxiety disorder, or psychotic disorder, and psychotherapy will help the patient sort out and improve her capacity to perceive and adapt. Psychotherapy has the potential to bring about long-term change, but might require "booster" experiences along the way, while psychopharmacology might be required for maintenance. Medication might reduce the patient's sense of blame and responsibility for her difficulties, but it might also decrease the feeling of having personally overcome and mastered her problems.

Phasing psychotherapy and psychopharmacology is a clinical art at this point, with little empirical data to guide us. Our approach is usually to educate the patient about what we know about psychotherapy and medication treatment for the problem they are dealing with, and offer the range of treatments when there are acute symptoms, whether depression or anxiety. When the patient requests combined treatment, we begin with weekly appointments and initiate and monitor the medication. We educate the patient about the presenting problem and the medication treatment. Support, behavioral management for acute symptoms, and family education are the psychotherapeutic interventions initially, while we set the stage for beginning an exploratory psychotherapeutic treatment when the patient is ready. Family members need to know what the problem is, and what the treatment plan will be, especially when the symptoms are significant. Often they are reassured when they meet the clinician.

If a patient is acutely agitated, it is unhelpful to explore and encourage even more intense affective experiences. When the patient starts to feel a little better, enough to be curious and to start to regain a sense of control, then the exploration can begin. Some patients are ready in the first session, some are not for a couple of months. Thus Sandra began to talk more about her relationships, history, and feelings and fantasies only when she was less depressed, more active, and a little more confident.

Just as one frequently waits for a psychopharmacology response to begin a more active psychotherapy, sometimes medication effects are limited by conflicts that get in the way. Some patients are so anxious and guilty about feeling better that they do not seem to get a full response until the therapy has helped them deal with this problem. Others are pleased with the relief of anxiety they may receive from medication, but worried that their decreased anxiety leaves them less vigilant about possible dangers, and this creates anxiety in response.

MEDICATION AND
THE THERAPEUTIC RELATIONSHIP

Education, discussion, informed consent, and a dispassionate evaluation of the risks and benefits of the medication are an essential aspect of the therapeutic alliance in combined treatment. Informed-consent decision making about medication is the rational ideal and must be pursued, but there are many emotional factors in taking medication that are driven by the patient's dynamics.

The patient's perspective on medication certainly has to do with specific factors in her own life, such as prior medication experience, medical history, experience of others, and media exposure. Riba and Tasman (2006) describe typical positive and negative medication transferences, and their thoughtful list categorizes these attitudes into good and bad reactions to medication. We have attempted to extend Riba and Tasman's ideas, identifying the positive and negative medication attitudes we observe are associated with each of the six common psychodynamic problems (Table 13.1). This will allow the clinician to anticipate patients' reactions and use dynamic understanding to advantage, increasing medication adherence and the patient's experience of medication as a positive intervention. This discussion cannot adequately cover the question of when psychopharmacology should and should not be used for patients with the six core problems, as that decision needs to take into account a variety of factors (e.g., family history, prior medication response, culture and other belief systems) and is outside the scope of this book. Instead, we address the meaning medications have to patients with each core problem.

PRESCRIBING FOR PATIENTS WITH DEPRESSION

Patients with depression feel hopeless, negative, and unloved, and they yearn for a prescribing doctor who is like a good parent—helpful, nurturing, supportive, giving them the sustenance they need so badly. They may be enormously appreciative of medication, as though it were good food on an empty stomach, desperately needed and in all-too-short supply. However, the opposite side of the coin is that medication may increase the feeling of stigma, punishment, and rejection. Patients may feel that medication marks them as damaged, worthy of rejection, and unredeemable. Instead of good food, the medication can be seen as poi-

TABLE 13.1. Common Medication Attitudes for Core Psychodynamic Problems

	Positive transference	Negative transferences	Techniques for managing
Depression	Nurturance, help, good food, love, support	Stigma, punishment, rejection, disappointment, poisoning	Caretaking, concern, carefulness, methodical attention
Obsessionality	Pleasure through compliance, pleasing the prescriber, resistance to transference	Controlled, intruded on, weak, shameful	Relinquish control, consultant/advisor to patient
Fear of abandonment	Love, interest, safety, security	Disinterest, don't care about person, inattention	Reassurance, attentiveness
Low self-esteem	Caring, admiration, enhancement, perfection, increased lovability	Defectiveness, inferiority, losing competition	Active, paternalistic stance
Panic	Gratitude, safe, caretaker	Abandonment, disappointment,	Active, advising, guiding
Trauma	Safety, protection, validation	Trauma, damage, invalidation, condoning trauma	Caretaking stance, active, respect for patient decisions

sonous, hurtful, and destructive. It is punishment for their inner badness.

When there are substantial side effects, or when the response is slow or not robust, this can tilt the medication transference toward the negative. When there is a rapid response, there is more likely a positive attitude. Because medication algorithms can take quite a while to work though, patience can be required to get to the point where the benefit begins to show. During this time, patients may feel more hopeless, rejected, and damaged.

A handsome, stylish man in his early 40s came for treatment, accompanied by his wife, when his depression recurred. His business was struggling, and he felt frustrated and disappointed with himself because he was depressed again after a long period of well-ness. He was ambivalent about medication, but felt from prior experience that it was necessary for him to get better. He was annoyed about having to restart medicine, and each dose and each side effect made him irritable.

It took 3 to 4 months before he began to feel better, and this sorely tried both his and his wife's patience. He was angry with the doctor, feeling that the medications were making him ill because of side effects. He felt that the seriousness of the medical treatment supported his fear that he would never be successful. He felt marked forever by his illness, and this resonated with earlier feelings that there was something deeply lacking about him. At times he was not only angry, but hopelessly negative and profoundly helpless.

It is essential for the prescriber to maintain some distance and objectivity from the painful symptoms of depression. The patient may be crying out in distress, intent on getting rapid relief, but the doctor must prescribe systematically and thoughtfully and not respond excessively to the pain. Responding overly quickly to the patient's suffering can lead to poor medical practice, such as switching drugs too quickly, escalating doses that may lead to unnecessary side effects, or using too many medications.

Concern, care, and patience are the hallmarks of good medical management of depression. Attention and empathic validation are good substitutes for impulsive action for the doctor, and the attempt to be caretaking will be more likely to evoke the positive transference than overly reactive prescribing. The patient described above responded to the medication after quite a while, and the doctor did her best to maintain a demeanor of patience, concern, affection, and caretaking while feeling under sustained attack and criticism. But since the patient was depressed and hopeless, it was not helpful to point out that his irritable and critical feelings were based on old patterns of feeling misunderstood and hurt. Instead, the doctor attempted to minimize the negative reactions through careful attention and made every attempt to provide the best and most effective medical care.

In chronic depression, the prescriber may develop an exclusive focus on medication, working intensely on drug combinations and doses while tending to disregard the patient's active responsibility in managing the symptoms. The patient and doctor can start to see the treatment as a biological puzzle and forget about important psychotherapeutic issues that should be dealt with. The opposite problem is when there is so much focus on working through conflicts that the clinician and patient forget to treat a syndrome that is right in front of them. It is hard to keep focused on mind and brain at the same time.

PRESCRIBING FOR OBSESSIONAL PATIENTS

The associated depression, anxiety, or obsessional intrusive thoughts and feelings are the pharmacologic target symptoms for obsessional patients. Because obsessional patients are preoccupied with control over inner thoughts and feelings, and therefore over relationships, the issue of control is paramount in the prescribing relationship. Taking medication can feel like a loss of control, being intruded upon and controlled internally by the doctor, and perhaps humiliating and shameful. On the positive side, the patient can take pleasure in being compliant, taking the medication just right, and eliciting the satisfaction of the doctor. Like a well-behaved child, the patient feels she has done well and will earn a reward. Taking medication may bolster the patient's feeling of strength and mastery.

Because obsessional patients need to keep distance from their feelings about others, especially powerful and potentially dangerous people like doctors, there is frequently a resistance to the transference. There is a defensive disavowal of having feelings about the medication and the treatment, whether the feelings are positive or negative. These patients often just do not want to think or talk about their feelings regarding the doctor, the prescribing, or the medication. They try to evaluate the medication from a purely rational perspective, one that does not take into account their ever-present emotions.

The prescriber will do best by using the traditional consultation model here. That is, the patient is coming to the doctor, inquiring about medication, and will use it or not based on the information learned, and it will be the patient's decision. Informed consent, patient autonomy, and respect for the patient's decision making are always important, but for these patients it is an absolute requirement. Any attempt to be paternalistic or manipulative in the service of symptom reduction will backfire sooner or later. The doctor should emphasize the patient's control and take the role of adviser. Inevitably, the patient will want the advice and will react to it either positively or negatively, depending on the dynamics and the status of the therapy. But the patient is most likely to make the best medication decision when the transference distortions are minimized by the doctor's taking a noncontrolling consultant role.

PRESCRIBING FOR PATIENTS
WITH FEAR OF ABANDONMENT

Insecure attachment is associated with depression and Cluster B personality disorder, and the pharmacologic interventions target depressive symptoms and the mood instability. Patients' positive reactions to medication include the feeling of being loved, cared for, or treated with special attention. Ingesting medication given to them by their doctor may promote a feeling of intimate attachment. On the negative side, psychopharmacology can stir up feelings of rejection, objectification, and stigma. The patient may feel disregarded, and just one of many patients, none of whom seem to be important to the doctor. Not infrequently the patient's attitudes can oscillate between these poles, needing and appreciating the medication and angry about the feeling of abandonment it stirs up.

The management approach here is to maintain clear boundaries, advocating for medication when it will really help the patient and expressing a consistent attitude of concern and attention to the patient's feelings. The need for continuing empathy and sensitive listening cannot be overemphasized, but the doctor must not overidentify with the patient's feelings and must maintain a consistent approach in the face of the patient's fluctuating reactions and feelings. Strengthening the experience of object constancy is the psychotherapeutic goal for those with insecure attachment, and the therapist's most powerful tool for this is maintaining a consistent demeanor. The prescribing doctor's stance attempts to strengthen this as well.

PRESCRIBING FOR PATIENTS
WITH SELF-ESTEEM PROBLEMS

The psychopharmacologic target symptom for patients with low self-esteem is rejection sensitivity. Patients with self-esteem problems respond to taking medication in terms of how it makes them feel about themselves. It can raise their self-esteem; positive reactions include the sense that medication reflects caring and admiration from the therapist. The patient feels special attention and regard in the discussions about alternatives, often feeling especially understood, supported, and attended to. The wishful feeling is that the medication may help the patient attain the perfection, desirability, and lovability they seek, and it feels like enhancement that will surely make them even better and more lovable.

The other side of this reaction is that medication reflects negatively on the patients and who they are. Some patients with self-esteem problems feel that taking medication is an acknowledgement of defectiveness and inferiority, and they are filled with shame. If they are competitive, they could feel that taking medication makes them less attractive, impressive, or intelligent than others (or whatever the fantasy may be).

> One patient commented that medication made him smarter and better than he had been before. Beyond the improvement in symptoms, he commented that the pill was like high-octane fuel in his tank, and he had never been as on top of his game as he was now. Some months later, the same patient had several setbacks at work, and he felt he was not able to keep up as he had in the past. Now he felt that the medication made him lose his edge. It was difficult to discern from observing him, from hearing about his situation, and from his wife's report whether there was any objective change in the medication response, but clearly his attitude had shifted dramatically from a positive medication transference to a negative one.

The management approach to medication for those with self-esteem problems is to keep an active advisory stance, letting suggestions and recommendations border on paternalism. The mood fluctuations and uncertainty these patients experience may make them uncertain about the value of medication and erode their motivation. If medication treatment is appropriate then a strong stance is helpful, and the patient feels it is supportive and empathic. That is, err on the side of pushing your opinion, and do not keep distance out of fear of hurting the patient's feelings.

An active stance is less likely to interfere with therapy for patients with self-esteem problems than for patients with obsessionality who are extremely sensitive to control, and for trauma patients to whom autonomy and safety are so important. Patients with self-esteem issues are more likely to want to be taken care of, but care must be taken that medication is not perceived as a substitute for close empathic attention in the psychotherapy.

PRESCRIBING FOR PATIENTS WITH PANIC

Panic is so acutely uncomfortable that patients are often desperate for symptom relief; this tends to induce a powerful dependent reaction. Patients with panic long for help from the doctor, and they will quickly step into a subordinate and supplicating position. When the medication is helpful, the patient will feel intense gratitude. Her safety is solely in the doctor's hands, and there is great confidence and conviction about the doctor's skills and power. The doctor is seen as a benign caretaker with powerful tools available. Alternatively, the medicine can be disappointing and ineffective, and the patient feels the negative aspect of dependency, which is abandonment and aloneness. The doctor's back is turned, and no one can help. Because patients with panic are so intently focused on internal sensations, they are particularly anxious about side effects. They worry that side effects presage more side effects or represent some kind of serious damage to the body. They can become terribly worried and seek reassurance.

It is a rule of thumb with these patients that there can never be too much reassurance and support during the initial phases of pharmacotherapy. It is hard to think clearly when you are seized by panic with little or no warning, and if the clinical situation warrants psychopharmacology, then it is appropriate to recommend the treatment in a decisive way, emphasizing the advantages and committing to helping the patient with side effects or difficulties along the way. The consultative distance that works so well with obsessional patients will just make patients with panic anxious and abandoned. Because the symptoms have been awful and the patients feel so dependent, not providing reassurance is tantamount to confirming the patient's worst fears, so specific recommendations about medication, dosing, and management of side effects are helpful. One should err on the side of lower doses followed by gradual increases; the more incremental the change, the more minimal the side effect, and the more likely the patient will be able to attain full therapeutic doses of medication.

PRESCRIBING FOR TRAUMATIZED PATIENTS

Psychopharmacology for traumatized patients focuses on symptoms of acute agitation, sleep problems, hyperarousal and activation, and associated depression. The patient may see the medication as affording safety and protection, decreasing the painful symptoms, and attending to the need to take the symptoms seriously and help.

These patients have so often felt ignored by others, and their trauma has not been taken seriously or validated. Because of this, medication directed at the symptoms can feel like a validation of the seriousness of what they have been through and what they are currently experiencing. But those with trauma are also acutely sensitive to feeling hurt again, whether it's through uncomfortable side effects, medical risks, or the prescriber's lack of attention to the process. They have been treated badly by those in more powerful positions than their own, and the context of the doctor–patient relationship and the perceived power differential can mirror this. Medication can feel like an attempt to silence the victim of abuse. These patients are already filled with shame and secrecy, and being given a pill may make them feel like their experience is being ignored. An attempt to "just treat symptoms" condones or at least inadequately recognizes the evil of the abuser and the unfairness of the trauma.

A caretaking stance that emphasizes respect for the patient's autonomy is the optimal approach. It is essential to respond appropriately to the severity of the patient's symptoms and try to intervene. The greatest damage of the trauma is to the patient's sense of integrity, autonomy, and empowerment, and healing this must be central to every aspect of the treatment. The patient is treated as the decision maker. Information is given and issues are discussed openly. But if the patient is so symptomatic as to make decision making difficult, the doctor should step in and actively guide the decision. Patient empowerment is essential, but compassionate care of the patient is also the doctor's responsibility.

PROBLEMS AND PITFALLS
IN PRESCRIBING MEDICATION

Just as patients have a variety of transference reactions based on their psychodynamic problems and specific life experiences, clinicians also have personal attitudes and feelings that are not based in current reality. These are medication countertransferences. Rescue fantasies about depressed patients, maternal urges toward those with abandonment fears, and aggressive feelings toward obsessional patients are all examples of these countertransference reactions that can be expressed in prescribing. For example, does the depressed patient really need a second antidepressant added, and does the abandonment-sensitive patient need more frequent sessions or more aggressive medication? It is incumbent on the doctor-therapist to examine these questions with as much self-reflection as other treatment decisions, understanding the ubiquity of enactments and the inevitable interplay between transference and countertransference.

Because prescribing is a real action, more tangible than many psychologically framed actions the therapist takes in the treatment, it may be outside the lens of self-reflection. Thus unrecognized and unacceptable feelings may come out in this area. For example, an angry and frustrated physician may withhold medication or impulsively change recommendations, or the need to keep a patient's admiration and affection may drive the doctor to make decisions that are not medically optimal.

At some point in treatment, the emotional meaning to the patient of taking medication should be explored. Analyzing the meaning of the medication with a patient does not suggest that the medicine is not needed and appropriate. The goal of this exploration is to clarify and free up the patient's and the doctor's decision-making process, so they are both guided by current and realistic considerations, not dynamic, historical ones.

It is confusing for the therapist-psychiatrist to keep track of two very different realms of data and action, and it requires a kind of compartmentalization. The interaction with the patient will tend to be in "therapy mode," or in "medication mode," and occasionally in the mode of reflecting on the meaning of medication decisions. The doctor must be able to move flexibly among these modes, responding to the patient's cues and the medical need for discussion.

We typically discuss medication issues either at the beginning of the session or the end. Some patients report on the medication response or side effects at the beginning; other patients will not bring it up, or bring it up at the end. The advantage of discussion at the beginning is that it leaves the remainder of the session open and does not require awkwardly closing down an open-ended emotional exchange to talk about side effects and doses. Medication talk at the beginning of the session can be a problem because the doctor has not yet gathered how the patient feels, and it may be hard to make recommendations about dosing and management without this information.

Discussion of medication at the end of the session is advantageous because it allows the patient to open the session with what is emotionally salient and get right into the important issues at hand without the sometimes distancing and rationalistic discussion about medication. The problem with a discussion at the end is that there may not be enough time, and the importance of the medication may be downplayed and avoided, treated as an afterthought. It may also be a sign that the medication is not being brought into the therapy and discussed in terms of its emotional meaning.

Many patients continue medication after the psychotherapy is over, and this causes a change in the doctor–patient relationship. Patients treated for recurrent depression with combined treatment may complete the therapy, but maintenance medication treatment continues. Thus the patient will come back for a medication visit, and this makes for a very different feel in the appointment.

The appointment schedule is much less frequent for medication review, for example every 3 to 6 months. Transference and countertransference feelings are likely to be present, less intense than previously, but active nonetheless. The transition in care also involves a departure from the traditional technique for handling termination. Before the advent of combined psychotherapy and psychopharmacology treatment, the end of the therapy was the end of the relationship. In combined treatment delivered by one psychiatrist, psychotherapy termination is the end of the frequent intense meetings, and the beginning of a new, more reality-oriented doctor–patient relationship. This new relationship may be helpful and consistent with the patient's improved outlook and functioning, but it might also be a nagging restimulation of issues and conflicts that were helped to some extent by treatment, but remain open and distressing. Discussion of the feelings about the transition may help the patient address it in a healthy way.

DUAL-PROVIDER SPLIT TREATMENT

All of the discussion until now has been about combined treatment offered by one doctor-therapist. But much more common is split treatment, where two providers work with the patient. Gabbard and Kay (2001) have written about the advantages and disadvantages of split treatment and suggest that single-provider care is better in a number of clinical settings, including the presence of schizophrenia or schizoaffective disorder, bipolar disorder with denial of illness, borderline patients who use frequent splitting, and patients with medical problems and psychiatric illness. Treatment in managed-care settings, community mental health centers, VA hospitals, and other health care centers is almost always split treatment. Single-provider treatment tends to be primarily available in private practice settings.[1]

---

[1] Although single-provider treatment is decreasing in frequency, a recent study suggested that 28.9% of outpatient visits to psychiatrists included psychotherapy (Mojtabai & Olfson, 2008).

A clinical vignette about split treatment described from the perspective of the psychodynamically oriented psychopharmacologist illustrates many of the issues involved in the therapist–pharmacologist collaboration.

Depressed, struggling with a crumbling marriage, and lonely, Karen was referred by her psychotherapist for a psychopharmacology evaluation. She had been treated with an antidepressant by a previous psychiatrist, which resulted in a little improvement but significant side effects. Karen felt her intensive psychotherapy was productive, though difficult, and both she and her therapist felt there was a strong therapeutic alliance. She was increasingly able to reflect on her feelings, naming and articulating experiences that she had heretofore needed to bury and disavow. But she was terribly sad and worried that she was not available to her preteen daughter during the separation and divorce. Although she was functioning well in her role as a professor, she found that it took more energy than usual to stay afloat.

The referring therapist and I had known each other for a while professionally, although we had not collaborated clinically. The initial phone call from therapist to psychopharmacologist included a synopsis of the patient's history and the current treatment, as well as the reason for the medication referral: reevaluation of the medication. The patient was quite motivated for the evaluation.

The initial contact was a consultation, organized around taking the history, identifying diagnoses, and discussing potential treatments. The frame of reference was descriptive diagnosis, which provides the best basis for making psychopharmacology decisions. I thought that the recurrent depression might be part of a bipolar type II mood disorder, and was concerned about excessive alcohol use. The consultation concluded with a discussion about these diagnoses and a recommendation to decrease and potentially stop alcohol use, switch antidepressants, and consider adding a mood-stabilizing agent. I discussed this with the patient, who agreed to proceed, and I informed the therapist of our conclusion by phone and in a follow-up letter, which was copied to the patient.

The course of treatment was favorable, and Karen began to feel less depressed and more stable in her mood with the medication changes. There was clearly (by both the therapist's and patient's report) an acceleration in her ability to work effectively in the therapy. She was less self-critical, more open, more self-reflective, and she began to feel better about herself, more engaged in her work, and more motivated to start dating.

About a year into the combined treatment, Karen reported she certainly felt better than she had before treatment, but she thought she had some continuing depression—there was nothing she really looked forward to, and life seemed gray and without interest. She was lonely and although she enjoyed her time with her daughter, now on a regular part-time custody arrangement, and she was productive and successful at work, it all seemed a little empty. At times, she stayed up late at night, needing less sleep, reading online. She wanted to change the medication and see whether there was anything that would work better.

Were Karen's continuing anhedonia and low-grade depression with intermittent sleep-cycle disturbance a result of partially effective medication or the important issues in self-esteem and intimacy that she was working on in psychotherapy? The therapist contacted me prior to the follow-up appointment, explaining her observations and describing this dilemma. The therapist definitely thought that more psychotherapy was needed to help Karen with her symptoms, but was not sure about medication change. She told the patient she would call and express this. Karen and I decided that she would benefit from adding a mood stabilizer, and I communicated this back to the therapist. The change did improve Karen's mood and sleep–wake cycle, and she began to report feeling better.

The next dilemma arose after Karen reported that she was worried that she was drinking too much alcohol. There was a family history of alcoholism, and both her father and brother were affected. The therapist and patient discussed this, and decided together that this was a problem. The therapist communicated this to me, so that at the next follow-up Karen and I discussed her drinking, genetic vulnerability, and mixing of medication and alcohol. The conclusion was that the continuing use probably contributed to her vulnerability to depression and constricted lifestyle, and there was a risk of escalating use and the complications of alcoholism. The patient and both clinicians agreed on a plan of a trial period of abstinence with follow-up and discussion. The patient agreed with the recommendations and committed to abstinence. She reported that although she struggled at times with cravings and missed the feeling of intoxication, she felt stronger, clearer, less depressed, and more motivated to make changes in her life.

This vignette illustrates a successful collaboration that involved well-defined therapist and pharmacologist roles, and effective, open, two-sided communication. The result was a good treatment plan, clarity and structure for the patient, and in this case, a good result. Interestingly, Karen later told her therapist that it was very important to her that the therapist and psychopharmacologist were in contact, and that they were in agreement with each other. She recalled her parents' dysfunctional communication and how scared and alone it had made her feel. She also found it very helpful to discuss her progress and her continuing symptoms with her therapist before each psychopharmacology visit to get the benefit of the therapist's perspective on how she was doing to inform her medication decisions.

CLINICIAN ROLES

In the field, clinicians may work together in a hierarchical or collaborative way. Hierarchical models, where the psychiatrist is the primary clinician and the therapist "reports" to the psychiatrist, are sometimes found in community mental health centers, inpatient services, or other complex institutions. On the other hand, psychotherapists are primary clinicians and psychiatrists serve as consultants in many group practice models. Both of these arrangements involve a hierarchical reporting relationship between the therapist and the prescriber.

We recommend whenever possible that the psychotherapist and prescriber work together in a collaborative model with clear roles (Moras & Summers, 2001). Collaborative arrangements involve shared responsibility, and they make use of the skills and expertise of each clinician more fully than the hierarchical arrangements. Making thoughtful clinical decisions about both the psychotherapy and psychopharmacology and how they interact requires the full input of both practitioners. All too often, the responsibilities and roles in the collaborative relationship are not clearly delineated, leading to disruption in the treatment when the patient is not doing well. Therefore, clear definitions of the respective roles and responsibilities are likely to be helpful (see Table 13.2).

The collaborative model requires that each practitioner do everything within her domain of responsibility, and that they communicate with each other to reach a consensus about a shared understanding of the patient. This means that both therapist and psychopharmacologist perform a full diagnostic evaluation; of course, the therapist will gather more extensive developmental, relationship, and functional data, and the psychiatrist's assessment will tend to focus more on symptoms, natural history of symptoms, genetic factors, and medical issues. But each must gather enough data to form an opinion about the diagnosis and treatment. Following the evaluation, both providers will communicate essential aspects of the clinical data and discuss the diagnosis (in most

TABLE 13.2. Psychotherapist–Psychiatrist Roles in Collaborative Care

Function	Psychotherapist	Psychiatrist	Communication
Data gathering	Gathers full historical and current database, including personal, family, and developmental history	Gathers full historical and current database, including medical history and complaints, medical database	Shared database
Diagnosis, formulation, and treatment goals	Makes clear diagnosis and formulation; identifies focal problems, treatment goals, and target symptoms	Makes clear diagnosis and formulation; identifies focal problems, treatment goals, and target symptoms	Consensus diagnosis and formulation; consensus regarding focal problems, treatment goals, and target symptoms; rationale for each component of treatment
Treatment selection	Selects appropriate form and frequency of psychotherapy	Selects appropriate psychopharmacology regimen	Agree on strategy with patient, interventions, potential pitfalls
Provision of treatment	Delivers psychotherapy	Delivers psychopharmacology	Coordination of therapeutic interventions
Evaluation of treatment	Assesses psychotherapy responses and inquires about psychopharmacology responses	Assesses psychopharmacology responses and inquires about psychotherapy response	Share observations about treatment responses and adjust ongoing treatment as needed
Crisis management	Shared primary responsibility, especially responsible for adjusting to acute psychosocial stressors, techniques for modulating affect and behavior (improve stability), support for and monitoring of basic safety issues	Shared primary responsibility, responsible for acute psychopharmacologic interventions, support for and monitoring of basic safety issues	Rapid communication, shared information, coordinated intervention with clear division of responsibility

Note. Adapted with permission of the authors from Moras and Summers (2001).

cases, this is brief and there is relatively easy agreement). When there is disagreement, it is important to share as much of the clinical data as possible, agree on what else needs to be learned, and discuss how the clinicians will resolve this disagreement. Nothing dooms a combined treatment more than significantly differing perspectives, as the patient will be confused about what is being treated and often tends to feel and function worse when this occurs. You cannot agree to disagree, because ultimately this will confuse the patient and undermine one or both clinicians.

The consensus diagnosis and the therapist's formulation will lead the way to treatment goals for each component of the treatment. The therapist and prescriber will emphasize what each will work on and what they hope to achieve. Karen's therapist focused more on her subjective experiences, relationships, self-esteem, and self-understanding. The psychopharmacologist paid attention to her depressive, agitated symptoms and her alcohol use. These approaches were coordinated rather than conflicting, and the communication between the two clinicians kept each focused on the appropriate domain of work and the specific treatment goals. Each functioned according to his or her role, and each could reference what the other was doing. The patient knew what to talk about where and knew that both clinicians were working together.

When Karen complained of residual depression and sleeplessness, the clinicians had to work together to evaluate the treatment and their work and its progress. They had to share observations, and find a way to reach consensus on what accounted for the limitations in progress—was it incomplete psychotherapy or incomplete psychopharmacology? The clinicians and the patient were open to the possibilities and aware that it was difficult to tease apart what symptoms might respond to more psychotherapy and what to additional medication. The patient wanted to try the medication and continue her work in the psychotherapy.

The greatest stress on the dual-provider relationship comes when the patient has a crisis. When there is an acute loss or personal crisis, or there is suicidality or homicidality, both clinicians typically become involved. Everyone is anxious about who has responsibility and for what. The psychotherapist has usually been meeting more frequently with the patient and has primary responsibility in a crisis for understanding and helping the patient deal with acute stressors and for improving techniques for behavioral stabilization. The psychopharmacologist's responsibility is to assess the degree of symptom severity and provide optimal pharmacology to promote stabilization. They are both responsible for decisions about hospitalization or emergency evaluation and will need to communicate, often on an urgent basis, until the crisis subsides. These danger situations are harrowing for the clinician practicing alone, and while the company of a colleague can sometimes add to the complexity, including finger-pointing and discontent, it can also be a source of support and validation in a difficult situation.

Of course, medical–legal anxieties develop when there is potential dangerousness. This is inevitably part of the clinicians' anxiety and may become more of a focus than when there are two clinicians treating a patient in crisis—they can disagree about decisions or roles or become anxious about who is supposed to do what. But the best medical–legal approach is the one that brings about the best patient outcome, and clear role definition with maximal help from both clinicians makes for the best outcome. Indeed, both clinicians are at medical–legal risk if a serious situation develops.

DUAL-PROVIDER TREATMENT PITFALLS

Dual-provider treatment works best when the two clinicians know and respect each other, have the same understanding of their collaborative and nonhierarchical roles and relationship, and communicate regularly. But threesomes are more complicated than twosomes, and problems can develop. Spotting the potential pitfalls is easier with the framework for the role relationships we have described, because it puts the clinicians' reactions to each other in the context of their roles and functions in a collaborative relationship, rather than personal qualities and skills. You can remember what you are supposed to do and encourage your colleague to follow her role expectations, and this makes the interaction less personal.

Sometimes therapists and psychiatrists stray from their responsibilities. Incomplete sharing of the clinical information—for example, one clinician learns about continuing obsessive–compulsive symptoms that the other clinician is unaware of—makes it hard for a thorough consensus diagnosis of the patient. Subtle or overt undermining of the other clinician's skills, expertise, or behavior throws the entire treatment into question for the patient. Unilateral assertions about the diagnosis, the need for treatment modifications, or conflicting assessments of the degree of progress cast doubt on the other provider's skill and trustworthiness.

Some clinicians find themselves collaborating because the patient requests it, or they happen into the situation. They may believe collaborative care is a less effective treatment model, and their ambivalence and doubt will likely come out at important moments. More insidious are the problems that come up when the clinicians are resolved to work together and observe the role expectations, but the countertransference experiences make this difficult. For example, patients who tend to split will often regard one clinician as better and more helpful than the other, or one treatment modality better than the other. Specific countertransference experiences in the psychotherapy—rescue fantasies, control struggles, hopelessness—may affect the therapist's view of the medication. This can cause noise in the collaborative relationship.

The "real relationship" between two providers affects the treatment as well. Close colleagues will tend to talk more frequently about their shared cases. Clinicians who do not get along for other reasons will tend to have more difficulty respecting their role divisions. Beliefs about each other's professional training and biases about the profession—physicians, psychologists, social workers, counselors, clergy—may creep into the communication, distorting and decreasing its effectiveness. The practice context may also affect the provider relationship. Clinic-based collaboration may be part of the culture and supported with group norms and ideals. In private practice, clinicians tend to select those they feel comfortable with for collaboration, but there is more difficulty finding the time to communicate, and lack of reimbursement for phone time may provide a disincentive for frequent contact. Close proximity helps the collaboration, as a brief discussion in the hallway is usually easier than repeated phone calls or voice mails.

SUMMARY

Combining psychopharmacology with psychotherapy adds another potential route of intervention. An integrated perspective on mind and brain allows us to see that interpersonal and biological therapies target the synapses as well as the soul. There is a bias in the clinical world that combined treatment is optimal, but this conviction may be more based on popular and cultural belief that more is better than on the strength of the evidence.

The overarching principles for combining treatments are: delineating a clear diagnosis and formulation, targeting specific problems with specific treatments, and transparent communication among multiple clinicians and the patient. Clearly defined roles and functions make the collaborative relationship between psychotherapist and psychopharmacologist function better. Attention to transference and countertransference is essential because these phenomena become even more complex when more players are involved. Attitudes of openness, humility, and empiricism, as well as a willingness to change plans based on results, result in the kind of flexibility many patients need.

~

CHAPTER 14

The Patient Is Part of a Family

with Ellen Berman

People change and forget to tell each other.
—LILLIAN HELLMAN

All "individual" problems, such as depression, low self-esteem, and abandonment anxiety, and indeed, all individual strengths, exist in a relational context, and recent work in social neuroscience reveals the complex neuroregulatory functions of relational attachments (Siegel, 2006). We are fundamentally social. Indeed, most problems cause trouble because of difficulties in relationships—either too much self-absorption to be attuned to others, distortions in reading cues and motives, or excessive awareness of other's needs. However, not all intrapsychic problems begin in or cause serious problems for important relationships. For many, the couple or family may buffer and heal. How do you treat an individual who is essentially part of a web of relationships? Traditional psychodynamic psychotherapy did not include meeting with a spouse or family members; in fact, it discouraged this. In this chapter we discuss how and when to combine psychodynamic psychotherapy with couple or family therapy.

Individual therapy will be necessary, helpful, and efficient the more the problem involves individual suffering and unconscious conflict in the midst of functional relationships, and the more the suffering seems

Ellen Berman, MD is Clinical Professor of Psychiatry at the University of Pennsylvania, where she directs couple and family therapy training in the adult psychiatry residency. She is a coauthor of *Marital and Family Therapy, Fourth Edition*.

discordant with the relationship system around it. PPP addresses the relationship problems from the individual perspective. Couple or family therapy is the place to start when the problem is manifested in relationship conflict, the suffering is defined as dissatisfaction with others rather than individual distress, and other people in the family are dysfunctional. It is common for a patient to start in individual therapy and then move to couple therapy later, or for couple therapy to become stalled until individual treatment begins. When used together the treatments can be synergistic, leading to greater symptom relief, change, and patient empowerment. We use the terms "couples," "family," and "systems" interchangeably in this chapter, referring to adult family systems in all of their permutations.

Marital or family problems do not always signal psychopathology in one of the individuals, although individual problems may stress the family. Marital or family tension may develop in generally well-functioning people when differences in temperament or goals are too great, or when a relationship is stressed beyond its ability to cope. Stressors may include a chronic and life-threatening illness, a complex step-family situation, or sudden job loss and financial stress. It is possible to have a great deal of marital tension when each partner alone appears symptom-free. Or marital stress may provoke symptoms in the individuals. Each member of the couple may react differently to marital conflict; one spouse may become depressed while the other may blithely ignore the tension.

There is potential for couple therapy to increase the power of the individual dynamic therapy; we describe this below. For the therapist, combining treatments requires humility and flexibility—trust and regard for approaches other than the ones you are expert in, and the openness to look at each patient and each problem in a fresh way. The collaboration issues are similar to those discussed in Chapter 13 between a psychotherapist and psychopharmacologist. Offering both individual and couple therapy could also be confusing, diluting the power of each approach and reflecting uncertainty and insecurity on the part of the clinician.

The following case demonstrates how, as a couple moves back and forth between therapies, the individual and marital factors become clearer.

Abby and Bob, a couple in their late 30s with one child, began marital therapy because of mutual feelings of tension, hurt, anger, and increasing alienation. Abby was petite, with a sad, faraway look, while Bob was lean and square-jawed, with an intense stare. Bob felt Abby was detached and unloving. Abby experienced Bob as angry, critical, demanding, and bullying, and twice in the past he had pushed her. Couple therapy in the early stages seemed to stall.

As with many couples, these young adults had begun their married life believing that their partner could meet their deepest needs. Abby was a shy, quiet, and lonely woman who was attracted to Bob because he appeared strong, powerful, helpful, and emotionally available. She believed he would protect her and give her love and liveliness.

Bob appeared to be a strong, confident man, but he had deep unmet longings for affection and approval, and he felt uncomfortable with these dependent feelings. He believed his job was to save, guide, and protect a woman who would then be grateful to him and make up for his insecurity.

But as time went on, their implicit emotional contract gave way to disappointment and resentment, as Abby felt overwhelmed and controlled by Bob's demands and responded passive–aggressively. He experienced her wish to control her own life and her subsequent depression as a rejection, so he began increasingly coercive attempts to get her attention and love. His anger dominated the couple's sessions and made it hard for the therapist to focus on Abby's indirectness and her quietly provocative behavior. The therapist was able to communicate more easily with Abby, whom she saw as victimized by Bob's anger, and this made Bob feel even more unsafe and mistrustful of the treatment.

The couple's therapist referred Abby for individual therapy because she became sad and depressed over the course of the marital treatment, and her issues about relationships and intimacy seemed to be an obstacle in the couple's work. They could not get past fighting in the shared session to discuss the deeper feelings behind the anger. The therapist also suggested individual therapy for Bob, who had difficulty controlling his anger, but he declined, feeling that he had had plenty of therapy in the past.

In her individual therapy, Abby worked on her feeling of rejection and detachment from her mother and the effect of this on her self-esteem. She was intensely self-critical and guilty and could begin to see that this had to do with the dynamics of her core problem of depression. The pair returned to couple therapy as her depression remitted following individual work on these issues as well as pharmacotherapy. She was more able to hold her own in the couple's meetings and began to give up the victim role and assert herself more effectively. Bob handled this with some ambivalence. He was able to think through what he had learned in his previous therapy and gave some support to this new way of relating. Communication between the two therapists allowed the couple therapist to rebalance her work and support Bob more effectively.

Abby's individual problems, primarily depression and low self-esteem, were intertwined with the marital problems. That is, they were manifested in and to some extent caused by the relationship. Bob was the perfectly fitting puzzle piece for her, with issues of rejection-sensitivity and anger when his needs were not met. But Abby's problems might have manifested differently if she had married a supportive and easygoing husband; then she might have presented with issues at work, or with her children. If she had married a quiet and passive man, she might have become the pursuer or emotionally demanding partner.

WHICH THERAPY FIRST?

The decision about whether to begin couple or individual therapy is often made by the couple as they begin to contemplate the possibility of treatment. Sometimes this occurs before the first contact with the therapist. If a coupled patient feels both individual upset and marital stress, a complex negotiation between the partners begins. Is the problem identified as the "fault" or "disease" of only one partner, or a problem for both? Who is most invested in change and willing to attempt therapy (which may be perceived as frightening or dangerous by either partner)? Who is willing to be identified as the patient? While it is common for both partners to have problems, often only one will be agreeable to therapy, usually the one who admits the most distress.

Sometimes one member is sent out to scout the therapist and report back about whether therapy is safe—that is, whether it will upset things too much. Gender is important in this determination. Women typically seek help from professionals earlier than men, who are more apt to insist they can "handle the problem on their own." Frequently, men see treatment as unwelcome and enter therapy as though it were an admission of failure, rather than an expression of hope and the possibility of change. The family member who presents for individual therapy is not necessarily the one who needs the most help.

Because of these complex negotiations, stated and unstated, it is very important to explore how the decision was made to seek help. For some individuals, opting for individual therapy aids their secret goal of ending the relationship; the patient can convince the individual therapist, and themselves, that this is the only possible outcome, without ever giving the partner a chance to understand the gravity of the situation. In these cases it is particularly important that the therapist see the spouse or send the couple for couple consultation.

Once therapy starts, either individual or couple, the treatment format may change, as it did with Abby and Bob. The therapist may recognize from the beginning that couple and individual dynamic therapy are both needed immediately, as in a situation where there is one very depressed partner who is on the verge of leaving the marriage. Sometimes it becomes clear after a while that one partner's individual symptoms fluctuate in response to the other's depression, and couple work is more appropriate.

Frequently, a patient begins individual therapy with the partner already in therapy with a different therapist. In these cases it is particularly important to consider the state of the marriage, since the dynamic therapy draws attention and emotional communication from the dyad to their relationships with the two individual therapists, who may have very strong opinions about their patients' partners. The alternatives here include a referral for couple therapy, frequent communication between the two individual therapists, or a periodic meeting of the four principals. The couple may be at increased risk for splitting, confusion, and increased stress if one of these options is not chosen.

In the end, whether the treatment takes the form of individual or family therapy, or both, is substantially a matter of patient choice and therapist–patient negotiation. The considerations above are important for us as therapists, but on this question the patient almost always carries the day in making the decision.

TYPICAL TREATMENT SCENARIOS

There are five common treatment scenarios for combining individual dynamic therapy and couple treatment: couple therapy leading to individual therapy, individual therapy leading to couple work, concurrent individual and couple therapy, individual therapy with a couple consultation by the individual therapist, and two individual therapists each seeing members of a couple. Our conceptual scheme was adapted for adults from Josephson and Serrano (2001). We will discuss some of the advantages and pitfalls of each clinical scenario and make specific management recommendations (summarized in Table 14.1).

TABLE 14.1. Combining Psychodynamic and Couple Therapy: Common Treatment Scenarios

Treatment sequence	Common clinical situations	Advantages	Pitfalls	Management strategies
Begin couple therapy; refer to individual therapy	Significant individual psychopathology that is an obstacle to couples/family work. Impasse in couple therapy.	Allows for more intensive focus of individual treatment when individual issues are compromising couple work.	Shame at being the "identified patient" unless both enter treatment. Emotional investment in individual therapy may decrease investment in relationship. If only one person changes, may increase possibility of divorce.	Concurrent vs. sequential therapy should be discussed. If sequential, a follow-up couple meeting should be arranged to determine when and if couple work should be resumed.
Begin individual therapy; refer to couple therapy	Problem turns out to be more relational than individual (e.g., questions of having a child, or possible divorce).	Allows for focus on relationship with both partners present. Decreases conflict that is undermining individual growth. Allows partner to acknowledge and participate in change.	Partners avoid dealing with internal issues or main secrets (e.g., affairs) in the couple work.	Individual therapist should not also be couple's therapist unless initial individual contact has been brief. Individual therapy can be continued concurrently if everyone is in agreement.
Concurrent couple and individual therapy	Urgent problem where both individual and couple issues need immediate attention. Not enough time in couple work to deal with	Allows for relationship support and exploration while allowing privacy for deeper individual work. If therapists work in concert,	Costly in time and money. Increased possibilities for splitting and therapist confusion. If only one person is in individual	Essential that all therapists remain in contact, which is often difficult when you have three therapists involved. Can be done sequentially.

	individual issues, but couple wants to continue the work.	can be strongly synergistic.	therapy, problem of "identified patient."	
Individual therapy with couple consultation	Problem is defined as individual, but in context of family relationships.	Practical and usually accepted by individual and couple. Provides very important data that can improve individual treatment. May facilitate beginning couple therapy if indicated.	May complicate alliance with individual patient by support for significant other. May solidify position of patient as "the problem" by not insisting on couple work. Sometimes difficult to recommend individual therapy for patient's partner even if clearly needed.	Couple consultation should be one to three sessions. Consultation is better done at the beginning of treatment. An occasional follow-up couple session may be scheduled later.
Two individual therapies	Each individual has long-standing personal issues, and relationship is basically functional.	Allows for intensive individual focus. Not as resource-intensive as concurrent individual therapies and couple therapy.	Therapists may unwittingly give directly contradictory advice to partners about handling situations. May direct couple's emotional commitments outward, decreasing potential for increased understanding and intimacy. Secrets are easier to keep.	Essential that therapists speak with each other to check that goals are similar and each has the same information about the relational problems.

Note. Adapted from Josephson and Serrano (2001). Copyright 2001 by Elsevier. Adapted by permission.

Begin Couple Therapy; Refer for Individual Therapy

We return to the case of Abby and Bob to discuss a few of these scenarios because there were consultations and referrals back and forth. Abby was referred for individual therapy because her individual problems, especially her depression, were contributing to and a response to the relationship problem.

> Abby's individual therapy helped her explore her early feelings of insecurity and loneliness, self-esteem vulnerability, and tendency to express her needs in an indirect way. She was no longer depressed, and she gained strength and insight from the experience and felt ready to try to make some changes in the marriage. Above all, she felt more able to be assertive.
>
> Abby and Bob returned to couple therapy while Abby continued in concurrent individual therapy. She was able to talk much more clearly about herself and her tendency to express her upset in a passive–aggressive manner. She saw how this fit perfectly with Bob's aggressiveness; her indirectness was a way of dealing with his implacable demands and provoking him at the same time, making him look even more wrong.
>
> Now she could use the individual sessions to discuss the interaction between them, including their interaction in the couple sessions. She saw her tendency to feel rejected, angry, and guilty, and how she expressed this by taking the role of victim in the relationship. She could really see the friction between them as a reflection of her older childhood-based conflicts about closeness, criticism, anger, and emotional withdrawal. This allowed her to keep her feelings and perceptions about Bob as current and adult as possible. Her self-awareness and ability to communicate what was going on with her helped the couple work on their interaction together, as they developed and practiced more effective ways of communicating and asserting their needs.
>
> With the rebalancing of attention in the couple therapy, the therapist could confront Bob's anger more effectively, and this along with Abby's increased availability, helped him to reflect on his angry behavior and make more effective attempts to work together.

In most couple therapy, the role of the past for each partner, including the core psychodynamic problem, beliefs about marriage, and old patterns of behavior are seen as contributing to the problem. The focus of individual dynamic therapy allows therapist and patient to look at the old unconscious patterns that may be less obvious in the couple setting than the more obvious legacies of family relationships and values. For Abby and Bob, this work reinvigorated the couple work, allowed Abby to put into practice what she had learned, and brought Bob back to a more constructive attempt to improve the relationship.

Begin Individual Therapy; Refer to Couple Therapy

Often the individual therapy comes before the couple's treatment, which raises a variety of technical issues.

> Mary was a married 35-year-old woman with four children under the age of 9. She entered individual treatment for depression when an antidepressant prescribed by her family doctor was deemed to be ineffective. Her initial concerns were that her children were "sick a lot," and her husband, Ron, was difficult to deal with.
>
> Although these stressors were noted, after about five sessions the therapist felt that "something was missing," and the therapy did not seem to be progressing. It was difficult to define the core psychodynamic problem and make a formulation. The therapist requested that Ron join them for a session, during which the couple reviewed their marital history and Ron's personal history.
>
> It turned out that Ron's father and two siblings had severe bipolar disorder, type I, and he himself had clear evidence of bipolar illness with both depression and mania. During manic periods he would overspend and engage in mildly risky behaviors. He was also very difficult at home, and in his depressed periods he needed constant reassurance. With a great deal of effort, Mary was able to keep his behavior within bounds. Her concern that "my kids are sick a lot" proved to be an understatement; three had serious asthma requiring a great deal of attention and frequent medical care. Mary's family had endured hardship and did not complain about it, and this perspective caused her to grossly understate her problems.
>
> Ron was referred for pharmacologic treatment, and the couple began marital therapy that focused on education and communications training. The couple's therapist supported Ron in becoming more emotionally available, helping his wife with the children, and becoming responsible for monitoring his condition.

The major problem here turned out to be Ron's illness and the stress on the couple. Mary's issues were primarily a reflection of this and not an individual problem that needed psychodynamic work. Because the couple's therapist was a psychiatrist (this is unusual), she saw Mary first, then the couple, and then periodically saw Ron individually for medication and support. Mary needed occasional support, but not much individual focus. Mary's depression remitted when her husband received appropriate psychopharmacology, and this is referred to as "medication by proxy."

Having one clinician perform all of these roles efficiently served the needs of the family. The transference of both partners was predominantly positive, there were no conflicting agendas, and the couple felt relieved that the therapist knew all the "players." In more complex cases where there is serious emotional conflict, the possibility of divorce, or issues of secrecy and jealousy, the therapist risks alienating one or both partners (or becoming completely confused) by trying to see both an individual and the couple. Typically, we recommend that the therapist see either the couple or one individual, and refer to colleagues with whom they can frequently communicate.

Individual Therapy with a Couple Consultation

Wachtel and Wachtel (1986) list several reasons for bringing other family members into the session: more accurate reconstruction of the patient's history, evaluating the current reality component of the patient's story, choosing a therapeutic direction (e.g., working with the patient toward changing a relationship vs. accepting it with greater equanimity), enabling the patient to see parents more positively, observing a sample of the patient's interactional style, and making the family more open to changes in the patient.

The traditional dynamic therapy model assumed that meeting with family members would complicate understanding of the patient's individual issues, confuse the transference relationship, and potentially compromise the therapeutic alliance by seeming to side with the other member of the couple. While each of these issues is genuine and has potential validity in particular cases, our view is that meeting a partner or family member is far more often valuable than it is hurtful.

Patients are just so different at home than they are in our offices. We forget the demand characteristics of the therapy situation (it is our home). Some patients are much more reasonable, reflective, and calm in the office than at home; some are less so. It is rare for family members to be aware of all of the communication that takes place, as so much is barely conscious or unconscious. We all miss important micro-level interaction. For example, when one spouse looks grim and worried, then the other reacts by moving away an inch and sitting up. This reflects a dynamic that is an essential part of the relationship, and individuals are often unable to describe these subtle but fundamental patterns. Of course, it is difficult to work on this in individual therapy when a patient cannot describe it.

Not only is it hard to see important couple and family interactional behavior in individual sessions, it is also hard for the patient to practice new perceptions and behaviors. For example, encouraging a passive person to become more assertive when other family members are not prepared to welcome the new behavior will likely increase conflict and set up a possible failure. This is what the Hellman quote at the beginning of the chapter referes to. Practicing new patterns of communication with the therapist present can improve the chances of success.

When Abby came for evaluation in individual dynamic therapy, her sadness had progressed to the point of significant sleep, appetite, and energy disturbance. She was passive, hopeless, and quietly angry. She felt the marital work was futile because Bob was not listening to her. The initial phase of treatment involved support and clarification of the situation, as well as pharmacotherapy. The individual therapist, however, began to feel that he also was siding with Abby in the frequent discussions of her interaction with Bob and requested that Bob come in for a consultation so that he could see them together and hear his perspective.

Faced with a different therapist and his own fear that Abby's individual therapy presaged a divorce, Bob was able to more calmly describe how he saw Abby's difficulty and his own. This included what she wanted from him, her provocative rejections, and his genuine attempt to make things better between them. He acknowledged his shame at having pushed her in the past and apologized for his impulsiveness. He was softer and more reasonable than he had appeared in the picture Abby had painted.

Following the meeting with Bob present, the individual therapist began to confront Abby harder about her own history and issues. Her difficult and critical relationship with her mother, lack of acknowledgement by her father, and her sense that her brother was favored, along with the family history of depression, seemed central to the origins of her fragile self-esteem, sensitivity to criticism, and avoidance of direct conflict. It was easier and more effective to work on her problems using the dynamic therapy model with the additional data that came from Bob's visit. The issues with Bob could be peeled away more easily, allowing her to look at what she brought to the relationship. This allowed her to return to the couple work with a fresh perspective.

Reality is fundamentally different from each partner's perspective. Where Abby felt criticized and victimized, resulting in withdrawal and anger, Bob felt set up and criticized, resulting in impotent frustration. The truth is that it is always easier to see the other person as the problem and see oneself as the victim, simply responding to unfairness. An intimate relationship can unfortunately bolster individuals' defenses against dealing with their problems honestly and directly. Abby's early attachment issues surely prefigured her role in the marriage. The same would be true for Bob. If the therapist really sees what is going on from all sides, there is greater potential for holding individual patients accountable for the dynamics they bring to the relationship.

We recognize that bringing others into individual psychotherapy does complicate transference reactions, but these reactions are usually pretty apparent and can withstand this influx of reality. The benefit in observing the partner and the interactions, and cementing the family members' support for the treatment, usually outweighs this concern. Temperance and care in supporting both parties will prevent the patient from feeling ganged up on.

Careful preparation of the patient is required for this kind of consultation. Confidentiality issues must be discussed in advance. When the patient is initially resistant, which is not uncommon, a discussion of concerns and fantasies about the meeting is useful as it leads to further understanding the patient's feelings about the relationship.

We recommend a specific format (Table 14.2) for couple consultation in the context of psychodynamic therapy. This will require slightly more time than the usual psychotherapy session. The implicit message of the consultation is that the family is important and the partner is an ally rather than the enemy. This model is easily modifiable for young

TABLE 14.2. Format for Couple Consultation in Individual Dynamic Psychotherapy

- Greet partner.
- Request a life history from the partner (approximately 15 minutes).
- Explore the partner's ideas and concerns about the patient's condition and his or her hopes for the patient's therapy.
- Ask the couple to give you a marital history as a shared task.
- Ask each partner to comment on the other's family and history and on the strengths of the marriage.
- Assess the couple's strengths and vulnerabilities.
- Thank the partner for coming.

adults meeting with parents or older patients in a consult with their adult children.

The purpose is to learn about the patient from the perspective of the partner and to see whether there is a couple problem, or if there are resources within the couple that can help the individual. Change is not expected.

- *Greet the partner,* reviewing the purpose of consultation, making it clear that this is not "therapy," but that you are interested in the partner's view of the situation. The partner is treated as a guest who has an interesting perspective rather than a problem.
- *Request a life history from the partner,* a description of the individual patient's strengths and vulnerabilities as the partner sees him or her, and an overview of his or her current work or life structure. Informally assess whether the partner has an Axis I diagnosis (do this as unobtrusively as possible, because you do not want this to look like a formal evaluation). A very brief history will facilitate an alliance and help develop some understanding of the partner's state of mind. We explain this is a "sound-bite" history and limit the time for this to 15 minutes.
- *Explore the partner's ideas and concerns* about the patient's condition, and the patient's hopes for therapy. This information will allow you and the patient to consider his behavior in a new way. This should be a three-way conversation, with the patient participating. A patient who has started therapy for depression and has trouble asserting himself might look at himself differently (as might his therapist) if his wife reports in a consultation that he is quite critical and demanding at home. If the patient already has a psychiatric diagnosis, ask what the partner knows about it. For example, the partner might know that the patient has attention-deficit disorder but not understand that his inability to carry out promised tasks is a symptom of the problem rather than lack of love.
- *Ask the couple to give you a marital history as a shared task.* You will get two different versions of the history, which is to be expected. What is of interest is where the differences are. During this time, ask the couple to talk to each other about shared events in their past. Ask about how the children, if any, are doing. Ask specifically about strengths in the relationship.
- *Ask each partner to comment on the other's family and history.* This will usually pick up obvious past issues and current in-law problems and add to your understanding of each person. If you are not sure

about the patient's family dynamics, the partner can usually tell you, and vice versa.

• *Assess the couple's strengths and vulnerabilities.* As the couple talks, consider their affective bonding, power relationships, boundaries, communication, and problem solving. How have they handled other stresses? How are they handling the current one? How do they understand the present problem? Does the relationship seem to be the cause of the problem, making it worse, or making it better? Ask specifically about what they see as current strengths in the marriage.

• *End the consult* by thanking the partner for coming in. Explain the individual treatment plan and highlight the couple's strengths and previous successes. If couple therapy is indicated, discuss it. If you believe the other partner could use therapy, consider whether it would be appropriate to gently suggest it.

Concurrent Individual and Couple Therapy

The Abby–Bob vignette raises the question of the potential advantages and disadvantages of concurrent individual and couple or family therapy. The integration of individual and couple treatments allows for more data—information about each person and how they are feeling, as well as the opportunity to see them together and understand how they interact. It also allows the spotlight to be on the relationship in the couple's therapy and on the individual psychodynamic problems in the individual therapy. Abby could focus on herself, her history, and what she brought to the relationship in the individual therapy. She could avoid getting caught in more conversation about the marital tension. The couple's work could avoid Bob's discussion of what was wrong with Abby and focus on getting along better. Couple therapy gives a chance to try out new ways of experiencing the partner and new behavioral responses. This synergy can occur if the individual and couple therapy happen concurrently, or if one follows the other.

Two Individual Therapies

It is very common for both members of a couple to be in individual therapy with different therapists. When the couple is stable and communicating well, they can share their learning and use it to improve their relationship. If the therapists do not speak to each other, however, or do not share each other's view of the world or the partner, difficulties may ensue. If the individual therapist sees the patient as the victim, there is a tendency, either by direct advice or by the way questions are posed, to encourage the patient to believe he or she has no responsibility for the problem. Frequently this leads to increased distance in the couple and sometimes even separation because the patient believes that the partner is hopeless and that there is no other way out.

Having two individual therapists is not the most effective way to track or alter marital communication. It does allow each of the partners time and space to work on their most troublesome problems. The two-therapist model works if the therapists communicate, and is most useful when each therapist meets the patient's partner at least once. In some cases, the two therapists and the patients meet periodically to make sure the relationship is being cared for. If the therapists are comfortable working with each other, this can be an effective way of dealing with relational and individual problems at the same time.

COLLABORATION BETWEEN THE INDIVIDUAL AND COUPLE THERAPISTS

The first principle sounds obvious, but is often not done. Open and frequent communication between the individual and couples therapist is very important. The therapists may be concerned about the time involved, or about the possibility of altering the transference or sharing secrets. The couple therapist's feeling about the patient may be very different from the individual therapist's, or he or she may be frustrated that the individual therapy is not covering areas that are important to the couple. Openness moves both treatments along, with judgment on all sides about what is essential and important to communicate, and what will quell difficulty rather than incite it. It is striking how often this type of communication helps to calm the couple down. When one member of the couple tries to limit the communication, this is a warning sign and must be dealt with carefully, but with an attempt to keep the lines of communication open.

The second principle in combined couple and individual therapy is that the individual therapy should not become a forum for complaining about the partner. It is natural enough for this to occur, as the patient may believe that the partner is the main source of his or her symptoms, but it is quite unproductive. The couple therapy is the outlet for those resentful feelings and the best place to handle them. The individual therapy should focus on the individual, and the therapist must be firm and clear about this; otherwise, time will be wasted and the couple therapy will be undermined. This requires trust by the individual therapist that the couple's work is moving along and fairly balanced.

Just as we have emphasized the importance of a clear formulation and treatment plan in individual treatment, this is true for combined treatment. The third principle is that the individual treatment plan should mesh with the couple plan. A coordinated plan orients the patient(s) and the therapists. Simply put, this means that the individual therapist works on a core psychodynamic problem and its manifestations in the patient's life, including in the relationship. The problem and the focus of that work should be communicated clearly to the couple therapist. When the couple therapist is aware of the central individual therapy focus and can refer to it, this will facilitate work on how this problem affects the couple's relationship.

PITFALLS IN COMBINING TREATMENTS

In contrast to the effective integration that occurs when the therapists communicate fully and regularly and keep the individual–couple treatment boundaries clear, there is much potential for confusion, disorganization, and damage when the coordination breaks down. Infrequent communication between the therapists is the mildest version of this problem. Patients may tell different stories to each therapist, promoting their own agendas differently in the two settings. For example, one patient insisted in couple therapy that she wanted to save the marriage, while discussing divorce with her individual therapist.

Perhaps one of the most difficult problems occurs when secrets are known to the individual therapist but not the couple's therapist, and the individual is not ready to allow these to be shared. An affair, strong homosexual feelings in a married partner, or impending plans for divorce are some examples of this. While the individual therapist is ethically bound not to reveal secrets, she should make clear to the patient that unless they are revealed, the couple's therapy may be compromised.

Therapists with different worldviews, values, therapeutic theories, or those who have specific disagreements create tremendous confusion and difficulty for their patients. For example, a therapist had seen a patient with fear of abandonment over a number of years, during which time the patient seemed to improve significantly. The couple's therapist thought the patient was still extremely disruptive within the marriage and requested that the individual therapist refer the patient back to the psychopharmacologist for a medication change. The individual therapist and the patient both saw this as an insult. The two therapists could not agree on a treatment plan, and the couple was finally faced with having to choose between plans themselves. The couple therapy nearly ended over this problem. This could have been avoided by a frank discussion between the two therapists where they resolved their differing perceptions and made a recommendation together.

It is hard enough for patients to sort out their problems and the complexity added by therapist–therapist conflict makes it much worse. While this situation is both frustrating and humbling to the therapists, it is also helpful to remember that well-trained therapists may differ enormously about the diagnosis and treatment of members of a system, depending on who in the family they are treating. Fortunately, Abby's and Bob's therapists had relative agreement about the nature of their difficulties, and respect for each other.

SUMMARY

Individual dynamic therapy and couple therapy can be synergistic, and there are a number of typical scenarios for how they are combined in clinical practice. Each scenario has particular advantages and pitfalls, and there are management approaches for each scenario. There are three principles for combining individual and couple work.

1. Communication and transparency between the two therapists is essential. Communication problems abound, and it is the therapists' responsibility to manage this and come to effective consensus.
2. The individual sessions should focus on individual psychodynamic problems, and the therapist must be active in maintaining this boundary.
3. A clear focus for individual therapy and for the couple therapy increases treatment effectiveness and decreases confusion for all involved.

PART V

ENDING

CHAPTER 15

Goals and Termination

> Freudian psychoanalysis is best for the young,
> Jungian analysis for the middle-aged, and
> when you are old, you need yoga.
> —MORRIS SCHWARTZ

Although less certain than death and taxes, the end of psychotherapy is inevitable. The term for the completion of therapy, termination, sounds more like a death than a new beginning, but ending therapy is actually a transition to greater independence and maturity. Termination signals the end of a relationship and a graduation from a personal development program; it also offers a new kind of relationship experience.

Feelings about ending psychotherapy run high for both the patient and therapist. For the patient it may be the loss of a benign and caretaking figure, and excitement and trepidation about flying solo. The special relationship and the undivided attention will be hard to replace, and there may be a powerful sense of sadness. The endings of earlier relationships will shape the emotional response to the end of this one.

Ending therapy means a return to traveling along life's developmental pathway without professional help. Ideally the patient will have greater self-awareness, new ways of perceiving experiences, and more adaptive behavior. There should be greater reflective capacity, use of more mature defenses, and greater strength. There will be future challenges and future conflict because maturation is never finished, and there will always be more adversity. One hopes that termination occurs at a time when the patient wants it and is ready for it. The quotation at the beginning of the chapter reminds us that working out emotional conflicts is only part of maturity, and in some ways is just the beginning. Knowing oneself and finding peace and acceptance is a lifelong task that requires various forms of attention; working through emotional problems only provides the platform for these subsequent growth opportunities.

For the therapist, ending the treatment is a loss, too. Patients figure prominently in our internal lives, and although the affective intensity of being a therapist is less than that of being a patient, termination is often a powerful emotional experience for us, too. The satisfaction of termination results from a job well done and vicarious enjoyment of another person's hard work and good results; unlike for the patient, for the therapist ending therapy does not have the satisfaction of personal change, the compensations of free time, and savings of money.

There is surprisingly little empirical study of termination in psychodynamic psychotherapy (see Joyce, Piper, Ogrodniczuk, & Klein, 2007). Some of the research has focused on patients who were thought to have terminated treatment too soon; this is a common phenomenon, and across psychotherapies the dropout rate is close to 50% (Roe, 2007). While some authors suggest that early dropout reflects poor patient outcome, other studies suggest that some "dropout" patients benefited from therapy (e.g., Roe, 2007). There has been no study of patients who may have stayed too long in therapy. Our discussion is about termination after a treatment of sufficient duration to identify problems, develop an alliance, work on a new narrative, and focus on making changes.

ENDING IS IN THE AIR:
PLANNED AND UNPLANNED TERMINATION

There is an intangible feeling in the air in the session when termination is imminent. Sometimes it is present early on, when the patient is feeling that the therapy will not be helpful or the therapist is not making her comfortable. This is an abortive treatment more than a termination proper.

Some patients feel they want to end and begin to consider their exit strategy well before they bring it up in a session. When a full treatment begins to move toward the phase of termination, often the patient has been feeling a sense of readiness (and the therapist, too) before it becomes conscious, and certainly well before the thought is articulated by either party.

When there is less new material, more working through of the same situations and interpretations, less distress for the patient, and more of a sense that the patient is reporting events and not breaking new ground, the treatment may be moving toward termination. The patient often tries to think of topics to discuss and seems pleased when there is a meaty or conflictual situation to bring up. There is less urgent need to get work done.

Sometimes the therapist becomes aware of the imminence of termination first. The patient is plowing forward, continuing to use the sessions in the same way, but the therapist senses that things are better for the patient, the goals have been accomplished, and the motivation for continuing is not clear. There is always something to talk about, always something to understand better or deal with in a better way. But the benefits of coming to treatment must be greater than the costs— of time, money, emotional involvement, distress—to justify it. If there is not genuine forward motion, the therapist will usually feel this and begin to wonder.

The challenge is to determine whether the therapy is slowing down because the work has largely been done, or whether there is an impasse in the treatment and the patient and therapist are stuck. There is always potential for transference and countertransference to interlock in such a way that the patient and therapist enact old scenarios from the patient's life. For example, a patient with fear of abandonment may handle this problem by rejecting closeness and leaving relationships prematurely. The therapist could be prone to feeling guilty about confrontation. This pair will be vulnerable to an impasse, where the patient could stop bringing in new material, and the therapist will let the patient go and support an early termination. The therapist and patient may not be able to get on top of this interlocking mutual fulfillment of unconscious need and free up the interaction to be able to talk about what is going on and enact it less. This is an example of a psychotherapeutic impasse.

We described the potential resistances, enactments, transferences, and countertransferences that could result in an impasse with each of the six core problems. The therapist is responsible for asking whether the feeling of termination "in the air" is a consequence of effective work done, or whether it reflects these phenomena. You will use your understanding of the core problem, formulation, and defined goals to consider this, and you will discuss it directly with the patient.

Although it is important to understand whether the impending termination is appropriate or the result of an impasse, much of the discussion in the psychodynamic and psychoanalytic literature presumes that the therapist has more control over the process than is actually the case. If starting the treatment and identifying the core problems is like taking a ski lift to the top of the mountain, rewriting the narrative with the patient is like skiing downhill. Termination is the last few minutes of the ride when you have built up so much speed that getting to the bottom is inevitable. We can raise questions, help to clarify what is going on about ending, but mostly we need to get out of the way and let the patient do whatever is necessary.

The only exception to this approach is when there has been an enactment where a patient abruptly and intensely wants to leave, and prior to this point there has been a good therapeutic alliance and good therapeutic work. The transference–countertransference may have built to a fever pitch, and the patient wants to leave because of it. The enactment may involve a negative transference with powerful feelings of anger or fear, or a positive transference that the patient is containing by leaving. In these situations the therapist must be clear and direct in interpreting the situation to the patient, supporting the reality, and explaining why it will help to stay and work this out.

> Carrie was the attractive twice-married woman in her early 50s described in Chapter 8. She had been previously treated with CBT for anxiety and mild depression. She was warm and friendly, with a very quick sense of humor that usually involved a rueful acknowledgement of her burdens in life.
>
> Carrie had lost her beloved father within the previous year and contended with an acrimonious relationship with her mother, a selfish and vain woman who felt increasingly alone and demanding as she aged. Carrie had two college-age daughters, one of whom had depression and a lot of interpersonal drama. The daughter was set to graduate from college, and Carrie was very worried about how she would do without the structure of college life. The daughter cried often and was alternately angry and needy. Carrie was glad that the daughter's long-suffering boyfriend was there to manage a lot of her emotional lability.
>
> The background, and ultimately the foreground, of the treatment was Carrie's worry that she was a bad mother, like her mother had been, and that's why her daughter was struggling so much. The psychotherapy took place on a weekly basis over a year and a half and was characterized by a strong alliance. We talked about her difficult early relationship with her mother, competitive older sister, and her fun-loving but intermittently unavailable father. Carrie

reexperienced many old emotions, including fear and anger toward her mother, a need to manage her mother's moods, worry about her criticism, and a feeling of helplessness and loss about not seeing her father much after the parents' divorce.

Carrie returned numerous times to the painful feeling of disappointing her mother, worrying about her mother's anger with her. This made her anxious and resulted in a characteristic compliant response. Over time, she learned to separate her feelings from her mother's and worry less about what her mother felt. She could decide what was an appropriate degree of responsiveness to her mother, tolerate her mother's disappointment, and be freer from guilt and self-criticism. Needless to say, this helped her with her relationship with her daughter, as well as other relationships.

Carrie felt that generally she functioned well in life and had made significant progress in feeling freed up from worrying so much about her mother and her reactions. She thought she might be ready to stop therapy. But she was worried she would start to feel the old feelings again if she stopped. She had felt well the last time she stopped therapy and later felt much worse.

My question about ending was whether it was true that Carrie's treatment had gone well and she was ready to stop, or whether she had only gone so far. Did the pleasant working relationship with me avoid conflict in the therapeutic relationship? In other words, was the positive transference a defense against more conflicted feelings about me, either as a cold mother or the unavailable father?

We had defined low self-esteem as Carrie's core problem and worked on this intensively in her relationship with her mother and at various times in her relationship with sister, husband, daughter, and colleagues at work. She did seem to feel much better, and was less upset when she spoke with or saw her mother. She seemed more even-keeled and happier. When there were glitches, she seemed to recognize the old patterns and correct them with a more contemporary perspective and response. She was appreciative about the therapy. But she was afraid to leave.

So I summarized all of the work we had done and wondered about how it felt to consider leaving. She worried I thought she was still "crazy," and felt sad that she would miss the sessions if she stopped because they had been so helpful. Mostly she wanted to know whether she could come back if she needed it. After probing further, I concluded that the dominant feeling about termination did seem to be a concern about losing support; this was likely connected to the old feeling of losing her close relationship with her father and her longing for a secure relationship with her mother. But I did not think these old feelings and the conflicts associated with them were resulting in an impasse. That is, it did not seem that there was a negative transference she was leaving treatment to defend against. There is always more to talk about, but Carrie seemed to have achieved the goals she had set out for herself: feeling freer in her relationship with her mother and less guilty about her daughter's difficulties.

I felt pleased at the progress, encouraged the termination, and asked Carrie how she would like to end. She wanted to switch to monthly appointments for a couple of months to be sure that she really did feel as well as she thought she did, and then stop from there. At the last appointment before moving to this monthly schedule, it was almost as though she were holding her breath as she left the office, excited about whether she would make it, but worried. In fact, she came back for four monthly appointments, weathering one small crisis during that time, and then she decided she would stop and hope for the best.

This example of a typical termination experience illustrates the attention to the criteria for termination, questioning of the decision (skeptical but respectful), attention to the transference meaning, and the expectation that the decision to end or continue belongs with the patient.

REASONS FOR TERMINATION

The psychodynamic psychotherapy literature emphasizes a variety of criteria for ending, such as symptom resolution, attainment of goals, internalization of the psychotherapy function, and resolution of the transference (Weiner, 1998). It is clear what is meant by symptom resolution and attainment of goals. The patient will be the best judge of this. The next criterion is interesting and important. It is variously referred to as identification with the therapist, development of self-reflective capacity, insight, and improved relationship skills. Each of these terms has a slightly different meaning and different connotation, but all speak to the patient's ability to do for herself what the therapy relationship helped her to do. Does the patient have the ability to continue the questioning, analyzing, self-assessing and self-correcting aspect of the work? This is essential because it is not possible (nor desirable, probably) to have a treatment that is so thorough that every possible issue is taken up and worked on. The patient should be able to function independently and manage problems as they come up.

The psychodynamic, and especially psychoanalytic, literature is focused on how termination can represent an acting out of unresolved transference (Greenson, 1967). Freud, however, seems to have had a rather pragmatic perspective, wondering in his classic work on the topic, *Analysis Terminable and Interminable,* "Is there such a thing as a natural end to an analysis?" (Freud, 1937) His point was that there is always more to do, and the timing of ending has some degree of arbitrariness. Indeed, Roe (2007) found that 60% of private practice dynamically oriented psychotherapy patients thought their treatment lasted too long or ended too soon.

Our view is that there is almost always a transferential aspect of the decision to end therapy, and if enough of the criteria for termination have been met and the patient really feels ready to go, you will probably not achieve more by pushing the patient to stay. A lot of life involves acting out of unresolved transference wishes, and our goal is to help the patient get some perspective on this, and determine how much is too much.

Some authors distinguish between forced and unforced terminations (Glick, 1987). Forced terminations come because the patient is leaving the area, there are financial or schedule limitations, or the therapist is no longer available. The determining event is something outside the treatment and outside the dynamic of the therapy. Unforced terminations occur when the internal logic of the treatment results in a decision to end, either because of effective resolution of the problems or an enactment. In our experience, it is much more common for patients to begin to consider ending than for therapists to propose it. Therapists tend to get involved and want to stay involved, and we experience less pressure to end than the patient does—after all, it's what we do, and for the patient therapy is an add-on to their lives.

BEYOND PATHOLOGY: ACHIEVING POSITIVE GOALS AS CRITERIA FOR TERMINATION

So far, we have mostly been discussing reduction in pathology as a marker for considering termination, but positive criteria may be even more important. If the goal of treatment is better adaptation, and not just symptom reduction, then perhaps the most important question is whether the patient's adaptation has improved and whether it could improve more. If each patient comes to the therapy with a set of characteristic defenses and usual coping strategies, by the end of the treatment the defenses should be healthier, employed more flexibly and smoothly, and there should be a greater inner sense of freedom. Is the obsessional patient using higher level defenses and employing them more effectively? Is the traumatized patient more empowered and more sure of herself? From this perspective, the termination question is: Has the mental health of the patient improved, not has the psychopathology diminished?

Andrew was a 49-year-old divorced graphic artist who came for therapy because of confusion about his bisexual interests. He was deeply attached to and even obsessed with a male friend who was an athletic companion. His marriage had been short-lived, and he felt very inadequate that his wife had left him, complaining that he was cold and unsympathetic. The divorce was 15 years ago, and she had remarried and now had three children. Andrew had had two enjoyable relationships with women since then, but when the possibility of marriage came up, he felt sure he would be rejected and humiliated and ended the relationships. He had a number of liaisons with men, but none became stable and intimate. He was depressed and thought constantly about how much he wanted a sexual relationship with his friend, how dishonest he was because he never expressed this, and how his friend would despise him if he knew.

In the therapy, there was a rich and thorough exploration of Andrew's early life, his relationships with his parents and brother, and his many friends. He understood a lot about his problems with self-esteem and his strategies for managing this. His male friend got married, and they saw each other less. He was less troubled because there was less contact. Andrew began to like himself more, and felt that his bisexuality was just the way he was—he was not twisted and sick. He wished he were simply straight, and wanted to find the right woman, but somehow he never felt as comfortable with women as with men.

There was no epiphany about his sexuality, and no clear solution to his problem. But he began to have a feeling of starting life anew. He changed jobs, moving to a smaller company where he took a leading creative role, and took a long vacation with some money he unexpectedly earned. He began to think about his future in a new way. He pondered the kinds of experiences and challenges he wanted to have. He was sad that he probably would not have the kind of relationship with a woman that he would have liked. Maybe he would find a man to be with, maybe the right kind of relationship with a woman. His dry sense of humor became more evident, and he was more playful. He had a number of excellent ideas at work that were recognized. His social life was more active.

He ended the therapy about 6 months after the vacation and move to the new job. He wrote a note less than a year later to say that he was feeling well, and was enjoying himself. He expressed his thanks for our work and wished me well.

This ending made sense from the perspective of symptom reduction, but it made even more sense in terms of the patient's return to a healthy life cycle progression. He certainly felt better, he was taking on the challenges of aging, and was using his characteristic strengths— creativity, persistence, vitality, social intelligence, and gratitude—to find fulfillment and closeness in the next phase of his life. He had learned a lot from the painful entanglement with his friend, and he found renewed engagement with his work. He was better adapted to his bisexual feelings and had more comfort with this, and more awareness of what kinds of relationships worked and didn't work. Andrew was more comfortably self-reflective, and from the defense perspective, he began to use less reaction formation and doing and undoing, and also less repression. There was more sublimation and humor.

LOSS OF THE THERAPY AND THE THERAPIST

So far, the picture we have painted of termination has a decidedly positive cast, and indeed positive feelings are often prominent at termination in longer-term dynamic psychotherapy (Roe, Dekel, Harel, & Fennig, 2006). Work has been done, goals are mostly met, and the patient is more or less ready to go. Both therapist and patient feel some degree of satisfaction. But ending will also stir up painful feelings of sadness and frustration. Patients may feel loss of the closeness with the therapist, disappointment about the extent of changes made, feelings of rejection, and reexperienced loss from long ago. These feelings will occur when there is an interruption in the natural progression of the treatment causing early termination, but they may be significant even when the termination is planned.

Psychodynamic psychotherapy allows the patient to experience these feelings of limitation, disappointment, and sadness, and explore them as fully as possible. Patients may be reluctant to discuss their negative feelings; after all, the treatment has to end sometime. They may be afraid to hurt the therapist's feelings and discuss how the relationship did not meet some of their expectations.

We have all had profound attachments, and loss or disappointment in those attachments is ubiquitous; it is part of normal and abnormal growing up. Because traumatic experiences repeat, childhood feelings of sadness, rejection, or abandonment will be triggered by the ending of the therapy. For example, a man whose father had died several years before, with whom he was especially close, was surprised at how much sadness and longing he had felt in the last couple of appointments before ending. A woman who had evolved a caretaking role with her mother to prevent fears of her mother's death wanted to avoid any sense of loss of the therapist; she was cheerful and focused on discussing her plans and the therapist's for the summer. Another woman whose father had died when she was a girl wanted to hold onto the therapy relationship and never finish, as she had always held onto her memories of her father.

Even if the patient wants to stop and is ready to stop, the end may be experienced as a rejection or disappointment. Transferential reactions are driven by timeless templates that do not obey the demands of current reality. That is why these feelings are so confusing to patients, and why exploring them and connecting them to the ongoing themes of the treatment (and the core psychodynamic problem) will help to complete the work.

Because the core psychodynamic problem is reflected in all areas of the patient's functioning, including endings, the patient's termination reaction can be anticipated. Depressed patients will likely react with ambivalence about losing the relationship, and this will be intermixed with guilt and self-criticism. Obsessional patients will feel the loss, and will tend to feel controlled by the therapist in the way the ending occurs; they will be angry and need to inhibit this aggression through the use of obsessional defenses. Patients with fears of abandonment will feel frankly bereft, and the loss will seem to them as real as the loss of a parent by a child. Patients with low self-esteem will commonly feel that the end of treatment, and the therapist's letting them go, means they were not so loved in the first place. It is a rejection, even if they initiated the ending. Patients with panic share the dependency and fear of separation that patients with fear of abandonment have, but they will likely anticipate a recurrence of panic and want to remain as dependent as possible. Traumatized patients will see the therapist as punitive, or as the bystander who stood by and did not help.

Thus the last task of psychodynamic psychotherapy is to help the patient see the connection between the negative feelings stirred up by termination and the main theme of the work. Carrie was able to connect her feeling of loss and worry that she would alienate the therapist by leaving with her feeling that being independent made her mother feel abandoned and angry. She was worried about leaving because something bad might happen and she would not be able to come back to therapy because she had burned her bridges. Once Carrie saw this as a transference reaction based on her relationship with her mother and connected to her main psychodynamic problem, she felt freer to leave. Andrew felt vaguely rejected by the therapist when he ended, although of course it was his decision. The therapist was male, and he felt such longing for and rejection by men.

Not all negative feelings at the end of treatment are based on transference. It is sad and disappointing for patients to realize that they are only able to change so much. Often they had hoped for more. Maybe the treatment was not more effective because there was more the therapist could have done, or more the patient could have contributed. Maybe it was all that could be accomplished. These are issues that most patients (and most therapists) ponder. It is necessary to validate the patient's feelings in this area and accept our own limitations as therapists as well.

TERMINATION AND THE THERAPIST

Although it is supposed to be the patient who regresses and gets in touch with old powerful feelings in the therapy, the therapist also gets deeply attached. It is painful and uncomfortable to say good-bye to patients at termination. It is worse because we feel we have no control over the process—it is supposed to happen when it does and how it does for the patient's greater good, not ours. Gabbard (2005) notes that, as therapists, we need to get used to a "professional life of constant loss" (p. 112).

We can become so set in our role as therapist that we ourselves might not notice how important the attachment to a particular patient has become. This attachment might reflect a powerful countertransference reaction or may just show the duration and intensity of a long-term relationship. You have spent more time in the last year with certain patients than you have with a lot of your good friends or relatives.

Therapists need to feel the end of the treatment relationship and in some way mourn the loss. If the end of a treatment fills you with feeling, then it will be important to sort out how much this has to do with losses and endings in your own life, or life cycle issues you are personally engaged with. Perhaps the patient's experience reminds you of some specific losses in your history. Just because you can interpret what is happening based on the patient's transference and conflicts does not mean it does not reflect your concerns as well. For example, patients with trauma often stir up guilt and anxiety in the therapist at the end of treatment because the therapist is no longer able to protect them. Patients with panic can be so dramatic and anxious at termination that therapists are relieved the treatment is over, and this leads to feelings of guilt. Like any mourning process, there is not much to do about it other than to know the meaning of what you are experiencing and try to let the feelings take their natural course.

If the problem is that you do not feel much about a termination, then it will be important to think more about the patient, the work together, the moments of emotional intensity, and try to think about the next chapter of the patient's life. This will likely bring up some of the unrecognized emotion you may have.

One of our trainees was excited about her graduation and beginning of a prestigious postgraduate fellowship. She had to refer several of her psychotherapy patients on to new trainees. She felt guilty about how well her life was going and how her patients were still struggling. This guilt caused her to delay telling her patients about her graduation—she thought they would be angry with her. One of the patients being transferred was a young woman who had been abused and was angry with women in general. The combination of the resident's guilty feelings and the patient's dynamics resulted in the resident's being especially avoidant. Not surprisingly, this made the patient especially hurt and angry when she heard without much notice that she would need to stop. The trainee then felt, of course, even more guilty.

We have become more interested in termination as the years go by, and see ending as more filled with emotion than in our years of training and early practice. Perhaps this has to do with aging, maturation, and awareness of loss, as younger people tend to focus more on the beginnings and the future and less on endings. Perhaps it just takes more experience to see these clinical phenomena at a moment in the relationship when there is so much going on. But the earlier you begin to attend to the feelings about termination the sooner you will see it.

MODELS OF TERMINATION

There are two different ways of conceptualizing the end of therapy: one based on the traditional techniques of psychodynamic psychotherapy, and one based on the primary care model of medicine and adapted for use in dynamic psychotherapy.

The traditional dynamic psychotherapy model sees treatment as a finite experience with a beginning, middle, and end, and regards the task of termination as the successful ending of the treatment, with the notion that the end of treatment should have a sense of finality. Treatment should be definitive, identify the key problems, and work them through to as successful a conclusion as possible. Maximal use should be made of the transference and what the patient can learn for herself from the transference experience of loss at the ending of treatment. Although the patient may have difficulty understanding the progress that has been made and also have an intense transference while ending, the working through of this experience is held to be highly therapeutic. The traditional model of termination is based on the idea that the patient will develop self-reflective functioning more fully when pushed to confront these transferential feelings and work on them. There will be subsequent life problems and life cycle issues to deal with, and patients will need to use the insight and changes they made during their finite course of therapy to manage these future challenges. This may explain the observation that patients continue to improve in the months after therapy (e.g., Blomberg, Lazar, & Sandell, 2001); that is, patients become increasingly adept at using the knowledge and self-awareness gained during treatment.

By contrast, the primary care model presumes that the work of therapy is never done and does not try to push it to a conclusion in the middle of the game, so to speak. In this model, patients come for bursts of treatment when they are experiencing symptoms, having difficulty functioning, or are lagging in their ability to manage some aspect of their life demands. This occurs at multiple points along the life cycle. Treatment is offered when needed, and as patients begin to feel better (whether this is in the symptom, subjective freedom, internalization of psychotherapy function, or mental health sense), they pull away from the therapy, aware that they may come back at some point in the future. The benefit of this model is that it may be more parsimonious in terms of therapy sessions because there is less pressure to make the treatment definitive and final (which may be unrealistic), it has a natural feel to it, and there is less concern about iatrogenically stirring the patient up to deal with transference feelings about ending that might not otherwise need much attention. The problem with this model is that issues can easily be left on the table and partially resolved, and it is easy to avoid confronting limitations and losses. This model presumes that the future is not knowable, and if there are problems later they can be dealt with then.

As you consider these two perspectives, you will see that they reflect two different ways of conceptualizing psychopathology. The traditional model is more consistent with treatment of a discrete and acute disease, while the primary care model presumes a chronic view of the problem and an appreciation of the need to develop strengths. It has become clear that depressive and anxiety syndromes often do not disappear, but tend to wax and wane during the lifespan. More important, though, when one sees a patient early in the development of his illness, one cannot know whether the problem will become chronic except in the cases of certain syndromal illnesses. We have some knowledge that helps us prognosticate about who will have what course of illness, but unfortunately we are not yet very good at predicting a priori the course of a specific individual. This may be especially true for patients with troubling but less severe problems.

Because there is little empirical research to guide us about whether to employ the traditional psychodynamic model for termination or the primary care model, a few orienting principles are useful. We consider how likely it is that the patient will need and want more treatment in the future. Patients with more chronic conditions are more likely to have future episodes of illness or difficulty than those who have more circumscribed emotional conflicts that can be more definitively worked on. Those more likely to return may not be best served by an attempt to make the treatment definitive. Those patients who have done more extensive and deeper work in therapy, especially using the treatment relationship, will benefit from an ending that takes full advantage of working with transferential feeling about ending, and will probably be left in some confusion and disarray if the transference feelings are not worked on. Patients who have a benign positive transference, and whose relationship with the therapist is more based on the actual relationship (or the therapeutic alliance) than on the transferential relationship, will probably be able to end more easily using when treated in the primary care model because conflictual aspects of the transference have not been brought to the surface.

Patients usually have feelings themselves about how they would like to end. Some want to end precipitously; having thought about it themselves, they will announce the decision and want that session to be the last. Others are very anxious about ending therapy and want to slowly titrate down the frequency, trying to minimize the impact and desensitize themselves to their feelings about stopping. These requests must be respected but questioned. Is the patient who wants to stop quickly defending against powerful feelings about ending that will plague her after the treatment and that would be better off being talked about? Or is she really ready to end and move on? Is the patient who is worried about leaving therapy quite able to stop but overly anxious about termination? Does she need encouragement to be more independent? These questions are best answered in the context of the issues you have worked on with the patient and can be fleshed out with direct discussion with the patient. Your job is to raise questions, slow down action, and encourage maximal reflection. This is the essence of therapy at any stage of treatment. Nevertheless, most of the time the patient (and the momentum of the treatment relationship) will determine how the ending is played out. Your job is to make as much as you can conscious and articulated and to express your understanding of what is going on in a constructive and therapeutic context.

Nicholas is the businessman discussed in Chapter 4 whose wife was planning to divorce him. He came for therapy to figure out how to win her back, and much of his thinking consisted of his using "chess-playing" logical strategic thinking to figure out what his wife wanted and give it to her. The work of therapy was in helping him to get in touch with the many feelings he had about being a husband and father so that he understood what he really felt and what kind of relationship he wanted to have.

Nicholas's parents divorced when he was 7 years old, and his mother became depressed and helpless. He remembers day after day coming home from school and finding her crying at the kitchen table. His father was living a bachelor's life, dating and driving a fancy car. Nicholas's younger sister was too young to really understand what was going on. He felt a tremendous amount of responsibility toward his mother, and also a lot of resentment about having to worry about her and take care of her (although he was not very aware of these latter feelings until the therapy because they made him feel quite guilty).

Nicholas's first round of therapy lasted 7 months, and he worked on understanding his relationship with his wife, why he experienced her as so demanding and difficult, and why he was so controlling and irritable with her. He realized that his superficially supportive demeanor hid his demands and frustration with her. In time, he understood more about his needs and was better at expressing them in a constructive way. As he became better able to do this, she was pleased and felt that he was easier to live with. He, in turn, was less angry because he felt less compelled to do whatever she wanted, and he felt he was getting more of her attention.

Nicholas felt very pleased with his work in therapy, and the marriage seemed patched up. He mentioned ending in a session, and then skipped the next appointment and did not call to reschedule. He did not return my phone calls asking him if he would like to come for a final appointment. I understood this as a return to business as usual for him, and an avoidance of saying good-bye. Perhaps it was connected to his early loss of his father, or maybe he was busy, not a natural communicator, and was finished with therapy.

A year and a half later, he called again and wanted to come back for some appointments. His wife had breast cancer and he was afraid he would lose her, and was also afraid for his two young children. This time he came for about 4 months on a weekly basis. His prior understanding that he related to his wife as though she were his unavailable childhood mother became even clearer this time. To Nicholas, his wife's breast cancer, emotional anguish, and the physical sequellae of her treatment were like his mother's depression. His wife was also drinking excessively at this point, and she wanted to spend time with a couple of friends who also enjoyed drinking. This also made him feel rejected and angry. Despite understanding that this was her attempt to deal with her feelings about the cancer, it was a tremendously sore spot in the marriage during this time. He could hardly stand all of the feelings of rejection, fear of loss, and resentment about being compelled to help her feel better. In addition, there seemed to be little he could really do to change things. But his ability to separate out the old template of his depressed mother from the current reality helped him ground himself.

The termination of this second round of treatment was different. This time, he did not disappear. He began to feel better and clearly was handling a tough situation better. He realized that his wife needed psychological help and needed treatment. He was able to step back and give her some space, and at the same time that he continued to appropriately express concern about her emotional state and her drinking. He asked to stop but left open the possibility of coming back. He planned a few final sessions, and left with a sense of clarity about what was ahead of him.

This vignette illustrates an intermittent course of treatment that is consistent with the primary care model. This was not the intended treatment, but it became the model de facto. The therapist did not push Nicholas to consider all of the transference implications of his decisions. While it is likely that there were conflictual roots to this decision— avoidance of the loss of the treatment, controlling the relationship with the therapist, avoidance of feelings of dependency—this was mentioned with the patient but not with a recommendation to stay in treatment and work on this until there was finality.

Despite the fact that in the primary care model there is no definitive termination, ending is a moment to tie up loose ends and help the patient summarize the work done together. The narrative is as full as it will be, and the therapist can reflect it back to the patient. A summary will pull both therapist and patient out of the emotion of ending, and so it should not be done at the same moment as when the patient is talking about sad feelings. But it will likely help to consolidate the benefits of the work.

The ending of treatment for Peter, the young man with depression discussed in Chapters 5 and 7, proceeded according to the traditional psychodynamic psychotherapy model. The goal was to definitively deal with his problems, so that he could try to manage psychological issues independently. The termination was planned several months in advance after an extended period of wellness. The feelings and conflicts around intimacy, loss, and self-esteem were well worked out, and the transference had long been a focus. With the end of the therapy looming, Peter felt a strong sense of loss, but he was pleased with his level of self-reflectiveness and self-sufficiency. Some of the old feelings of self-criticism, anger, guilt, and low self-esteem did crop up toward the end of the appointments, but they were understandable and interpreted as transferential reactions to the loss of the therapist. Because Peter had found his new career interest, and he considered it to be similar in seriousness and status to the therapist's, he seemed to be managing the loss through a healthy identification. After the end of the treatment, Peter communicated every couple of years with his therapist, reporting on his progress and successes and frustrations.

This type of ending feels more rigorous and difficult for both patient and therapist. The worry about the patient's ability to do it all without help is paramount in both people's minds. But a great degree of respect of the patient's strength and resilience is implied in trying to end the relationship in a definitive way.

Although a full discussion of the medical–legal issues surrounding psychotherapy, including informed consent, ethical requirements regarding boundaries, collaboration, coverage, and privacy, is beyond the scope of this book, it is important to recognize that the end of treatment requires particular attention to these issues (see, e.g., Barnett, 1998). The problem of abandonment, in the legal not the emotional sense, is an area of vulnerability for therapists. Clinicians have a responsibility to treat those in their care, and they cannot dismiss patients from their practices willy-nilly. Terminations must be well documented, and patients who drop out of treatment without discussion need to be contacted, and alternatives to returning to you should be reviewed and then spelled out in a letter.

TERMINATION FOR TRAINEES

Ending therapy is often a particularly emotional experience for trainees. They have never done it before, and it is often forced by circumstances. A common problem is that patients in training clinics are passed on from trainee to trainee as people graduate or change location. This puts young therapists in the difficult position of beginning treatment with patients who were treated by older trainees whom the new therapist may know and have great respect for. Also, this system confronts a new therapist with a patient who is sometimes more experienced than they are. This is certainly a stressful undertaking, and understanding what is going on and doing the best job possible is the best antidote to these anxieties.

A forced termination, where the therapist leaves, is particularly likely to stir up feelings of loss and rejection in the patient and guilt in the therapist. When this has happened before to the patient (some patients work with several trainees over the course of their treatment), it is harder to elicit a fresh reaction to what is going on. The patient becomes a "professional" in dealing with transfers, and the issues are harder to discuss. This in turn makes it harder for the therapist to learn about the situation and to focus on the patient's feelings and needs. When the patient becomes inured to the loss of multiple therapists but remains connected to the clinic, the concept of "institutional transference" is invoked. This is the notion that the patient forms an attachment to something larger than the individuals, to the organization itself. More likely, this "institutional transference" reflects a quasi-adaptive detachment from the losses and disappointments about multiple individuals.

Training clinics tend to promote the traditional psychodynamic model of termination because they want to teach the time-honored concept—this is seen as the "real thing." That is well and good, but the actual practice is likely closer to the primary care model. This disparity between ideals and practice can make therapists-in-training feel they are not living up to the expectations of their supervisors and mentors.

However, a wonderful benefit of being in a training clinic is that you are made to think about termination. We are all somewhat avoidant of the pain of loss, and when the treatment is going to be over soon there is a tendency to move one's attention on to something else. In clinical practice there is very little stimulus to think about termination except when the patient is upset. So the training clinic facilitates learning about termination, but the excessive application of the traditional psychodynamic model for patients makes for confusion at times.

Bostic, Shadid, and Blotchy (1996) make excellent practical sugges-tions about forced terminations in training, including giving patients 3 to 6 months' notice, not divulging the specifics of the reasons for the ter-mination too quickly in order to facilitate discussion, active collabora-tion about plans for transfer, support and encouragement for the patient, erring on the side of accepting gifts that are offered, and frequent discus-sion in supervision about termination.

SUMMARY

Termination provides the patient and the therapist with closure on an important experience. We know more about beginning treatments than ending them, and the two main ways of conceptualizing termination, the traditional psychodynamic model and the primary care model, both offer meaningful approaches to a successful ending. Opening up the decision to end, and exploration of the feelings involved, allows for a last piece of work on the therapeutic relationship, sorting out the trans-ferential and alliance components, and lets the patient include this in the final psychotherapy narrative. Personal emotional reactions are frequent during the end of treatment, and therapists, like patients, need to reflect on the ending of the relationship.

References

Abraham, K. (1923). Contributions to the theory of the anal character. *International Journal of Psychoanalysis, 4*, 400–418.

Akiskal, H. S. (2001). Dysthymia and cyclothymia in psychiatric practice a century after Kraepelin. *Journal of Affective Disorders, 62*, 17–31.

Akkerman, K., Lewin, T. J., & Carr, V. J. (1999). Long-term changes in defense style among patients recovering from major depression. *Journal of Nervous and Mental Disease, 187*(2), 80–87.

Alexander, F., & French, T. M. (1946). *Psychoanalytic therapy.* New York: Ronald Press.

Alon, N., & Omer H. (2004). Demonic and tragic narratives in psychotherapy. In A. Lieblich, D. P. McAdams, & R. Josselson (Eds.), *Healing plots: The narrative basis of psychotherapy* (pp. 29–48). Washington, DC: APA Books.

American Psychiatric Association. (2000). *Diagnostic and statistical manual of mental disorders* (4th ed., text rev.). Washington, DC: Author.

Anderson, E. M., & Lambert, M. J. (1995). Short-term dynamically oriented psychotherapies: A review and meta-analysis. *Clinical Psychology Review, 15*, 503–514.

Andrews, G., Stewart, C., Morris-Yates, A., Holt, P. & Henderson, S. (1990). Evidence for a general neurotic syndrome. *British Journal of Psychiatry, 157*, 6–12.

APA Presidential Task Force on Evidence-Based Practice. (2006). Evidence-based practice in psychology. *American Psychologist, 61*, 271–285.

Badgio, P. C., Halperin, G., & Barber, J. P. (1999). Acquisition of adaptive skills: Psychotherapeutic change in cognitive and dynamic therapies. *Clinical Psychology Review, 19*, 721–737.

Baker, H. S., & Baker, M. N. (1987). Heinz Kohut's self psychology: An overview. *American Journal of Psychiatry, 144*, 1–9.

Barber, J. P. (2009). Towards a working through of some core conflicts in psy-
    chotherapy research. *Psychotherapy Research, 19*, 1–12.

Barber, J. P., Connolly, M. B., Crits-Christoph, P., Gladis, M., & Siqueland, L.
    (2000). Alliance predicts patients' outcome beyond in-treatment change
    in symptoms. *Journal of Consulting and Clinical Psychology, 68*, 1027–
    1032.

Barber, J. P., & Crits-Christoph, P. (Eds.). (1995). *Dynamic therapies for psy-
    chiatric disorders (Axis I)*. New York: Basic Books.

Barber, J. P., Crits-Christoph, P., & Luborsky, L. (1996). Effects of therapist
    adherence and competence on patient outcome in brief dynamic therapy.
    Journal of Consulting and Clinical Psychology, 64(3), 619–622.

Barber, J. P., & DeRubeis, R. (1989). On second thought: Where the action is
    in cognitive therapy for depression. *Cognitive Therapy and Research, 13*,
    441–457.

Barber, J. P., & DeRubeis, R. J. (2001). Change in compensatory skills in cog-
    nitive therapy for depression. *Journal of Psychotherapy, Practice, and
    Research, 10*, 8–13.

Barber, J. P., & Ellman, J. (1996). Advances in short-term dynamic psycho-
    therapy. *Current Opinion in Psychiatry, 9*(3), 188–192.

Barber, J. P., Gallop, R., Crits-Christoph, P., Barrettt, M. S., Klostermann, S.,
    McCarthy, K. S., et al. (2008). The role of the alliance and techniques in
    predicting outcome of supportive–expressive dynamic therapy for cocaine
    dependence. *Psychoanalytic Psychology, 25*, 461–482.

Barber, J. P., Gallop, R., Crits-Christoph, P., Frank, A., Thase, M. E., Weiss, R.
    D., et al. (2006). The role of therapist adherence, therapist competence, and
    the alliance in predicting outcome of individual drug counseling: Results
    from the NIDA Collaborative Cocaine Treatment Study. *Psychotherapy
    Research, 16*, 229–240.

Barber, J. P., Khalsa, S-R., & Sharpless, B. A. (in press). The validity of the
    alliance as a predictor of psychotherapy outcome. In J. C. Muran & J. P.
    Barber (Eds.), *The therapeutic alliance: An evidence-based approach to
    practice and training*. New York: Guilford Press.

Barber, J. P., Morse, J. Q., Krakauer, I., Chittams, J., & Crits-Christoph, K.
    (1997). Change in obsessive–compulsive and avoidant personality disor-
    ders following time-limited supportive-expressive therapy. *Psychotherapy,
    34*, 133–143.

Barber, J. P., & Muentz, L. R. (1996). The role of avoidance and obsessiveness in
    matching patients to cognitive and interpersonal psychotherapy: Empirical
    findings from the Treatment for Depression Collaborative Research Pro-
    gram. *Journal of Consulting and Clinical Psychology, 64*(5), 951–958.

Barber, J. P., Sharpless, B. A., Klostermann, S., & McCarthy, K. S. (2007).
    Assessing intervention competence and its relation to therapy outcome: A
    selected review derived from the outcome literature. *Professional Psychol-
    ogy: Research and Practice, 38*(5), 493–500.

Barlow, D. H., Gorman, J. M., Shear, M. K., & Woods, S. W. (2000). Cognitive-behavioral therapy, imipramine, or their combination for panic disorder: A randomized controlled trial. *Journal of the American Medical Association 283,* 2529–2536.

Barnett, J. E. (1998). Termination without trepidation. *Psychotherapy Bulletin, 33*(2), 20–22.

Baron-Cohen, S. (1997). *Mindblindness: An essay on autism and theory of mind.* Cambridge, MA: MIT Press.

Barrett, M. S., & Berman, J. (2001). Is psychotherapy more effective when therapists disclose information about themselves? *Journal of Consulting and Clinical Psychology, 69,* 597–603.

Bartlett, F. C. (1932). *Remembering: A study in experimental and social psychology.* Cambridge, UK: Cambridge University Press.

Basoglu, M., Marks, I. M., Kilic, C., Brewin, C. R., & Swinson, R. P. (1994). Alprazolam and exposure for panic disorder with agoraphobia: Attribution of improvement to medication predicts subsequent relapse. *Canadian Journal of Psychiatry, 164,* 652–659.

Bateman, A., & Fonagy, P. (2008). 8-year follow-up of patients treated for borderline personality disorder: Mentalization-based treatment versus treatment as usual. *American Journal of Psychiatry, 165,* 631–638.

Beahrs, J. O., & Gutheil, T. G. (2001). Informed consent in psychotherapy. *American Journal of Psychiatry, 158*(1), 4–10.

Beck, A. T. (1976). *Cognitive therapy and the emotional disorders.* New York: International Universities Press.

Beck, A. T., Freeman, A., Davis, D., & Associates (2004). *Cognitive therapy of personality disorders* (2nd ed.). New York: Guilford Press.

Beck, A. T., Rush, A. J., Shaw, B. I., & Emery, G. (1979). *Cognitive therapy of depression.* New York: Guilford Press.

Beck, J. S. (2005). *Cognitive therapy for challenging problems: What to do when the basics don't work.* New York: Guilford Press.

Bein, E., Anderson, T., Strupp, H. H., Henry, W., Schacht, T. E., Binder, J. L., et al. (2000). The effects of training in time-limited dynamic psychotherapy: Changes in therapeutic outcome. *Psychotherapy Research, 10*(2), 119–132.

Beutel, M. E., Stern, E., & Silbersweig, D. (2003). The emerging dialogue between psychoanalysis and neuroscience: Neuroimaging perspectives. *Journal of the American Psychoanalytic Association, 51*(3), 773–801.

Beutler, L. E., Malik, M., Alimohamed, S., Harwood, T. M., Talebi, H., Noble, S., et al. (2003). Therapist variables. In M. Lambert (Ed.), *Bergin and Garfield's handbook of psychotherapy and behavior change* (pp. 227–306). New York: Wiley.

Bibring, E. (1953). The mechanics of depression. In P. Greenacre (Ed.), *Affective disorders: Psychoanalytic contributions to their study* (pp. 13–48). New York: International Universities Press.

Biederman, J., Hirshfeld-Becker, D. R., & Rosenbaum, J. F. (2001). Further evidence of association between behavioral inhibition and social anxiety in children. *American Journal of Psychiatry, 158*(10), 1673–1679.

Biederman, J., Rosenbaum, J. F., Bolduc-Murphy, E. A., Faraone, S. V., Chaloff, J., Hirshfeld D. R., et al. (1993). A 3-year follow-up of children with and without behavioral inhibition. *Journal of the American Academy of Child and Adolescent Psychiatry, 32*(4), 814–821.

Blatt, S. J., Sanislow, C. A., Zuroff, D. C., & Pilkonis, P. A. (1996). Characteristics of effective therapists: Further analyses of data from the National Institute of Mental Health Treatment of Depression Collaborative Research Program. *Journal of Consulting and Clinical Psychology, 64,* 1276–1284.

Blomberg, J., Lazar, A., & Sandell, R. (2001). Outcome of patients in long-term psychoanalytical treatments. First findings of the Stockholm Outcome of Psychotherapy and Psychoanalysis (STOPP) study. *Psychotherapy Research, 11,* 361–382.

Book, H. E. (1998). *How to practice brief dynamic psychotherapy: The CCRT method.* Washington, DC: American Psychological Association.

Bordin, E. S. (1979). The generalizability of the psychoanalytic concept of the working alliance. *Psychotherapy: Theory, Research, and Practice, 16*(3), 252–260.

Borkovec, T. D., & Sharpless, B. (2004). Generalized anxiety disorder: Bringing cognitive behavior therapy into the valued present. In S. Hayes, V. Follette, & M. Linehan (Eds.) *Mindfulness and acceptance: Expanding the cognitive-behavioral tradition.* New York: Guilford Press.

Bostic, J. Q., Shadid, L. G., & Blotchy, M. J. (1996). Our time is up: Forced terminations during psychotherapy training. *American Journal of Psychotherapy, 50,* 347–359.

Bowlby, F. (1958). The nature of the child's tie to his mother. *International Journal of Psychoanalysis, 39,* 350–373.

Bowlby, J. (1988). *A secure base.* New York: Basic Books.

Brenner, C. (1974). *An elementary textbook of psychoanalysis.* New York: Anchor.

Brom, D., Kleber, R. J., & Defares, P. B. (1989). Brief psychotherapy for post-traumatic stress disorders. *Journal of Consulting and Clinical Psychology, 57,* 607–612.

Brown, T. E. (2000). *Attention-deficit disorders and comorbidities in children, adolescents, and adults.* Washington, DC: American Psychiatric Press.

Busch, F. N., Ruden, M., & Shapiro, T. (2004). *Psychodynamic treatment of depression.* Washington, DC: American Psychiatric Press.

Carey, B. (2008, September 30). Psychoanalytic therapy wins backing. *New York Times,* p. A18.

Casement, P. (2002). *Learning from our mistakes: Beyond dogma in psychoanalysis and psychotherapy.* New York: Guilford Press.

Castonguay, L. G., & Hill, C. E. (Eds). (2007). *Insight in psychotherapy*. Washington, DC: APA Press.

Charney, D. (2004). Psychobiological mechanisms of resilience and vulnerability: Implications for successful adaptation to extreme stress. *American Journal of Psychiatry, 161*(2), 205.

Charon, R. (2006). *Narrative medicine: Honoring the stories of illness*. New York: Oxford University Press.

Chess, S., & Thomas, A. (1996). *Temperament: Theory and practice*. New York: Brunner/Mazel.

Clarkin, J. F., Yeomans, F. E., & Kernberg O. F. (1999). *Psychotherapy for borderline personality*. New York: Wiley.

Coleman, D. (2005). Psychodynamic and cognitive mechanisms of change in adult therapy: A pilot study. *Bulletin of the Menninger Clinic, 69*(3), 206–219.

Connolly-Gibbons, M. B., Crits-Christoph, P., de la Cruz, C., Barber, J. P., Siqueland, L., & Gladis, M. (2003). Pretreatment expectations, interpersonal functioning, and symptoms in the prediction of the therapeutic alliance across supportive–expressive psychotherapy and cognitive therapy. *Psychotherapy Research, 13*, 59–76.

Cooper, A. M. (1989). Concepts of therapeutic effectiveness in psychoanalysis: A historical review. *Psychoanalytic Inquiry, 9*, 4–25.

Coyne, J. C. (1976). Toward an interactional description of depression. *Psychiatry, 39*, 28–40.

Crits-Christoph, P. (1992). The efficacy of brief dynamic psychotherapy: A meta-analysis. *American Journal of Psychiatry, 149*, 151–158.

Crits-Christoph, P., & Barber, J. P. (2007). Psychological treatments for personality disorders. In P. E. Nathan & J. M. Gorman (Eds.), *A guide to treatments that works* (3rd ed., pp. 641–658). New York: Oxford University Press.

Crits-Christoph, P., Barber, J. P., & Kurcias, J. S. (1991). Historical background of short-term dynamic therapy. In P. Crits-Christoph & J. P. Barber (Eds.), *Handbook of short-term dynamic psychotherapy* (pp. 1–16). New York: Basic Books.

Crits-Christoph, P., Barber, J. P., & Kurcias, J. S. (1993). The accuracy of therapists' interpretations and the development of the therapeutic alliance. *Psychotherapy Research, 3*, 25–35.

Crits-Christoph, P., Connolly Gibbons, M. B., Crits-Christoph, K., Narducci, J., Schamberger, M., & Gallop, R. (2006). Can therapists be trained to improve their alliances? A preliminary study of alliance-fostering psychotherapy. *Psychotherapy Research, 16*, 268–281.

Crits-Christoph, P., Connolly Gibbons, M. B., Narducci, J., Schamberger, M., & Gallop, R. (2005). Interpersonal problems and the outcome of interpersonal–psychodynamic treatment of generalized anxiety disorder. *Psychotherapy: Theory, Research, Practice, Training, 42*, 211–224.

Crits-Christoph, P., Cooper, A., & Luborsky, L. (1988). The accuracy of therapists' interpretations and the outcome of dynamic psychotherapy. *Journal of Consulting and Clinical Psychology, 56*, 490–495.

Csikszentmihalyi, M. (1991). *Flow.* New York: Harper.

Damasio A. (2000). *The feeling of what happens: Body and emotion in the making of consciousness.* New York: Harcourt.

Davanloo, H. (Ed.). (1980). *Short-term dynamic psychotherapy.* New York: Aronson.

Davenport, B. R., & Ratliff, D. (2001). Alliance ratings as a part of trainee evaluations within family therapy training. *Contemporary Family Therapy, 23*(4), 441–454.

Dunkle, J. H., & Friedlander, M. L. (1996). Contribution of therapist experience and personal characteristics to the working alliance. *Journal of Counseling Psychology, 43*, 456–460.

Eagle, M. N. (1984). *Recent developments in psychoanalysis.* New York: McGraw-Hill.

Eells, T. T. (Ed.) . (2006). *Handbook of psychotherapy case formulation* (2nd ed.). New York: Guilford Press.

Ehrlich, F. M. (1998, December). Psychoanalysis and couple therapy. *Psychiatric Times, XV*(12).

Elliot, R. (2001). Contemporary brief experiential therapy. *Clinical Psychology: Science and Practice, 8*, 38–50.

Erikson, E. (1964). *Childhood and society.* New York: Norton.

Erickson, M., & Rossi, E., (1981). *Experiencing hypnosis: Therapeutic approaches to altered state.* New York: Irvington.

Etkin, A., Pittenger, C., Polan, H. J., & Kandel, E. R. (2005). Toward a neurobiology of psychotherapy: Basic science and clinical applications. *Journal of Neuropsychiatry and Clinical Neuroscience, 17*(2), 145–158.

Evans, L. A., Acosta, F. X., Yamamoto, J., & Skilbeck, W. M. (1984). Orienting psychotherapists to better serve low-income and minority patients. *Journal of Clinical Psychology, 40*, 90–96.

Feeley, M., DeRubeis, R. J., & Gelfand, L. A. (1999). The temporal relation of adherence and alliance to symptom change in cognitive therapy for depression. *Journal of Consulting and Clinical Psychology, 67*(4), 578–582.

Ferenczi, S. (1926). The further development of an active therapy in psychoanalysis. In E. Jones (Ed.) & J. I. Suttie (Trans.), *Further contributions to the theory and technique of psychoanalysis* (pp. 198–217). London: Hogarth Press, 1950.

Foa, E. B., Franklin, M. E., & Moser, J. (2002). Context in the clinic: How well do cognitive-behavioral therapies and medications work in combination? *Biological Psychiatry, 52*, 987–997.

Foa, E. B., & Rothbaum, B. O. (1998). *Treating the trauma of rape: Cognitive-behavioral therapy for PTSD.* New York: Guilford Press.

Foa, E. B., Hembree, E. A., & Rothbaum, B. O. (2007). *Prolonged exposure for PTSD: Emotional processing of traumatic experiences, A therapist's guide.* New York: Oxford University Press.

Frank, J. D., & Frank, J. B. (1991). *Persuasion and healing.* Baltimore: Johns Hopkins University Press.

Frankl, V. E. (1946). *Man's search for meaning.* London: Hodder and Stoughton, 1964.

Fredrickson, B. L. (2001). The role of positive emotions in positive psychology. *American Psychologist, 56*(3), 218–226.

Freud, A. (1936). *The ego and the mechanisms of defense: The collected works of Anna Freud, Vol. 2.* New York: International Universities Press.

Freud, A. (1966). Obsessional neurosis: A summary of psycho-analytic views as presented at the congress. *International Journal of Psycho-Analysis, 47,* 116–122.

Freud, S. (1895). Studies in hysteria. In J. Strachey (Ed. and Trans.), *The standard edition of the complete psychological works of Sigmund Freud* (Vol. 2, pp. 1–323). London: Hogarth Press, 1955.

Freud, S. (1905). Fragment of an analysis of a case of hysteria. In J. Strachey (Ed. and Trans.), *The standard edition of the complete psychological works of Sigmund Freud* (Vol. 7, pp. 1–22). London: Hogarth Press, 1953.

Freud, S. (1908). Character and anal erotism. In J. Strachey (Ed. and Trans.), *The standard edition of the complete psychological works of Sigmund Freud* (Vol. 9, pp. 167–175). London: Hogarth Press, 1959.

Freud, S. (1912a). The dynamics of transference. In J. Strachey (Ed. and Trans.), *The standard edition of the complete psychological works of Sigmund Freud* (Vol. 12, pp. 97–108). London: Hogarth Press, 1958.

Freud, S. (1912b). Recommendations to physicians practicing psycho-analysis. In J. Strachey (Ed. and Trans.), *The standard edition of the complete psychological works of Sigmund Freud* (Vol. 12, pp. 109–120). London: Hogarth Press, 1958.

Freud, S. (1914). On narcissism. In J. Strachey (Ed. and Trans.), *The standard edition of the complete psychological works of Sigmund Freud* (Vol. 14, pp. 67–102). London: Hogarth Press, 1963.

Freud, S. (1916). Introductory lectures on psycho-analysis: Parts I, II. In J. Strachey (Ed. and Trans.), *The standard edition of the complete psychological works of Sigmund Freud* (Vol. 15, pp. 9–239). London: Hogarth Press, 1961.

Freud, S. (1917a). Introductory lectures on psycho-analysis: Part III. In J. Strachey (Ed. and Trans.) *The standard edition of the complete psychological works of Sigmund Freud* (Vol. 16, pp. 243–463). London: Hogarth Press, 1953.

Freud, S. (1917b). Mourning and melancholia. In J. Strachey (Ed. and Trans.), *The standard edition of the complete psychological works of Sigmund Freud* (Vol. 14, pp. 237–258). London: Hogarth Press, 1963.

Freud, S. (1918). From the history of an infantile neurosis. In J. Strachey (Ed.

and Trans.), *The standard edition of the complete psychological works of Sigmund Freud* (Vol. 17, pp. 7–122). London: Hogarth Press, 1955.

Freud, S. (1926). Inhibitions, symptoms and anxiety. In J. Strachey (Ed. and Trans.), *The standard edition of the complete psychological works of Sigmund Freud* (Vol. 20, pp. 77–178). London: Hogarth Press, 1959.

Freud, S. (1937). Analysis, terminable and interminable. In J. Strachey (Ed. and Trans.), *The standard edition of the complete psychological works of Sigmund Freud* (Vol. 23, pp. 216–253). London: Hogarth Press, 1964.

Gabbard, G. O. (2000). *Psychodynamic psychiatry in clinical practice* (3rd ed.). Washington, DC: American Psychiatric Association.

Gabbard, G. O. (2005). *Psychodynamic psychiatry in clinical practice* (4th ed.). Washington, DC: American Psychiatric Publishing.

Gabbard, G. O., Horwitz, L, Allen, J. G., Frieswyk, S., Newsom, G., Colson, D. B., et al. (1994). Transference interpretation in the psychotherapy of borderline patients: A high-risk, high-gain phenomenon. *Harvard Review of Psychiatry, 2,* 59–69.

Gabbard, G. O., & Kay, J. (2001). The fate of integrated treatment: Whatever happened to the biopsychosocial psychiatrist? *American Journal of Psychiatry, 158,* 1956–1963.

Gabbard, G. O., & Westen, D. (2003). Rethinking therapeutic action. *International Journal of Psychoanalysis, 84,* 823–841.

Gallagher, D. E., & Thompson, L. W. (1982). Treatment of major depressive disorder in older adult outpatients with brief psychotherapies. *Psychotherapy: Theory, Research, and Practice, 19,* 482–490.

Gardner, H. (1993). *Frames of mind: The theory of multiple intelligences.* New York: Basic Books.

Geller, J. D., & Farber, B. A. (1993). Factors influencing the process of internalization in psychotherapy. *Psychotherapy Research, 3*(3), 166–180.

Glick, R. A. (1987). Forced terminations. *Journal of the American Academy of Psychoanalysis, 15,* 449–463.

Goldapple, K., Segal, Z., Garson, C., Lau, M., Bieling, P., Kennedy, S., et al. (2004). Modulation of cortical-limbic pathways in major depression. *Archives of General Psychiatry, 61,* 34–41.

Goleman, D. (2006). *Emotional intelligence: 10th anniversary edition: Why it can matter more than IQ.* New York: Bantam.

Grace, M., Kivlighan, D. M., Jr., & Kunce, J. (1995). The effect of nonverbal skills training on counselor trainee nonverbal sensitivity and responsiveness and on session impact and working alliance ratings. *Journal of Counseling and Development, 73,* 547–552.

Greenberg, J., & Mitchell, S. (1983). *Object relations in psychoanalytic theory.* Cambridge, MA: Harvard University Press.

Greenberg, L. S. (2002). *Emotion-focused therapy: Coaching clients to work through feelings.* Washington, DC: American Psychological Association Press.

Greenberg, L. S., & Watson, J. (2005). *Emotion-focused therapy for depression*. Washington, DC: American Psychological Association

Greenberg, R. P., Constantino, M. J., & Bruce, N. (2006). Are expectations still relevant for psychotherapy process and outcome? *Clinical Psychology Review, 26*, 657–678.

Greenson, R. R. (1967). *The technique and practice of psychoanalysis*. New York: International Universities Press.

Gunderson, J. G. (2000). Psychodynamic psychotherapy for borderline personality disorder. In J. G. Gunderson & G. O. Gabbard (Eds.), *Psychotherapy for personality disorders* (pp. 33–64). Washington, DC: American Psychiatric Press.

Gunderson, J. G., & Gabbard, G. O. (1999). Making the case for psychoanalytic therapies in the current psychiatric environment. *Journal of the American Psychoanalytic Association, 47*, 679–704.

Habl, S., Mintz, D. Bailey, A. (2009). *The role of personal psychotherapy in psychiatry residency training: A survey of psychiatry training directors*. Manuscript accepted for publication.

Harrington, A. (Ed.). (1997). *The placebo effect: An interdisciplinary exploration*. Cambridge, MA: Harvard University Press.

Herman, J. L. (1997). *Trauma and healing*. New York: Basic Books.

Hersen, M., Bellack, A. S., Himmelhoch, J. M., & Thase, M. E. (1984). Effects of social skills training, amitriptyline, and psychotherapy in unipolar depressed women. *Behavior Therapy, 15*, 21–40.

Hersoug, A. G., Sexton, H. C., Høglend, P. (2002). Contribution of defensive functioning to the quality of working alliance and psychotherapy outcome. *American Journal of Psychotherapy, 56*(4), 539–554.

Hersoug, A. G., Bøgwald, K. P., Høglend, P. (2005). Changes of defensive functioning. Does interpretation contribute to change? *Clinical Psychology and Psychotherapy, 12*, 288–296.

Høglend P., Amlo, S., Marble, A., Bøgwald, K. P., Sorbye, O., Sjasstad, M. C., et al. (2006). Analysis of the patient–therapist relationship in dynamic psychotherapy: An experimental study of transference interpretations. *American Journal of Psychiatry, 163*, 1739–1746.

Høglend, P., Bøgwald, K. P., Amlo, S., Marble, A., Ulberg, R., Sjaastad, M. C., et al. (2008). Transference interpretations in dynamic psychotherapy: Do they really yield sustained effects? *American Journal of Psychiatry, 165*, 763–771.

Horowitz, M. J. (1976). *Stress response syndromes*. Northvale, NJ: Aronson.

Horowitz, M. J., Marmar, C., Krupnick, J., Kaltreider, N., Wallerstein, R., & Wilner, N. (1984). *Personality styles and brief psychotherapy*. New York: Basic Books.

Horvath, A. O., & Symonds, B. D. (1991). Relation between working alliance and outcome in psychotherapy: A meta-analysis. *Journal of Counseling Psychology, 38*, 139–149.

Hupert, J. D., Bufka, L. F., Barlow, D. H., Gorman, J. M., Shear, M. K., & Woods, S. W. (2001). Therapists, therapist variables, and CBT outcome for panic disorder: Results from a multicenter trial. *Journal of Consulting and Clinical Psychology, 69,* 747–755.

Josephson, A., & Serrano, A. (2001). The integration of individual therapy and family therapy in the treatment of child and adolescent psychiatric disorders. *Child and Adolescent Psychiatric Clinics of North America, 10,* 431–450.

Josselson, R. (2004). On becoming the narrator of one's own life. In A. Lieblich, D. P. McAdams, & R. Josselson (Eds.), *Healing plots: The narrative basis of psychotherapy* (pp. 111–129). Washington, DC: APA Books.

Joyce, A. S., Piper, W. E., Ogrodniczuk, J. S., & Klein, R. H. (2007). *Termination in psychotherapy: A psychodynamic model of processes and outcomes.* Washington, DC: American Psychological Association.

Kandel, E. (1999). Biology and the future of psychoanalysis. *American Journal of Psychiatry, 156,* 505–524.

Keller, M. B., McCullough, J. P., Jr., Klein, D. N., Arnow, B. A., Dunner, D. L., Gelenberg, A. J., et al. (2000). A comparison of nefazodone, the cognitive behavioral analysis system of psychotherapy, and their combination for the treatment of chronic depression. *New England Journal of Medicine, 342,* 1462–1470.

Kendall, P. C., & Chu, B. C. (2000). Retrospective self-reports of therapist flexibility in a manual-based treatment for youths with anxiety disorders. *Journal of Clinical Child Psychology, 29,* 209–220.

Kendler K. S. (2005). Toward a philosophical structure for psychiatry. *American Journal of Psychiatry, 162*(3), 433–440.

Kernberg, O. F. (1975). *Borderline conditions and pathological narcissism.* New York: Aronson.

Kernberg, O. F. (1988). Object relations theory in clinical practice. *Psychoanalytic Quarterly, 57,* 481–504.

Kernberg, O. F. (1993). *Severe personality disorders: Psychotherapeutic strategies.* New Haven: Yale University Press.

Kernberg, O. F. (1999). Psychoanalysis, psychoanalytic psychotherapy, and supportive psychotherapy: Contemporary controversies. *International Journal of Psychoanalysis, 80,* 1075–1091.

Kernberg, O. F., Selzer, M. A., Koenigsberg, H. W., Carr, A. C., & Appelbaum, A. H. (1989). *Psychodynamic psychotherapy of borderline patients.* New York: Basic Books.

Klerman, G. L., Weissman, M. M., Rounsaville, B. J., & Chevron, E. S. (1984). *Interpersonal psychotherapy of depression.* New York: Basic Books.

Kohut, H. (1971). *The analysis of the self: A systematic approach to the psychoanalytic treatment of narcissistic personality disorders.* New York: International Universities Press.

Kohut, H. (1977). *The restoration of the self.* New York: International Universities Press.

Kohut, H. (1984). *How does analysis cure?* New York: International Universities Press.

Konner, M. (2007). Trauma, adaptation, and resilience: A cross-cultural and evolutionary perspective. In L. J. Kirmayer, R. Lemelson, & R. Barad (Eds.), *Understanding trauma: Integrating biological, clinical, and cultural perspectives* (pp. 295–299). New York: Cambridge University Press.

Kurcias, J. (2000, June). *Therapy trainees and developmental changes in the alliance.* Dissertation Abstracts International: Section B: the Sciences & Engineering; 60(11-B), Jun 2000, 5779, US: Univ. Microfilms International.

Lazarus, R. S., & Folkman, S. (1984). *Stress, appraisal, and coping.* New York: Springer.

LeDoux, J. E. (1996). *The emotional brain.* New York: Simon & Schuster.

Leichsenring, F. (2001). Comparative effects of short-term psychodynamic psychotherapy and cognitive-behavioral therapy in depression: A meta-analytic approach. *Clinical Psychological Review, 21,* 401–419.

Leichsenring, F., & Rabung, S. (2008). Effectiveness of long-term psychodynamic psychotherapy: A meta-analysis. *Journal of the American Medicial Association, 300,* 1551–1565.

Leichsenring, F., Rabung, S., & Leibing, E. (2004). The efficacy of short-term psychodynamic psychotherapy in specific psychiatric disorders: A meta-analysis. *Archives of General Psychiatry, 61*(12), 1208–1216.

Levy, K. N., Meehan, K. B., Kelly, K. M., Reynoso, J. S., Weber, M., Clarkin, J. F., et al. (2006). Change in attachment patterns and reflective function in a randomized control trial of transference-focused psychotherapy for borderline personality disorder. *Journal of Consulting and Clinical Psychology, 74,* 1027–1040.

Lieblich, A., McAdams, D. P., & Josselson, R. (Eds.). (2004). *Healing plots: The narrative basis of psychotherapy.* Washington, DC: American Psychological Association.

Lilliengren, P., & Werbart, A. (2005). A model of therapeutic action grounded in the patients' view of curative and hindering factors in psychoanalytic psychotherapy. *Psychotherapy: Theory, Research, Practice, Training, 42*(3), 324–339.

Linehan, M. (1993) *Cognitive-behavioral treatment of borderline personality disorder.* New York: Guilford Press.

Loewald, H. W. (1960). On the therapeutic action of psycho-analysis. *International Journal of Psychoanalysis, 41,* 16–33.

Luborsky, L. (1977). Measuring a pervasive psychic structure in psychotherapy: The Core Conflictual Relationship Theme. In N. Freedman & S. Grand (Eds.), *Communicative structures and psychic structures* (pp. 367–395). New York: Plenum Press.

Luborsky, L. (1984). *Principles of psychoanalytic psychotherapy: A manual for supportive–expressive (SE) treatment.* New York: Basic Books.

Luborsky, L., & Crits-Christoph P. (Eds.). (1990). *Understanding transference: The CCRT method.* New York: Basic Books.

Luborsky, L., & Crits-Christoph, P. (Eds.). (1998). *Understanding transference: The Core Conflictual Relationship Theme method* (2nd ed.). Washington, DC: American Psychological Association.

Luhrmann, T. M. (2000). *Of two minds: The growing disorder in American psychiatry*. New York: Knopf.

MacKinnon, R. A., & Michels, R. (1971). *The psychiatric interview in clinical practice*. Philadelphia: Saunders.

MacKinnon, R. A., & Yudofsky, S. (1991). *Principles of psychiatric evaluation*. New York: Lippincott, Williams and Wilkins.

Mahler, M. (1972). On the first three subphases of the separation-individuation process. *International Journal of Psychoanalysis, 53,* 333–338.

Maina, G., Ross, G., Bogetto, F. (2009). Brief dynamic therapy combined with pharmacotherapy in the treatment of major depressive disorder: Long-term results. *Journal of Affective Disorders, 114,* 200–207.

Malan, D. H. (1976a). *The frontier of brief psychotherapy*. New York: Plenum Press.

Malan, D. H. (1976b). *Toward the validation of dynamic psychotherapy: A replication*. New York: Plenum Press.

Malan, D. H. (1979). *Individual psychotherapy and the science of psychodynamics*. Woburn, MA: Butterworth.

Mallinckrodt, B., & Nelson, M. L. (1991). Counselor training level and the formation of the psychotherapeutic working alliance. *Journal of Counseling Psychology, 38*(2), 133–138.

Maltsberger J. T., & Buie, D. H. (1974). Countertransference hate in the treatment of suicidal patients. *Archives of General Psychiatry, 30,* 625–633.

Mann, J. (1973). *Time-limited psychotherapy*. Cambridge, MA: Harvard University Press.

Martin, D. J., Garske, J. P., & Davis, M. K. (2000). Relation of the therapeutic alliance with outcome and other variables: A meta-analytic review. *Journal of Consulting and Clinical Psychology, 68,* 438–450.

May, R. (1969a). *Existential psychology*. New York: Random House.

May, R. (1969b). *Love and will*. New York: Delta.

Mayberg, H. S., Silva, J. A., Brannan, S. K., Tekell, J. L., Mahurin, R. K., McGinnis, S., et al. (2002). The functional neuroanatomy of the placebo effect. *American Journal of Psychiatry, 159,* 728–737.

McAdams, D. P. (1990). *The person: An introduction to personality and psychology*. San Diego: Harcourt Brace Jovanovich.

McCarthy, W. C., & Frieze, I. H. (1999). Negative aspects of therapy: Client perceptions of therapists' social influence, burnout, and quality of care. *Journal of Social Issues, 55,* 33–50.

McCullough, J. P. (1999). *Treatment for chronic depression: Cognitive behavioral analysis system of psychotherapy (CBASP)*. New York: Guilford Press.

McCullough, L., Kuhn, N., Andrews, S., Kaplan, A., Wolf, J., & Hurley, C. L.

(2002). *Treating affect phobia: A manual for short-term dynamic psychotherapy.* New York: Guilford Press.

McGuff, R., Gitlin, D., & Enderlin, M. (1996). Clients' and therapists' confidence and attendance at planned individual therapy sessions. *Psychological Reports, 79,* 537–538.

McHugh, P. R., & Slavney, P. R. (1998). *The perspectives of psychiatry.* Baltimore: Johns Hopkins University Press.

McLean, P. D., & Hakstian, A. R. (1979). Clinical depression: Comparative efficacy of outpatient treatments. *Journal of Consulting and Clinical Psychology, 47,* 818–836.

McWilliams, N. (1999). *Psychoanalytic case formulation.* New York: Guilford Press.

McWilliams, N. (2004). *Psychoanalytic psychotherapy: A practitioner's guide.* New York: Guilford Press.

Messer, S. B., & Wampold, B. E. (2002). Let's face facts: Common factors are more potent than specific therapy ingredients. *Clinical Psychology— Science and Practice, 9*(1), 21–25.

Milrod, B. L., Busch, F. N., Cooper, A. N., & Shapiro, T. (1997). *Manual of panic-focused psychodynamic psychotherapy.* Washington, DC: American Psychiatric Press.

Milrod, B., Leon, A. C., Barber, J. P., Markowitz, J. C., & Graf, E. (2007). Do comorbid personality disorders moderate psychotherapy response in panic disorder? A preliminary empirical evaluation of the APA Practice Guideline. *Journal of Clinical Psychiatry, 68,* 885–891.

Milrod, B. L., Leon, A. C., Busch, F., Rudden, M., Schwalberg, M., Clarkin, J., et al. (2007). A randomized controlled clinical trial of psychoanalytic psychotherapy for panic disorder. *American Journal of Psychiatry, 164*(2), 265–272.

Minuchin, S., & Fishman, H. C. (2004). *Family therapy techniques.* Harvard University Press.

Mitchell, J. (1986) (Ed.). *The selected Melanie Klein.* New York: Free Press.

Mitchell, S. M. (1988). *Relational concepts in psychoanalysis.* Cambridge, MA: Harvard University Press.

Mojtabai, R., & Olfson, M. (2008). National trends in psychotherapy by office-based psychiatrists. *Archives of General Psychiatry, 65*(8), 962–970.

Moras, K., & Strupp, H. H. (1982). Pretherapy interpersonal relations, patients' alliance, and outcome in brief therapy. *Archives of General Psychiatry, 39,* 405–409.

Moras, K., & Summers, R. F. (2001, March). *A manualized model for dual-provider combined psychotherapy and psychopharmacology.* Workshop presented at the American Association of Directors of Psychiatry Residency Training, Seattle, WA.

Mundo, E. (2006). Neurobiology of dynamic psychotherapy: An integration possible? *Journal of the American Academy of Psychoanalysis, 34,* 679–691.

Muran, J. C., & Safran, J. D. (2002). A relational approach to psychotherapy: Resolving ruptures in the therapeutic alliance. In F. W. Kaslow (Series Ed.) & J. J. Magnavita (Vol. Ed.), *Comprehensive handbook of psychotherapy: Vol. 1. Psychodynamic/object relations* (pp. 253–282). New York: Wiley.

Orlinsky, D. E., Ronnestad, M. H., Willutzki, U. (2004). Fifty years of psychotherapy process-outcome research: Continuity and change. In M. Lambert (Ed.), *Handbook of psychotherapy and behavior change* (pp. 307–389). New York: Wiley.

OPD Task Force. (Ed.). (2008). *Operationalized psychodynamic diagnosis OPD-2: Manual of diagnosis and treatment planning.* Cambridge, MA: Hogrefe.

PDM Task Force. (2006). *Psychodynamic diagnostic manual (PDM).* Silver Spring, MD: Alliance of Psychoanalytic Organizations.

Perls, F. S., Hefferline, R. F., & Goodman, P. (1951). *Gestalt therapy.* New York: Julian Press.

Perry, J. C. (1989). Scientific progress in psychodynamic formulation. *Psychiatry, 52*(3), 245–249.

Perry, S., Cooper, A. M., & Michels, R. (1987). The psychodynamic formulation: Its purpose, structure, and clinical application. *American Journal of Psychiatry, 144*(5), 543–550.

Peterson, C. (2006). *A primer of positive psychology.* New York: Oxford University Press.

Peterson, C., & Seligman, M. E. P. (2004). *Character strengths and virtues.* New York: Oxford University Press.

Piper, W. E., Joyce, A. S., Azim, H. F., & McCallum, M. (1998). Interpretive and supportive forms of psychotherapy and patient personality variables. *Journal of Consulting and Clinical Psychology, 66*(3), 558–567.

Piper, W., McCallum, M., Joyce, A. S., Azim, H. F., & Ogrodniczuk, J. S. (1999). Follow-up findings for interpretive and supportive forms of psychotherapy and patient personality variables. *Journal of Consulting and Clinical Psychology, 67*(2), 267–273.

Popper, K. (1962). *Conjectures and refutations.* New York: Basic Books.

Propst, A., Paris, J., & Rosberger, Z. (1994). Do therapist experience, diagnosis, and functional level predict outcome in short-term psychotherapy? *Canadian Journal of Psychiatry, 39*(3), 168–176.

Pulver, S. E. (1970). Narcissism: The term and the concept. *Journal of the American Psychoanalytic Association, 18,* 319–341.

Rank, O. (1929). *Will therapy.* New York: Knopf, 1936.

Rathod, S., Kingdon, D., Weiden, P., & Turkington, D. (2008). Cognitive-behavioral therapy for medication-resistant schizophrenia: A review. *Journal of Psychiatric Practice, 14*(1), 22–33.

Renik, O. (1993). Analytic interaction: Conceptualizing technique in light of the analysts's irreducible subjectivity. *Psychoanalytic Quarterly, 62,* 553–571.

Riba M. B., & Tasman, A. (2006). Psychodynamic perspective on combining therapies. *Psychiatric Annals, 36*(5), 353–360.

Rizzolatti, G. (2005). The mirror neuron system and its function in humans. *Anatomy and Embryology, 210,* 419–421.

Rockland, L. H. (2003). *Supportive therapy: A psychodynamic approach.* New York: Basic Books.

Roe, D. (2007). The timing of psychodynamically oriented psychotherapy termination and its relation to reasons for termination, feelings about termination, and satisfaction with therapy. *The Journal of the American Academy of Psychoanalysis and Dynamic Psychiatry, 35*(3), 443–453.

Roe, D., Dekel, R., Harel, G., & Fennig, S. (2006). Clients' feelings during termination of psychodynamically oriented psychotherapy. *Bulletin of the Menninger Clinic, 70*(1), 68–81.

Rogers, C. R. (1959). A theory of therapy, personality and interpersonal relationships, as developed in the client-centered framework. In S. Koch (Ed.), *Psychology: A study of science* (pp. 184–256). New York: McGraw-Hill.

Rogers, C. R. (1961). *On becoming a person: A therapist's view of psychotherapy.* Boston: Houghton Mifflin.

Rogers, C. R. (1965). *Client-centered therapy.* Boston: Houghton Mifflin.

Roose, S. P., & Stern, R. H. (1995). Medication use in training cases: A survey. *Journal of the American Psychoanalytic Association, 43,* 163–170.

Rutter, M. (1987). Temperament, personality and personality disorder. *British Journal of Psychiatry, 150,* 443–458.

Sadler, J. Z. (2002). *Descriptions and prescriptions: Values, mental disorders, and the DSMs.* Baltimore: Johns Hopkins University Press.

Safran, J. D., Crocker, P., McMain, S., & Murray, P. (1990). Therapeutic alliance rupture as a therapy event for empirical investigation. *Psychotherapy, 27*(2), 154–165.

Safran, J. D., & Muran, J. C. (2000). *Negotiating the therapeutic alliance: A relational treatment guide.* New York: Guilford Press.

Salminen, J. K., Karlsson, H., Hietala, J., Kajander, J., Aalto, S., Markkula, J., et al. (2008). Short-term psychodynamic psychotherapy and fluoxetine in major depressive disorder: A randomized comparative study. *Psychotherapy and Psychosomatics, 77,* 351–357.

Salzman, L. (1968). *The obsessive personality: Origins, dynamics, and therapy.* New York: Science House.

Satterfield, W. A., & Lyddon, W. J. (1995). Client attachment and perceptions of the working alliance with counselor trainees. *Journal of Counseling Psychology, 42,* 187–189.

Schafer, R. (1981). *Narrative actions in psychoanalysis (The Heinz Werner lectures).* Worcester, MA: Clark University, Heinz Werner Institute.

Schottenbauer, M. A., Glass, C. R., Arnkoff, D. B., & Gray, S. H. (2008). Contributions of psychodynamic approaches to treatment of PTSD and trauma: A review of the empirical treatment and psychopathology literature. *Psychiatry: Interpersonal and Biological Processes, 71*(1), 13–34.

Seligman, M. E. P. (2002). *Authentic happiness*. New York: Free Press.

Seligman, M. E. P., Steen, T. A., Park, N., & Peterson, C. (2005). Positive psychology progress: Empirical validation of interventions. *American Psychologist, 60*, 410–421.

Selzer, M. A., Koenigsberg, H. W., & Kernberg, O. F. (1987). The initial contract in the treatment of borderline patients. *American Journal of Psychiatry, 144*, 927–930.

Shakespeare, W. *The tempest*. New York: Oxford University Press.

Shapiro, D. (1965). *Neurotic styles*. New York: Basic Books.

Sharpless, B. A., & Barber, J. P. (2009). Psychodynamic therapy. In R. E. Ingram (Ed.), *The international encyclopedia of depression* (pp. 460–465). New York: Springer.

Shear, M., Cooper, A., Klerman, G., Busch, M., & Shapiro T. (1993). A psychodynamic model of panic disorder. *American Journal of Psychiatry, 150*, 859–866.

Siegel D. (2006). An interpersonal neurobiology approach to psychotherapy. *Psychiatric Annals, 36*, 248–258.

Sifneos, P. (1979). *Short-term dynamic psychotherapy: Evaluation and technique*. New York: Plenum Press.

Singer, J. A. (2004). A love story: Self-defining memories in couples therapy. In A. Lieblich, D. P. McAdams, & R. Josselson (Eds.), *Healing plots: The narrative basis of psychotherapy* (pp. 189–208). Washington, DC: American Psychological Association.

Slap, J. W., & Slap-Shelton, L. (1991). *The schema in clinical psychoanalysis*. London: Analytic Press.

Solms, M. (1995). New findings on the neurological organization of dreaming: Implications for psychoanalysis. *Psychoanalytic Quarterly, 64*, 43–67.

Spence, D. (1982). Narrative truth and theoretical truth. *Psychoanalytic Quarterly, 51*, 43–69.

Strachey, J. (1934). The nature of the therapeutic action of psychoanalysis. *International Journal of Psychoanalysis, 15*, 127–159.

Strupp, H. H., & Binder, J. L. (1984). *Psychotherapy in a new key: A guide to time limited dynamic psychotherapy*. New York: Basic Books.

Sullivan, H. S. (1947). *Conception of modern psychiatry*. Washington, DC: William Alanson White Psychiatric Foundation.

Summers, R. F. (2002). The psychodynamic formulation updated. *American Journal of Psychotherapy, 57*, 39–51.

Summers, R. F., & Barber, J. P. (2003). Therapeutic alliance as a measurable psychotherapy skill. *Academic Psychiatry, 27*, 160–165.

Svartberg, M., & Stiles, T. C. (1991). Comparative effects of short-term psychodynamic psychotherapy: A meta-analysis. *Journal of Consulting and Clinical Psychology, 59*, 704–714.

Thase, M. E. (1999). When are psychotherapy and pharmacotherapy combinations the treatment of choice for major depressive disorder? *Psychiatric Quarterly, 70*(4), 333–346.

Thase, M. E., Greenhouse, J. B., Frank, E., Reynolds, C. F., Pilkonis, P. A., Hurley, K., et al. (1997). Treatment of major depression with psychotherapy or psychotherapy–pharmacotherapy combinations. *Archives of General Psychiatry, 54,* 1009–1015.

Thompson, C. E., Worthington, R., & Atkinson, D. R. (1994). Counselor content orientation, counselor race, and Black women's cultural mistrust and self-disclosures. *Journal of Counseling Psychology, 41,* 155–161.

Thompson, L. W., Gallagher-Thompson, D., & Steinmetz Breckenridge, J. (1987). Comparative effectiveness of psychotherapies for depressed elders. *Journal of Consulting and Clinical Psychology, 55,* 385–390.

Thorne, A., & Klohnen, E. (1993). Interpersonal memories as maps for personality consistency. In D. C. Funder, R. D. Parke, C. Tomlinson-Keasey, & K. Widaman (Eds.), *Studying lives through time: Personality and development* (pp. 223–253). Washington, DC: American Psychological Association.

Tyrer, P., Seivewright, N., Ferguson, B., & Tyrer, J. (1992). The general neurotic syndrome: A coaxial diagnosis of anxiety, depression, and personality disorder. *Acta Psychiatrica Scandinavica, 85,* 201–206.

Ursano, R. J., Sonnenberg, S. M., & Lazar, S. G. (1998). *Psychodynamic psychotherapy: Principles and techniques in the era of managed care.* Washington, DC: APPI.

Vaillant, G. E. (1992). The beginning of wisdom is never calling a patient a borderline; or, the clinical management of immature defenses in the treatment of individuals with personality disorders. *Journal of Psychotherapy Practice and Research, 1,* 117–134.

Vaillant, G. E. (2008). *Spiritual evolution.* New York: Broadway.

Vinnars, B., Barber, J. P., Norén, K., Thormählen, B., Gallop, R., & Weinryb, R. M. (2005). Supportive–expressive psychotherapy in personality disorders: An outpatient randomized controlled trial. *American Journal of Psychiatry, 162,* 1933–1940.

Wachtel, E., & Wachtel, P. (1986). *Family dynamics in individual psychotherapy: A guide to clinical strategies.* New York: Guilford Press.

Wachtel, P. L. (1997). *Psychoanalysis, behavior therapy, and the relational world.* Washington, DC: American Psychological Association.

Wade, P., & Bernstein, B. L. (1991). Culture sensitivity training and counselor's race: Effects on black female clients' perceptions and attrition. *Journal of Counseling Psychology, 38,* 9–15.

Waelder, R. (1936). Principle of multiple functions: Observations on overdetermination. *Psychoanalytic Quarterly, 5,* 45–62.

Watson, D., Clark, L. A., & Tellegen, A. (1988). Development and validation of brief measures of positive and negative affect: The PANAS Scales. *Journal of Personality and Social Psychology, 54,* 1063–1070.

Weiden, P., & Havens, L. (1994). Psychotherapeutic management techniques in the treatment of outpatients with schizophrenia. *Hospital and Community Psychiatry, 45*(6), 549–555.

Weiner, I. B. (1998). *Principles of Psychotherapy*. New York: Wiley.

Weiss, J., Sampson, H., & the Mount Zion Psychotherapy Research Group. (1986). *The psychoanalytic process: Theory, clinical observation, and empirical research*. New York: Guilford Press.

Westen, D., & Gabbard, G. (2002). Developments in cognitive neuroscience: I. Conflict, compromise, and connectionism. *Journal of the American Psychoanalytic Association, 50*, 53–98.

Williams, K. E., & Chambless, D. L. (1990). The relationship between therapist characteristics and outcome of in vivo exposure treatment for agoraphobia. *Behavior Therapy, 21*, 111–116.

Winnicott, D. W. (1953). Transitional objects and transitional phenomenon: A study of the first not-me possession. *International Journal of Psychoanalysis, 34*, 89–97.

Winnicott, D. W. (1965). *The maturational processes and the facilitating environment: Studies in the theory of emotional development*. London, UK: Hogarth Press.

Wiseman, H., & Barber, J. P. (2008). *Echoes of the trauma: Relationship themes and emotions in the narratives of the children of holocaust survivors*. London, UK: Cambridge University Press.

Wright, J. H., & Hollifield, M. (2006). Editorial: Combining pharmacotherapy and psychotherapy. *Psychiatric Annals, 36*, 320–328.

Yalom, I. D. (1980). *Existential psychotherapy*. New York: Basic Books.

Zetzel, E. R. (1956). Current concepts of transference. *Journal of Abnormal and Social Psychology, 53*, 16–18.

Index